Maternity and Women's Health Care

Maternity and Women's Health Care

Editor: Nicole McConnell

AMERICAN
MEDICAL PUBLISHERS
www.americanmedicalpublishers.com

AMERICAN
MEDICAL PUBLISHERS
www.americanmedicalpublishers.com

Cataloging-in-Publication Data

Maternity and women's health care / edited by Nicole McConnell.
p. cm.
Includes bibliographical references and index.
ISBN 978-1-63927-155-9
1. Maternity nursing. 2. Gynecologic nursing. 3. Maternal health services. 4. Women's health services.
5. Pregnancy--Complications. 6. Motherhood. I. McConnell, Nicole.
RG951 .M38 2022
610.736 78--dc23

American Medical Publishers,
41 Flatbush Avenue,
1st Floor, New York,
NY 11217, USA

ISBN 978-1-63927-155-9 (Hardback)

Contents

Preface

Every book is a source of knowledge and this one is no exception. The idea that led to the conceptualization of this book was the fact that the world is advancing rapidly; which makes it crucial to document the progress in every field. I am aware that a lot of data is already available, yet, there is a lot more to learn. Hence, I accepted the responsibility of editing this book and contributing my knowledge to the community.

Maternity refers to the time period during pregnancy and soon after childbirth. It presents various health risks to a woman. It comes with major changes and challenges in the physical, emotional and social health of a woman. It is necessary to provide appropriate health care to the woman going through the maternity period. The conditions such as hemorrhage, eclampsia, sepsis and obstructed labor often lead to maternal death. Maternal health is affected by several factors such as early marriage, home birth and various cultural attitudes towards sexuality. The woman going through pregnancy often deals with various non-fatal health problems such as ectopic pregnancy, preterm labor, gestational diabetes, hyperemesis gravidarum, obstetrical fistulae, and anemia. This book contains some path-breaking studies in the field of maternity and women's health care. It will also provide interesting topics for research which interested readers can take up. Those in search of information to further their knowledge will be greatly assisted by this book.

While editing this book, I had multiple visions for it. Then I finally narrowed down to make every chapter a sole standing text explaining a particular topic, so that they can be used independently. However, the umbrella subject sinews them into a common theme. This makes the book a unique platform of knowledge.

I would like to give the major credit of this book to the experts from every corner of the world, who took the time to share their expertise with us. Also, I owe the completion of this book to the never-ending support of my family, who supported me throughout the project.

Editor

1

Better than nothing? maternal, newborn, and child health services and perinatal mortality, Lubumbashi, democratic republic of the Congo

Abel Mukengeshayi Ntambue[1*], Françoise Kaj Malonga[1], Michele Dramaix-Wilmet[2], Roger Nlandu Ngatu[3] and Philippe Donnen[2,4]

Abstract

Background: The Democratic Republic of Congo (DRC) has a high rate of perinatal mortality (PMR), and health measures that could reduce this high rate of mortality are not accessible to all women. Where they are in place, their quality is not optimal. This study was initiated to assess the relationship between these suboptimal maternal, newborn and child health (MNCH) services and perinatal mortality (PM) in Lubumbashi, DRC's second-largest city.

Methods: We conducted a prospective cohort study, comparing women who had no, low, moderate, or high numbers of antenatal care (ANC) visits; three different levels of delivery care; and who did or did not attend postnatal care (PNC). Women were followed for 50 days after delivery, with PM as the primary endpoint.

Results: Uptake of recommended prenatal interventions was between 11-43 % among ANC attenders, regardless of the frequency of their visits. PM was 26 per 1000. ANC attendance was associated with PM. Newborns of mothers who had the lowest attendance had a mortality two times higher than newborns of women who had not attended ANC (low visits: adjusted odds ratio (aOR) = 2.2; 95 % confidence interval (CI) = 1.4-3.8). However, moderate (aOR = 1.4; 95 % CI =0.7–2.2) and high (aOR = 1.3; 95 % CI 0.7–2.2) attendance were not statistically significantly associated with PM. PNC attendance was not significantly associated with lower PM (relative risk 0.4, 95 % CI 0.1–2.6). Emergency obstetric and newborn care (EmONC) was significantly associated with a reduction in mortality (aOR = 0.2; 95 % CI = 0.2–0.8), with an 84.4 % reduction among newborns at risk, and an overall reduction in mortality of 10 % for all births.

Conclusion: Perinatal mortality was high among the infants of women in the cohort under study (26 per 1000 live births). Availability of MNCH, specifically EmONC, was associated with lower perinatal mortality, and if this association is causal, might avert 84.4 % of perinatal deaths among newborns at high-risk.

Keywords: Perinatal mortality, Maternal health services, Perinatal care, Postnatal care, Emergency obstetric and neonatal care, Democratic Republic of the Congo

* Correspondence: abelntambue@yahoo.fr
[1]Université de Lubumbashi: École de Santé Publique, Unité d'Epidémiologie et de Santé de la Mère, du Nouveau-né et de l'enfant, Lubumbashi, Democratic Republic of the Congo (DRC)
Full list of author information is available at the end of the article

Background

The Democratic Republic of Congo (DRC) has one of the highest perinatal mortality rates (PMR) in the world (>40 per 1000) [1]; maternal, neonatal, and child health (MNCH) services are rarely used and are of poor quality [2, 3]. As in other countries [4], there are differences between rural and urban areas [3]. Lubumbashi, the second largest city, has a PMR greater than 27 per 1000, with mediocre MNCH utilization [5]. Complicated delivery and low birth weight are the main risk factors for perinatal death [5, 6].

MNCH includes antenatal care (ANC), skilled attendance at delivery and postnatal consultations (PNC), and integrated management of newborn and childhood illnesses (IMCI) [4]. Although the individual impact of certain interventions in the MNCH package remains to be shown, as a whole, this package is an effective intervention to reduce maternal and perinatal mortality (PM) [7–10]. Thus, MNCH care is most effective when the interventions are offered, not as isolated interventions, but in the form of a package on the continuum: pregnancy, delivery, and postpartum [11–13].

In 2008, a meta-analysis by Bhutta et al. [11] showed that quality ANC and appropriate care at delivery and during the neonatal period could reduce maternal mortality by more than 65 %, and PM by 80 %. Here, as elsewhere [4, 7–10, 13, 14], the authors mentioned that the impact of MNCH interventions could only be attained if the care — quality ANC with skilled attendance at delivery and postnatal care (PNC)— was offered as a 'package' and on a continuum rather than through isolated interventions. In South Africa, Pattinson et al. [15] observed similar results when women had received appropriate care at each critical phase.

In several settings in Africa, it is still rare for all the components of this package to be offered to all women and newborns throughout the continuum [4]. In Lubumbashi in 2009, while over 90 % of pregnant women used ANC at least once during their pregnancies, less than 30 % received the recommended and/or necessary interventions during these visits (iron, folic acid, sulphadoxine-pyrimethamine, tetanus toxoid, and HIV, syphilis, and intrauterine growth restriction screening) [2]. Although almost all women (97.2 %) had an assisted delivery, the utilization and quality of emergency obstetric and newborn care (EmONC) remained inadequate. Only 7.6 % of births in 2010 took place in health facilities that offered Comprehensive EmONC. Moreover, only 35 % of women had attended PNC at 42 days, and PNC services were restricted to simply weighing and vaccinating the child [2, 16].

These data illustrate the insufficient quantity and quality of MNCH care in this environment, and are consistent with the high PMR observed, as well as with the maternal mortality due to direct obstetric causes and intrapartum and very early neonatal death – indicators of EmONC – which, instead of being below 1.5 %, have generally been higher, above 3 %. They beg the question of what, if any, impact on PM, MNCH care may have in this precarious context. This study was conducted to assess the relation between the MNCH package as currently provided with PM in Lubumbashi.

Methods

Study setting

Lubumbashi is the capital of the province of Katanga. In 2010, its population was estimated at 1,548,923 inhabitants in an area of 747 square kilometers [17]. It has 11 health zones (HZ) and 267 health facilities, of which only 180 have a maternity ward [18]. Each HZ has a hospital and comprises both urban and rural areas. Within each HZ, facilities were purposively chosen for inclusion in the study. Each of the ten general reference hospitals (GRH) and the one provincial reference hospital was chosen, and in the corresponding HZ, one health center or private clinic (≥30 deliveries per month) in an urban setting and one in a rural (or urban-rural) setting was selected. Thus, apart from Lubumbashi (1 GRH, 1 provincial hospital, two health centers) and Kowe HZ (one health center), each HZ had 3 facilities participating in the study.

Study population

Selection of subjects

We conducted a prospective cohort study, comparing women who delivered in one of the study facilities and had received various levels of ANC with women who delivered in those same facilities but had not received ANC. The study took place over a 5-month period from October 2010 to February 2011.

Women who did not use ANC were recruited at their admission to the maternity unit. Those who attended ANC were recruited at their first prenatal visit. They were followed at ANC visits. At the end of scheduled prenatal visits, they were sought in the maternity wards where they had planned to give birth according to their expected date of delivery. Women were also encouraged to contact the research team in case of premature birth. Women who had not attended the ANC were recruited at the time of their admission during the same period and in the same maternity units as women of the ANC group.

At the ANC, like in the maternity unit, women were recruited by nurses and doctors trained in the study procedures. The admission of a woman to a maternity unit did not automatically guarantee her inclusion in the study; written informed consent was first obtained.

All women included in the study were followed until 50 days after delivery. The follow-up consisted of verification of care received during the stay in the maternity unit, and, after the stay, use of postnatal care and assessment of maternal and neonatal survival.

In the ANC group, women were monitored to assess the quality of care received during pregnancy. They were recruited during ANC; only pregnant women attending their first visit were enrolled in the study. In Lubumbashi, the minimum number of women expected at ANC annually is about 60,000. Allowing for a significance level of 5 % and loss to follow-up of 20 %, with a power of 80 % to detect a reduction of PM with ANC attendance of ≈ 22.1 % [5], we needed to recruit at least 1812 pregnant women (906 per group). However, taking into account the analysis in subgroups planned to assess the impact of ANC on the maternal-fetal prognosis, the number of women was multiplied by 3 (number of ANC subgroups), which gave a minimum number of 2745 pregnant women to be recruited [19]. The number of women enrolled by each health facility was proportional to the ANC capacity of the facility (in 2009), relative to the total number of women attending ANC during the same year, across all selected health facilities [19, 20].

These women were followed by the research team according to the WHO ANC program [21], operating in the health facilities. During this monitoring period, meetings were held with women in the health facilities on the occasion of their prenatal visits. Women were not sought at home when they were absent from the appointment given by the health personnel. There was no interference from investigators in the organization of activities at a prenatal visit. No intervention was proposed to the women during this period. The fiftieth day postpartum marked the end of this monitoring period.

During the monitoring period, the investigators interviewed women to obtain information about the date of their last menstrual periods (LMP), their use of home health practices, and advice and examinations they received during ANC visits. Investigators also reviewed ANC records to record which recommended interventions were administered, obstetric history, and morbidity during pregnancy.

A total of 2823 pregnant women was recruited into this group. During the follow-up period, 5 women (0.2 %) experienced a miscarriage, and 424 (15 %) were lost to follow-up (not found even at home). There was no statistically significant difference in the profile of the women who remained in the study and those lost to follow-up. No maternal deaths were recorded before delivery. At delivery, the remaining 2,394 women were compared with those who had not attended ANC.

According to the model of focused ANC, women should make at least four prenatal visits [21, 22]. The interventions received depend not only on the frequency of these visits, but on when the visits occur. For most developing countries, the recommended gestational ages for ANC attendance are ≤ 16 weeks, ≤ 28 weeks, ≤32 weeks, and ≤ 36 weeks since LMP [21, 22].

Thus, if a woman gives birth prematurely, at 34 weeks, she would be expected to have made three visits to ANC. We calculated the adequacy of visits according to gestational age at delivery to classify women as low, moderate, or high ANC attenders. A low ANC attender was one who attended only one of either 3 or 4 expected visits, for an adequacy of 25 or 33 % (912 women, 38.1 %). A moderate ANC attender was one who attended one of two or three of 3 or 4 expected visits, for an adequacy of 50, 66, or 75 % (748 women, 31.2 %). A high ANC attender was one who attended all, or more than, the expected visits (734 women, 30.7 %). There were 1,910 women who delivered at a study facility but who had not attended ANC, for a total of 4,304 women in the study.

Written informed consent was obtained from each woman prior to inclusion in the study and was reassessed at each contact. Literacy is low in DRC (a recent estimate put it at 67 %), especially among women (52 %), and especially among those with less education and lower socioeconomic status [3]. For those whose reading ability and understanding of French were low, the consent form was read and explained to the woman in one of the local languages (Swahili, Tshiluba or Lingala), in the presence of a witness. This protocol was approved by the Comité d'Éthique Medicale (CEM; Medical Ethics Committee) of the University of Lubumbashi (CEM-UNILU: UNILU/CEM/010/2011).

Monitoring of women and data collection

The women were followed from their admission to the maternity unit until 50 days after delivery. Women in the ANC group were sought in maternity facilities where they had followed the ANC program at the time of their estimated date of delivery. Those with a telephone were contacted at this date to confirm their stay in the maternity facility. Women not found in the facility where they had attended ANC (11.8 %) were sought at their homes.

At the maternity facility, we interviewed women to get data relating to pregnancy for women who had not attended ANC, and the circumstances in which the woman had arrived at the facility, including time of leaving home, means of transport, and difficulties at admission for both groups of women. From maternity records, we collected data related to the diagnosis at admission, type of pregnancy, fetal presentation, mode of delivery, the occurrence of complications, the weight of the newborn and the fetal-maternal prognosis. During an interview with the health staff who managed the delivery, a table with information on the organization and access to obstetric and neonatal care in the health facility, as well as the availability of care at the time of delivery, was filled in. This table evaluated the availability of staff with surgical skills, as well as the availability of drugs and equipment (blood, oxytocin, antibiotics, surgical kits, oxygen, an incubator, magnesium sulfate, phototherapy, nasogastric tube, a partograph, an 'Ambu' bag, a bulb syringe and vacuum extraction cup) for each delivery. The availability of these latter varied according to the ability of the woman or her family to pay for (≥ US $20–60) and obtain them, and were not characteristics of the facility.

After women and their infants returned home, the study team visited them 8, 30, and 50 days after delivery. At these visits, we assessed the vital status of mother and child and the use of postnatal care at 7, 21 and 42 days after delivery.

Data management and definition of variables

The study data were double-entered and analyzed using Stata v.11.0 (College Station, TX). As described above, the use of ANC was evaluated in terms of the number of visits. A woman was considered at high risk of PM if she had at least one complication occurring before, during, or after delivery. Also, a fetus or a newborn was considered to be at high risk of dying if born to a woman at risk, or if it experienced a complication at birth or during the neonatal period [21, 23–25]. To study the impact of the management of delivery on maternal-fetal and neonatal survival, we identified three care groups. The first we called Essential Care–Low Risk (EC-LR), which was the general care given to women and newborns at low risk. This care included clean birth practices, labor monitoring using a partograph, the active management of the third stage of labor (AMTSL), hygienic methods to cut and tie off the cord, basic thermal care, immediate breastfeeding, prevention of mother-to-child transmission of HIV (PMTCT), and increasing the satisfaction and comfort of the mother. The second group received the same care, but were determined to be high-risk; this group was called Essential Care-High Risk (EC-HR). The third group was that which received emergency obstetric and neonatal care (EmONC), as defined by WHO [23, 24]. The PNC visits were evaluated according to whether the women had attended them or not [4].

The level of risk of the pregnancy was determined by the presence during pregnancy of at least one factor of poor prognosis for mother and child. The criteria were those of the WHO, as well as others observed by us previously in Lubumbashi [5, 23]. They included age < 20 and > 37 years, primigravidity, miscarriage of the previous pregnancy, previous infant born at less than 2500 g, fetal or neonatal death at previous delivery, the occurrence of complications or Caesarean section at previous delivery, hypertension, diabetes, maternal malnutrition, sexually transmitted infections, or HIV during the current pregnancy, and type of pregnancy (singleton vs. multiple pregnancy). Thus, every woman having least one of these factors or complications was considered as having a high-risk pregnancy [23].

PM was defined as all stillbirths (≥28 weeks gestational age) and early neonatal deaths (≤7 days) [26]. For women who had multiple pregnancies, only one infant was selected at random to be included in the univariate and multivariate analyses.

Data analysis

Usual descriptive statistics were used to describe groups. Comparisons of the mean or median between groups involved ANOVA or Kruskal-Wallis tests, as appropriate [20]. The association between use of MNCH services and PM was measured by calculating a relative risk (RR), the significance of which was tested using a chi-square test, with a significance level of 5 %. The adjusted odds ratios (aOR) were calculated by forward stepwise logistic regression. Confidence intervals at 95 % were calculated for crude RR and aOR. All variables with an unadjusted p-value ≤ 0.10 had the opportunity to enter into the multivariable logistic regression analysis. Model fit was checked by the Hosmer-Lemeshow test [27].

The impact of each MNCH component in reducing PM was assessed by the fraction of risk prevented in newborns at high risk (FRP_c) and the fraction of risk prevented in all births (FRP_A) for all variables significantly associated with the reduction of PM. The total fraction of risk prevented, FRP_t, for all MNCH was calculated using the following formula:

$$FRP_t = 1\text{-}[(1\text{-}FRP_{S1})(1\text{-}FRP_{S2})(1\text{-}FRP_{S3})\ (1\text{-}FRP_{S4})]$$

Where FRP_{Si} = fraction of risk prevented with a given MNCH service [28–31].

Results

Characteristics of subjects

At delivery, 4,304 women were included in this study (Fig. 1). Of these, 2,394 (55.6 %) were in the group followed during ANC, while 1,910 others (44.4 %) had not received ANC and were recruited in the delivery room. No maternal deaths occurred during or within 42 days of childbirth.

A total of 4,315 children were born to these women; 1,921 (44.5 %, including 22 twins from 11 multiple pregnancies), were born to mothers who had not attended the ANC program, and 2,394 (55.5 %) were born to mothers who had attended.

The total number of fetal deaths in this cohort was 63 (14.6 per 1000 births), 9 in women who had not attended the ANC program (0.47 %), and 54 in those who had attended (2.3 %). A total of 48 early neonatal deaths occurred; 28 of these deaths (58.3 %) occurred

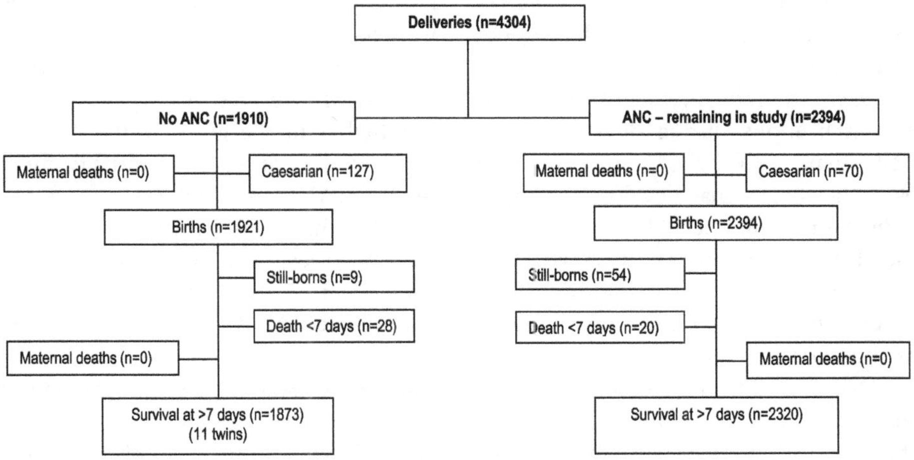

Fig. 1 Numbers of women and newborns according to their prognosis at childbirth and during the neonatal period

among infants born to women who did not attend the ANC (28/1910 = 1.5 %; 20/2394 = 0.84 %). The PMR was 25.3 per 1000 births. At the end of the first week of neonatal life, the total number of surviving infants was 4,204. This number consisted of 1,884 (1884/1921 = 98.1 %) neonates born to mothers who had not attended the ANC program and 2,320 (2320/2394 = 96.9 %) to mothers who had attended (Fig. 1).

The mean age of women in both groups was 26 years (standard deviation (SD) 6). Women who had not attended ANC were on average a year or two younger than those who had (no ANC, 25.1 (SD 6.7) years vs low visits, 26.9 (SD 6.2), moderate visits, 26.4 (SD 5.9), and high visits 26.4 (SD 5.9) years). In Table 1, it can be seen that there were more unmarried women among those who had not attended ANC than those who had. Similarly, the proportion of women working at home was higher in the group with high attendance than in women who did not attend ANC.

Women who had high attendance were more highly educated than those who did not receive ANC. The proportion of women with high-risk pregnancies was lowest in the moderate-attendance group. Among the factors associated with high-risk pregnancies were early motherhood (<18 years), high parity, and poor obstetric history in the preceding pregnancy and delivery. Early motherhood was twice as high in the group without ANC as in the one with ANC. In contrast, the high parity and poor outcomes of previous pregnancy were more frequent in the group with ANC than in the one without ANC. Only 11 of the 4,304 women enrolled had a twin pregnancy, all of whom were in the group with no ANC attendance.

During pregnancy, it was the women who had high ANC attendance who received more recommended prenatal health interventions. However, even among women at the highest level of ANC attendance, interventions such as HIV screening and tetanus vaccination were well

Table 1 Socio-demographic and obstetric characteristics of women by level of antenatal care (ANC) attendance, Lubumbashi, DRC, 2010–11

Characteristics	No ANC (n = 1910) %	ANC Visits			
		Low (n = 912) %	Moderate (n = 748 %	High (n = 734) %	p
Age (Years)					<0.001
<20	23.6	11.5	11.0	10.9	
20–34	64.7	73.9	77.2	77.1	
≥35	11.7	14.6	11.8	12.0	
Marital status					<0.001
Married	95.2	97.7	97.5	98.5	
Unmarried	4.8	2.3	2.5	1.5	
Education					<0.001
None or primary	27.6	25.9	24.7	21.8	
Secondary school	69.5	68.5	69.4	69.6	
University	2.9	5.6	5.9	8.6	
Occupation					0.032
Housework	54.9	59.4	55.9	60.1	
Other	45.1	40.6	44.1	39.9	
High-risk pregnancy	43.3	43.3	32.5	42.5	<0.001
<18 yrs	17.5	8.3	7.1	7.0	<0.001
>37 yrs	7.4	8.1	6.8	6.1	<0.001
≥6 previous deliveries	12.8	20.3	16.8	17.0	<0.001
Poor OH[a]	10.6	12.1	9.6	15.3	<0.001
Multiple pregnancy	0.6	0.0	0.0	0.0	

OH obstetrical history

[a]: poor obstetrical history (low birth weight, stillborn, abortion)

below 50 %. Overall, nearly 60 % of all women were recruited in the general referral hospitals. The place of delivery was not significantly associated with the adequacy of prenatal visits (Table 2). In Table 3, it can be seen that there were more complications during delivery in the group without ANC than with ANC. Similarly, there were more fetuses or newborns that developed complications at birth or in the neonatal period among women who had not attended ANC than among those who had. The nature of the complications varied according to the adequacy of visits. Among women who had not attended ANC, post-partum hemorrhage was the most common complication observed, followed by prolonged labor (4.3 %) and eclampsia (1.8 %). Prolonged labor and eclampsia were the most often observed complications among women who had low or moderate ANC attendance. Besides the complications commonly seen in women who had low attendance, uterine rupture was frequently seen in women who had high attendance. There was no post-partum hemorrhage in women who had received ANC.

Maternal and neonatal complications were used to determine the proportion of fetuses and/or newborns at high risk. Considering complications occurring in the mother and those occurring in newborns together, the proportion of fetuses or newborns at risk was 21.3 % (917 of 4304). It was higher in the group without ANC than for those with any ANC. Low birth weight (LBW), defined as < 2500 g, and respiratory distress syndrome (RDS) were frequently observed complications. The proportion of newborns with LBW was nearly two times higher in the group without ANC than in the one with any ANC. There was no statistically significant difference in the proportion of newborns with RDS among newborns of women who had attended ANC and women who had not.

Regarding the management of care, the proportion of women who received emergency obstetric care (EmOC) was higher in the group without ANC than in the one with ANC. Similarly, newborns of mothers who had not received ANC received more emergency neonatal care (EmNC) than those of mothers who had received ANC (all categories). The proportion of women who had used PNC within 7 days was higher among women who had not followed the ANC than among those with ANC.

Relation between MNCH and fetal and neonatal prognosis

From the unadjusted analysis in Table 4, it appears that women who had occupations other than housework had 1.5 times the PMR as those who were only occupied in the home. The PMR was twice as high among infants of mothers who had previously experienced a high-risk pregnancy compared with those whose mothers had no risk in previous pregnancies, and newborns of mothers who experienced birth complications also had 4 times the PMR as mothers who did not. Newborns who had complications at birth or during the first week of life were at 5.4 times higher PMR than those who had not.

In Table 5, we note that women who had low attendance had twice the PMR as those who did not attend ANC. The PMR was reduced by two-thirds among infants at high risk whose mothers had received EmOC compared to infants at high risk whose mothers had received only EC-HR. Similarly, newborns at high risk who received EmNC were more likely to survive than those at high risk who received standard care. Although the difference was not significant, the PMR was lower

Table 2 Properties of the ANC program and the place of delivery by level of antenatal care (ANC) attendance, Lubumbashi, DRC, 2010–11

Characteristics	No ANC ($n = 1910$) %	ANC Visits Low ($n = 912$) %	Moderate ($n = 748$) %	High ($n = 734$) %	p
Health interventions during ANC					
Sulfadoxine- Pyrimethamine	0.0	22.5	35.3	37.6	<0.001
Iron	0.0	24.8	31.0	29.0	0.015
Folic acid	0.0	17.9	21.1	22.1	0.08
ITN	0.0	19.5	23.8	17.9	0.013
Mebendazole	0.0	29.7	29.0	27.7	0,65
Antitetanus Vaccination	0.0	35.1	43.1	41.8	0.002
HIV screening	0.0	11.8	13.6	11.2	0.32
Place of delivery					0.39
Health center	42.6	45.3	42.2	41.4	
General Referral Hospital	57.4	54.7	57.8	58.6	

ITN Insecticide-treated net

Table 3 Adequacy of prenatal care based on maternal and neonatal complications and use of obstetric, neonatal and postnatal care by level of antenatal care (ANC) attendance, Lubumbashi, DRC, 2010–11

Characteristics	No ANC ($n = 1910$) %	ANC Visits			
		Low ($n = 912$) %	Moderate ($n = 748$ %	High ($n = 734$) %	p
Maternal complications	15.2	5.9	6.6	11.6	<0.001
Fever	2.1	0.5	0.8	0.8	<0.001
Premature rupture of membranes	0.6	0.8	1.1	1.1	<0.001
Severe anemia	0.4	0.6	1.1	1.1	<0.001
Dystocia (prolonged labor)	4.3	1.2	1.6	3.3	<0.001
Eclampsia	1.8	1.1	0.8	0.5	<0.001
Placenta abruptio	0.1	0.1	0.1	0.3	<0.001
Placenta Prævia	0.0	1.0	0.6	2.5	<0.001
Uterine rupture	0.2	0.6	0.5	2.0	<0.001
Postpartum hemorrhage	5.4	0.0	0.0	0.0	[a]
Neonatal Complications	26.5	16.9	13.9	20.6	<0.001
Respiratory distress (Apgar < 7)	17.2	11.9	11.1	15.1	
Low birth weight	9.3	5.0	2.8	5.5	
Obstetrical care					<0.001
EC-LR	84.8	94.1	93.5	88.4	
EmOC	9.9	2.7	2.1	6.3	
EC-HR	5.6	3.2	4.4	5.3	
Neonatal Care					<0.001
EC-LR	73.5	88.1	86.1	79.4	
EmNC	15.2	6.7	4.9	10.5	
EC-HR	11.3	10.2	9.0	10.1	
Postnatal consultation[b]	6.9	3.4	5.2	5.9	0.003

[a]not calculated; [b]$n = 4241$

among infants whose mothers had attended the PNC compared to those whose mothers had not attended this service. The type of facility in which delivery occurred was not associated with mortality.

From the multivariate analysis (Table 6), it can be seen that women who had low ANC attendance had a higher PMR than those who had not attended ANC, while the risk did not differ significantly for those who were moderate or high attenders. EmOC for women who had complications reduced PMR by more than half. There was 62.3 % less PMR for such women than for those who had not. Similarly, newborns at high risk who received EmNC had 58.7 % less PMR than those who did not receive such care.

By calculating the fraction of risk prevented in infants at high risk, it appears that 84.4 % of perinatal deaths were avoided by EmONC, which accounts for 10 % of deaths avoided among all births.

Discussion

In our results, we observed an elevated PMR among newborns of women who attended ANC compared to those of women who did not. We noted, however, that the newborns who had received emergency neonatal care and those of women who had received EmOC had a lower PMR than those of women who had not received EmOC. These results corroborate the estimates provided by Darmstadt et al. [12] regarding the prevention of PM from the model for MNCH continuity. They are also in line with the observations of Bhutta [11] and Pattinson [15] who showed that MNCH services, when continuously available, reduce PM by more than 35 % in the general population, or by 85 % among infants at high risk. Nonetheless, it remains debatable whether we can evoke a causal role for MNCH care in the reduction of PM.

In fact, even with intervention studies, evidence is insufficient concerning the individual impact – in terms of a causal role – of each component of prenatal, perinatal, and postnatal care on the reduction of PM, even if globally this reduction is observed among the women and newborns who receive a high-quality package of MNCH care [7–12, 32]. Such is the case for our study, in which the low PMR was observed among the newborns who

Table 4 Perinatal mortality based on maternal characteristics and maternal and neonatal complications: unadjusted analysis, by level of antenatal care (ANC) attendance, Lubumbashi, DRC, 2010–11

Factors	Total	Rate (per 1000)	RR	95 % IC	p
Marital status					0.85
Married	4162	26.0	1		
Unmarried	142	28.2	1.1	0.4–2.9	
Education					0.07
None or primary	1108	31.6	1.3	0.8–1.9	
Secondary school	2983	25.1	1		
University	213	5.0	0.2	0.1–1.3	
Occupation					0.030
Housework	2450	21.2	1		
Other[a]	1854	32.0	1.5	1.1–2.2	
Status of pregnancy					<0.001
High risk	1778	36.6	2.0	1.4–2.9	
Low risk	2526	18.2	1		
Maternal complications					<0.001
Yes	478	77.4	4.0	2.7–5.9	
No	3826	19.3	1		
Neonatal Complications					<0.001
Yes	916	72.1	5.4	3.7–7.9	
No	3388	13.3	1		

RR Relative Risk
[a]civil servant, agriculture, sales, works in business or industry

Table 5 Perinatal mortality in terms of the services available to the mother, to the newborn and to the child: unadjusted analyses

Factors	Total	Rate (per 1000)	RR	95 % CI	p
Type of maternity facility					0.39
Health center	1846	28.2	1.2	0.8–1.7	
General Referral Hospital	2458	24.0	1		
ANC (adequacy of visits)					0.006
None	1910	19.4	1		
Low	912	41.7	2.1	1.4–3.4	
Moderate	748	24.1	1.2	0.7–2.2	
High	734	24.5	1.3	0.7–2.2	
Obstetrical care					<0.001
EC-LR	3826	19.3	0.1	0.08–0.2	
EmOC	270	44.4	0.3	0.2–0.7	
EC-HR	208	120.2	1		
Neonatal Care					<0.001
EC-LR	3388	13.3	0.1	0.08–0.2	
EmNC	466	42.9	0.4	0.2–0.8	
EC-HR	450	102.2	1		
PNC ≤ 7 days[a]					0.27
Yes	243	4.1	0.4	0.1–2.6	
No	3998	11.8	1		

RR Relative Risk
[a]$n = 4241$

had received adequate care. The package of neonatal and maternal care was put in place based on the convergence of expert opinion about the averred or presumed effectiveness of the interventions and their synergy, although solid scientific evidence, in terms of the specific contribution of each one, is yet to be found [32–37].

During pregnancy

The impact of interventions offered through ANC (screening for high-risk pregnancy, micronutrient supplementation, intermittent presumptive treatment (IPT) and long-lasting insecticide treated bed nets (LLIN), management of chronic hypertension, screening and treatment of syphilis) on the reduction of PM has not been proven for some and remains to be qualified for others [32–44].

On the other hand, screening for syphilis, IPT and LLIN, screening and treatment of diabetes over the course of pregnancy, prenatal corticoids as well as screening and induction of labor in cases of intrauterine growth retardation (IUGR) are, of all these interventions, the ones for which there is some proof in terms of impact on reduction of PM [45–52].

As to screening and management of diabetes mellitus, some prospective studies have shown that adequate glycemic control and follow-up during pregnancy are a reasonable means to reduce stillbirth and numerous other complications like congenital anomalies and macrosomy [51–53]. The effect of prenatal corticosteroids on fetal maturity has been extensively documented and it has been observed that this intervention reduced respiratory distress syndrome (RDS) by 34 %, cerebroventricular hemorrhage by 46 %, and neonatal death by 31 % [54]. Induction of labor for pregnancies past 41 weeks of gestation has been associated with a 69 % reduction in PM as well as the aspiration of meconium [55, 56].

In the DRC and in the province of Katanga, the prevalence of syphilis among pregnant women is 1.9 and 0.8 %, respectively [57]. This infection is not yet systematically detected during pregnancy [2], which means that whether women have attended ANC or not, the risk of fetal death from the infection remains unchanged because ANC services have not been financed to test for it. This is also the case for malaria, which affects more than 30 % of pregnant women and for which only 30 % receive IPT [5], gestational diabetes and IUGR, which are still rarely screened during pregnancy in Lubumbashi. Since this factor is significantly associated with PM [16], and as long as women who have them fail to receive

Table 6 Perinatal mortality according to MNCH: adjusted analyzes and risk in infants at high risk and among all births

Factors	aOR	95 % CI	p	Surviving % ($n = 4193$)	FRP_C	FRP_A
Education			0.07			
None or primary vs Secondary school	0.8	0.5–1.2				
University vs Secondary school	0.2	0.1–1.1				
ANC (adequacy of visits)			0.010			
Low vs No ANC	2.2	1.4–3.8				
Moderate vs No ANC	1.4	0.7–2.2				
High vs No ANC	1.3	0.7–2.2				
Presence of partograph (Yes vs No)	1.1	0.7–1.7	0.58			
General Reference Hospital vs. Health Center	0.8	0.5–1.2	0.23			
High-risk pregnancy vs low risk	1.9	1.3–2.9	0.002			
Obstetrical care			<0.001			
EC-LR vs EC-HR	0.3	0.2–0.5		89.5	71.3	63.8
EmOC vs EC-HR	0.4	0.2–0.8		6.1	62.3	3.8
Neonatal care			<0.001			
EC-LR vs EC-HR	0.2	0.1–0.3		79.7	83.3	66.4
EmNC vs EC-HR	0.4	0.2–0.8		10.6	58.7	6.2
EmONC					84.4	10.0

proper care, it is clear that ANC cannot make a difference to the level of PM between those who attend and those who do not.

However, apart from the particular interventions highlighted above, the impact of ANC on PM appears indirect. Women who attend ANC are more likely to give birth in the presence of skilled health personnel than those who do not [58]. Given that delivery complications occurred as often in women who attended ANC as in those who did not, ANC alone is not likely to reduce this mortality. Thus, if the woman attended ANC and gives birth in the presence of skilled health personnel, she is more likely to receive appropriate care during delivery and postpartum, which helps to improve her prognosis and that of her newborn.

Delivery and the postnatal period

In Lubumbashi, more than 70 % of perinatal deaths occurred between birth and the 7th postnatal day, whereas for stillbirths, half of the deaths were during delivery [5]. This implies that the interventions most likely to significantly reduce PM are those given during the delivery and up to the 7th post-natal day rather than before delivery [9, 32–37, 59–62]. This is especially true as, during this period, these deaths are usually due to complications of delivery, including prolonged labor, eclampsia, *placenta abruptio*, *placenta previa*, and umbilical cord prolapse [63], prematurity and low birth weight, and infections [64].

At this critical moment, the impact of care on the reduction of PM, varies from one intervention to the other. For example, the available results on the use or not of the partogram for surveillance of spontaneous labor at term, or different versions of the partogram with different positioning of the line of action on the results of labor have not shown significant differences in terms of the rate of cesareans and the perinatal or maternal prognosis [65]. However, studies evaluating the impact of EmONC abound. Even though intervention studies are rare, observational studies, taken as a whole, indicate that skilled birth attendance with providers capable of safe and timely provision of all the signal functions of EmONC are essential to reduce the PMR [59, 66, 67]. The quality of EmONC, rather than its simple availability, is essential in the prevention of PM. The available data show that emergency cesarean and assisted vaginal delivery by ventouse contribute enormously to the reduction of stillbirth. This interventions are signal functions of EmONC with a high impact in the prevention of PM tied to direct delivery complications [68, 69].

During the neonatal period, interventions include prevention of hypothermia, management of RDS, pneumonia, infection, hyperbilirubinemia, as well as early initiation of breastfeeding [69]. This package offered in a hospital setting to newborns, especially those with LBW, is associated overall with a 51 % reduction in neonatal mortality; 58 % by antibiotic administration, and 77 % by prevention of hypothermia [8]. Neonatal resuscitation in health facilities reduces PM by more than 30 % [32, 70].

Evidence from low-income countries show that prevention and management of hypothermia reduces early neonatal mortality by about 25 % [32, 70–72].

In our study, we observed that a significant proportion of women and newborns with complications receive inadequate care in Lubumbashi. This was due to lack of consumables, medicines and equipment, inadequate training, and lack of protocols for the management of complicated deliveries. Further, many women who arrive late in the reference hospital maternity unit often come from primary care facilities after a significant delay from the onset of complications. To the extent that, even in reference hospital maternity units emergency kits are often lacking (it is the families who have to buy them, at a cost of ≈ US $20–60), it is obvious that not all referred women receive appropriate care. Thus it has happened that, in the same delivery room, of 2 infants with severe respiratory distress, only one survived because oxygen was available, and the other died because the oxygen had run out. Also, since kangaroo mother care is not widely disseminated in health care facilities, the staff tend to keep the very low birth weight (less than1500 g) infants in the incubator, while those between 1500–2500 g are not kept warm well. If the complications of extreme prematurity will kill the very low birth weight infant, it's often hypothermia that kills those between 1500 and 2500 g.

Regarding PNC, although the difference was not significant, we also found that the PMR tended to be higher in women who had not attended PNC than for those who had attended PNC. This lack of significant association may result from the low power of the tests given the very small number of perinatal deaths among women who followed PNC (Table 5).

All the above observations concerning MNCH care show that it is precarious in Lubumbashi and that the packages are not offered in such a way as to attain their maximum impact. But our observations also call attention to the fact that when the recommended care is given to mothers and newborns, even in this context where organization and work are difficult, it contributes nonetheless to reduction of PM [32, 72]. However, as stated above, it is not easy or possible to determine which interventions in the package of EmONC and care of ill and LBW infants has contributed most to reduce PM in Lubumbashi. It is likely that there exists a synergy of mutual reinforcement among the interventions, while others had an indirect role in the reduction of PM through an effect on factors intimately associated with it. For example, the administration of prenatal corticosteroids is associated with reduced need for ventilation, and reduces the mortality attributable to RDS up to 53 % in settings where oxygen and ventilation is not always available, as in Lubumbashi [70–72]. Synergy between interventions thus reinforces the idea by which, the more the interventions are offered as a package, all along the continuum and at critical points in the life of the mother and child, the more likely they are to be effective and to reduce PM.

Limitations

This work, which is an observational study, has limitations that are important to present. Although the research team did not interfere in the organization of activities during ANC sessions, or in the use of health interventions by pregnant women, it is unclear to what extent our presence in structures where women were recruited may have been perceived as an audit by the personnel, leading them to change their practices. Likewise, we cannot tell whether the interviews conducted with women at each visit influenced their behavior vis-a-vis the ANC. However, taking into account the organizational constraints of ANC observed in Lubumbashi, such as lack of consumables, drugs and equipment, and also the inaccessibility to pregnant women of certain interventions for financial reasons, despite their availability [2], we believe that the presence of the investigators had no significant influence, in that it did not change either the organization or the financial ability of women to access recommended treatments.

As to the 11 sets of twins born only to women who did not attend ANC, we believe this is a chance finding; we have no particular explanation for it. The same is true of post-partum hemorrhage, which occurred only among women who had not attended ANC. Worldwide, incidence of PPH is 6 %; it is 10 % in Africa [63]. The low incidence of PPH observed in Lubumbashi in this study, compared to that reported in Africa, may be due to differential access to health care. In Lubumbashi, ≈94 % of women have an institutional delivery and ≈ 70 % undergo active management of the third stage of labor. The higher use of this practice may have an effect on the reduction of PPH, which could explain the difference between the incidence reported in our study and that observed at the level of Africa as a whole.

Conclusion

Perinatal mortality was high among the infants of women in the cohort under study (26 per 1000 live births). MNCH was associated with a reduction in perinatal mortality, specifically through EmONC, which might account for a reduction of 84.4 % in perinatal deaths among newborns at high-risk.

Ethics approval and consent to participate

Written informed consent was obtained from each woman prior to inclusion in the study and was reassessed at each contact. The study protocol was approved by the Comité d'Éthique Medicale (CEM; Medical Ethics Committee) of the University of Lubumbashi (CEM-UNILU: UNILU/CEM/010/2011).

Abbreviations

AMTSL: active management of the third stage of labor; ANC: antenatal care; ANOVA: analysis of variance; aOR: adjusted odds ratios; CEM: Comité d'éthique médicale; CI: confidence interval; DRC: Democratic Republic of the Congo; EC-HR: essential care-high risk; EC-LR: essential care–low risk; EmNC: emergency neonatal care; EmOC: emergency obstetric care; EmONC: emergency obstetric and newborn care; FRP: fraction of risk prevented in newborns with complications; FRP_P: risk prevented in all births; GRH: general referral hospitals; HC: health center; HIV: human immunodeficiency virus; HZ: health zone; IMCI: integrated management of newborn and childhood illnesses; IPT: intermittent presumptive treatment; IUGR: intrauterine growth retardation; LBW: low birth weight; LLIN: long-lasting insecticide treated bed nets; LMP: last menstrual period; MNCH: Mother Newborn and Child Health; PM: perinatal mortality; PMR: perinatal mortality rate; PMTCT: prevention of mother-to-child transmission (of HIV); PNC: postnatal consultations; PPH: postpartum hemorrhage; PROM: premature rupture of membranes; RDS: respiratory distress syndrome; RPR: rapid plasma reagin; RR: relative risk; SD: standard deviation; UNILU: Université de Lubumbashi; US $: United States dollars; WHO: World Health Organization.

Competing interests

The authors declare that they have no competing interests in the present research.

Authors' contributions

AMN, FKM, MDW, RNN and PD conceptualized the research question. AMN conceived of the study, its design and participated in its coordination, conducted the statistical analysis, wrote the methods, results, helped to draft the manuscript and incorporated comments from co-authors for the final draft. FKM participated in the design of the study and coordination (collection of data) and helped to draft the manuscript. MDW conducted the statistical analysis, wrote the methods and proof read the manuscript critically. RNN wrote the methods and proof read the manuscript critically. PD wrote the first draft of the paper, wrote the background information, discussion and proof-read the drafts before submission. All authors read and approved the final draft of the manuscript.

Acknowledgements

We sincerely thank the Belgium "Académie de Recherche et d'Enseignement Supérieur" (ARES), formerly CCD, for funding our research, and KD Cowgill, Fulbright Scholar at the University of Lubumbashi School of Public Health, for review and translation assistance. Our thanks also go to the coordination of scientific cooperation of the University of Lubumbashi, for having facilitated the implementation of our research activities.

Funding

This research was funded by the l'*Académie de Recherche et d'Enseignement Supérieur" (ARES)* in the P3-Lub03 program. Funding concerned only the collection of data and the initial English translation of this manuscript.

Author details

[1]Université de Lubumbashi: École de Santé Publique, Unité d'Epidémiologie et de Santé de la Mère, du Nouveau-né et de l'enfant, Lubumbashi, Democratic Republic of the Congo (DRC). [2]Université Libre de Bruxelles: École de Santé Publique: Centre de recherche en Epidémiologie, Biostatistiques et recherche clinique, Brussels, Belgium. [3]Graduate School of Health and Nursing Sciences & Disaster Nursing Global Leader doctoral program (DNGL), University of Kochi, Kochi, Japan. [4]Université Libre de Bruxelles: École de Santé Publique: Centre de Recherche en Politiques et systèmes de santé-Santé internationale, Brussels, Belgium.

References

1. Wang H, Liddell CA, Coates MM, Mooney MD, Levitz CE, Schumacher AE, et al. Global, regional, and national levels of neonatal, infant, and under-5 mortality during 1990–2013: a systematic analysis for the Global Burden of Disease Study 2013. Lancet. 2014;384:957–79.
2. Ntambue MA, Malonga KF, Dramaix-Wilmet M, Donnen P. Determinants of maternal health services utilization in urban settings of the Democratic Republic of Congo – A Case study of Lubumbashi City. BMC Pregnancy Childbirth. 2012;12:66.
3. Ministère de la santé publique. Rapport par grappes à indicateurs multiples: Rapport Final. Kinshasa: DRC; 2011
4. Lawn J, Kerber K. Donnons Sa chance à chaque nouveau-né de l'Afrique: données pratiques, soutien programmatique et de politiques pour les soins du nouveau-né en Afrique. Partenariat pour la Santé maternelle, néonatale et infantile, Cap Town 2006
5. Ntambue MA, Malonga KF, Dramaix-Wilmet M, Donnen P. Ampleur et causes de la mortalité périnatale à Lubumbashi en République démocratique du Congo. Rev Epidemiol Sante Publique. 2013;61:519–29.
6. Ntambue AM, Donnen P, Dramaix-Wilmet M, Malonga KF. Facteurs de risque de la mortalité périnatale dans la ville de Lubumbashi en République démocratique du Congo. Rev Epidemiol Sante Publique. 2012;60:167–76.
7. Carolli G, Rooney C, Villar J. How effective is antenatal in preventing maternal mortality and serious morbidity? An overview of the evidence. Paediatr Perinat Epidemiol. 2001;15:1–42.
8. Bhutta, Zulfiqar A, Darmstadt GL, Hassan BS, Haws RA. Outcomes in developing countries: An review of the evidence community-based interventions for improving perinatal and neonatal Health. Pediatrics. 2005;115:519–617.
9. Yakoob MY, Ali MA, Ali MU, Imdad A, Lawn JEBN, et al. The effect of providing skilled birth attendance and emergency obstetric care in preventing stillbirths. BMC Public Health. 2011;11:S7.
10. Yakoob MY, Menezes EV, Soomro T, Haws RA, Darmstadt GLBZ. Reducing stillbirths: behavioural and nutritional interventions before and during pregnancy. BMC Pregnancy Childbirth. 2009;9:S3.
11. Bhutta ZA, Ali S, Cousens S, Ali TM, Haider BA, Rizvi A, Okong P, Bhutta SZ, Black RE. Interventions to address maternal, newborn, and child survival : what difference can integrated primary health care strategies make ? Lancet. 2008;372:972–89.
12. Darmstadt GL, Bhutta ZA, Cousens S, Adam T, Walker N, De Bernis L, et al. Evidence-based, cost-effective interventions : how many newborn babies can we save ? Lancet. 2005;365:977–88.
13. Kerber KJ, De Graft-johnson JE, Bhutta ZA, Okong P, Starrs A, Lawn JE. Continuum of care for maternal, newborn, and child health : from slogan to service delivery. Lancet. 2007;370:1358–69.
14. Unicef. La Situation Des Enfants Dans Le Monde 2009: La Santé Maternelle et Néonatale. New York 2009
15. Pattinson R, Kerber K, Buchmann E, Friberg IK, Belizan M, Lansky S, et al. Stillbirths : how can health systems deliver for mothers and babies ? Lancet. 2015;377:1610–23.
16. Ntambue AM, Malonga KF, pour l'UNFPA. Evaluation de la disponibilité, utilisation et qualite des soins obstetricaux et néonatals d'urgence dans les zones de santé Kampemba et Sakania: rapport d'enquête. Lubumbashi: DRC; 2012.
17. Institut National des Statistiques. RDCKatangaInfo 1.0: Indicateurs Clés. DevInfo. Lubumbashi: RDC; 2010.
18. District Sanitaire de Lubumbashi. Plan de Développement Sanitaire Du District Sanitaire de Lubumbashi 2010-2015. Lubumbashi: DRC; 2010.
19. Rabe-Hesketh S, Everitt B. A Handbook of Statistical Analyses Using Stata. Third Edit, New York: CRC Press LLC; 2004
20. Falissard B. Comprendre et utiliser les statistiques dans les sciences de la vie. Paris: Masson; 2005.
21. WHO. WHO Antenatal Care Randomized Trial: Manual for the Implementation of the New Model. Geneva 2001
22. Programme National de la Santé de la Reproduction. Normes de la zone de santé relatives aux interventions de santé de la mère, du nouveau-né et de l'enfant en Republique Démocratique du Congo: soins obstetricaux éssentiels. Ministère de la santé. DRC: Kinshasa; 2012.
23. OMS. Prise en charge des complications de la grossesse et de l'accouchement : guide destine à la sage-femme et au médecin. Geneva 2004
24. OMS. Prise en charge intégrée de la grossesse et de l'accouchement; Soins liés à la grossesse, à l'accouchement, au post-partum et à la période néonatale: guide de pratiques essentielles. Geneva 2009
25. OMS. Soins lies à la grossesse, à l'accouchement et à la periode néonatale: guide de pratiques essentielles. Geneva 2003
26. WHO. Neonatal and Perinatal Mortality Country: Regional and Global Estimates 2004. Geneva: WHO; 2007.

27. Bagley SC, White H, Golomb BA. Logistic regression in the medical literature : Standards for use and reporting, with particular attention to one medical domain. J Clin Epidemiol. 2001;54:979–85.
28. Steenland K, Armstrong B. An Overview of Methods for Calculating the Burden of Disease Due to Specific Risk Factors. Epidemiology. 2006;17:512–9.
29. Barendregt JJ, Veerman JL. Categorical versus continuous risk factors and the calculation of potential impact fractions. J Epidemiol Community Health. 2010;64:209e212.
30. Ollivier L, Michel R, Spiegel A, Boutin JP. Mesures d'impact en épidémiologie. Med Trop. 2004;64:71–4.
31. Rowe AK, Powell KE, Flanders WD. Why Population attributable fractions can sum to more than one. Am J Prev Med. 2004;26:243–9.
32. Bhutta ZA, Das JK, Bahl R, Lawn JE, Salam RA, Paul VK, et al. Can available interventions end preventable deaths in mothers, newborn babies, and stillbirths, and at what cost? Lancet. 2014;384:347–70.
33. Darmstadt GL, Yakoob MY, Haws RA, Menezes EV, Soomro TBZ. Reducing stillbirths: interventions during labour. BMC Pregnancy Childbirth. 2009;9:S6.
34. Jabeen M, Yakoob MY, Imdad A, Bhutta ZA. Impact of interventions to prevent and manage preeclampsia and eclampsia on stillbirths. BMC Public Health. 2011;11:S10.
35. Lee ACC, Cousens S, Darmstadt GL, Blencowe H, Pattinson R, Moran NF, et al. Care during labor and birth for the prevention of intrapartum-related neonatal deaths: a systematic review and Delphi estimation of mortality effect. BMC Public Health. 2011;11:S10.
36. Lee ACC, Cousens S, Wall SN, Niermeyer S, Darmstadt GL, Carlo WA, et al. Neonatal resuscitation and immediate newborn assessment and stimulation for the prevention of neonatal deaths: a systematic review, meta-analysis and Delphi estimation of mortality effect. BMC Public Health. 2011;11:S12.
37. Menezes EV, Yakoob MY, Soomro T, Haws R, Darmstadt GL, Bhutta ZA. Reducing stillbirths: prevention and management of medical disorders and infections during pregnancy. BMC Pregnancy Childbirth. 2009;9:S4.
38. Hofmeyr GJ, Atallah AN, Duley L. Calcium supplementation during pregnancy for preventing hypertensive disorders and related problems. Cochrane Database Syst Rev. 2006;3, CD001059.
39. Magee LA, Duley L. Oral beta-blockers for mild to moderate hypertension during pregnancy. Cochrane Database Syst Rev. 2003;3:CD002863.
40. Gyorkos TW, Larocque R, Casapia M, Gotuzzo E. Lack of risk of adverse birth outcomes after deworming in pregnant women. Pediatr Infect Dis J. 2006; 25(9):791–4.
41. Torlesse H, Hodges M. Albendazole therapy and reduced decline in haemoglobin concentration during pregnancy (Sierra Leone). Trans R Soc Trop Med Hyg. 2001;95(2):195–201.
42. Duley L, Henderson-Smart D. Magnesium sulphate versus diazepam for eclampsia. Cochrane Database Syst Rev 2003;4:CD000127.
43. Kenyon S, Boulvain M, Neilson J. Antibiotics for preterm rupture of membranes. Cochrane Database Syst Rev 2003;2:CD001058.
44. Majoko F, Nystrom L, Munjanja S, Lindmark G. Usefulness of risk scoring at booking for antenatal care in predicting adverse pregnancy outcome in a rural African setting. J Obstet Gynaecol. 2002;22(6):604–9.
45. Temmerman M, Gichangi P, Fonck K, Apers L, Claeys P, Van Renterghem L, et al. Effect of a syphilis control programme on pregnancy outcome in Nairobi, Kenya. Sex Transm Infect. 2000;76(2):117–21.
46. Di Mario S, Say L, Lincetto O. Risk factors for stillbirth in developing countries: a systematic review of the literature. Sex Transm Dis. 2007;34:S11–21.
47. Ishaque S, Yakoob MY, Imdad A, Goldenberg RL, Eisele TP, Bhutta ZA. Effectiveness of interventions to screen and manage infections during pregnancy on reducing stillbirths: a review. BMC Public Health. 2011;11:S3.
48. Blencowe H, Cousens S, Kamb M, Berman S, Lawn JE. Lives Saved Tool supplement detection and treatment of syphilis in pregnancy to reduce syphilis related stillbirths and neonatal mortality. BMC Public Health. 2011;11 Suppl 3:S9.
49. Garner P, Gulmezoglu AM. Drugs for preventing malaria in pregnant women. Cochrane Database Syst Rev. 2006;4:CD000169.
50. Gamble C, Ekwaru JP, ter Kuile FO. Insecticide-treated nets for the prevention of malaria in pregnancy: A systematic review of randomized controlled trials. PLoS Med. 2007; 4(3):e107.
51. Jarrett RJ, Castro-Soares J, Dornhorst A, Beard RW. Should we screen for gestational diabetes? BMJ. 1997;315(7110):736–9.
52. Langer O, Rodriguez DA, Xenakis EM, McFarland MB, Berkus MD, Arrendondo F. Intensified versus conventional management of gestational diabetes. Am J Obstet Gynecol. 1994;170(4):1036–46.
53. Crowther CA, Hiller JE, Moss JR, McPhee AJ, Jeffries WS, Robinson JS. Effect of treatment of gestational diabetes mellitus on pregnancy outcomes. N Engl J Med. 2005;352(24):2477–86.
54. Waters TP, Mercer BM. The management of preterm premature rupture of the membranes near the limit of fetal viability. Am J Obstet Gynecol. 2009; 230–239.
55. Imdad A, Yakoob MY, Siddiqui S, Bhutta ZA. Screening and triage of intrauterine growth restriction (IUGR) in general population and high risk pregnancies: a systematic review with a focus on reduction of IUGR related stillbirths. BMC Public Health. 2011;11:S3.
56. Hussain AA, Yakoob MY, Imdad A, Bhutta ZA. Elective induction for pregnancies at or beyond 41 weeks of gestation and its impact on stillbirths: a systematic review with meta-analysis. BMC Public Health. 2011;11 Suppl 3:S5.
57. Programme National de Lutte contre le VIH/SIDA. Rapport épidemiologique de surveillance du VIH chez les femmes enceintes fréquentant les structures des CPN. Kinshasa: DRC; 2007.
58. Tann CJ, Kizza M, Morison L, Mabey D, Muwanga M, Grosskurth H, et al. Use of antenatal services and delivery care in Entebbe, Uganda: a community survey. BMC Pregnancy Childbirth. 2007;7:23.
59. Graham WJ, Bell JS, Bullough CHW. L'assistance qualifiée à la naissance peut-elle réduire la mortalité maternelle dans les pays en développement? In De Brouwere V, Van Lerberghe W, editors. Réduire les risques de la mortalité: stratégies et évidence scientifique. Studies in Health Services organisation& Policy 2001, 18: 105–137
60. Ronsmans CCM, Koblinsky MAA. Care seeking at time of childbirth, and maternal and perinatal mortality in Matlab, Bangladesh. Bull World Health Organ. 2010;88:289–96.
61. Pasha O, Goldenberg RL, Elizabeth M, Saleem S, Goudar SS, Althabe F, et al. Communities, birth attendants and health facilities: A continuum of emergency maternal and newborn care (The Global Network's EmONC Trial). BMC Pregnancy Childbirth. 2010;10:82.
62. Crowe S, Utley M, Costello A, Pagel C. How many births in sub-Saharan Africa and South Asia will not be attended by a skilled birth attendant between 2011 and 2015? BMC Pregnancy Childbirth. 2012;12:4.
63. Khan K, Wojdyla D, Say L, Gulmezoglu M, Van Look PF. WHO analysis of causes of maternal death: a systematic review. Lancet. 2006;367:1066–74.
64. Lawn JE, Blencowe H, Oza S, You D, Lee ACC, Waiswa P, et al. Every Newborn: progress, priorities, and potential beyond survival. Lancet. 2014; 384:189–205.
65. Lavender T, Hart A, Smyth RM. Effect of partogram use on outcomes for women in spontaneous labour at term. Cochrane Database Syst Rev. 2013; (7):CD005461
66. Rautava L, Lehtonen L, Peltola M, Korvenranta E, Korvenranta H, Linna M, et al. The effect of birth in secondary- or tertiary-level hospitals in Finland on mortality in very preterm infants: a birth-register study. Pediatrics. 2007; 119(1):e257–63.
67. Lansky S, Franca E, Kawachi I. Social inequalities in perinatal mortality in Belo Horizonte, Brazil: the role of hospital care. Am J Public Health. 2007; 97(5):867–73.
68. McClure EM, Wright LL, Goldenberg RL, Goudar SS, Parida SN, Jehan I, et al. The global network: a prospective study of stillbirths in developing countries. Am J Obstet Gynecol. 2007;197(3):247: e241–245.
69. Goldenberg RL, McClure EM, Bann CM. The relationship of intrapartum and antepartum stillbirth rates to measures of obstetric care in developed and developing countries. Acta Obstet Gynecol Scand. 2007;86(11):1303–9.
70. Barros FC, Bhutta ZA, Batra M, Hansen TN, Victora CG, Rubens CE, et al. Global report on preterm birth and stillbirth (3 of 7): evidence for effectiveness of interventions. BMC Pregnancy Childbirth. 2010;10 Suppl 1:S3.
71. Crowley P. Prophylactic corticosteroids for preterm birth. Cochrane Database Syst Rev. 2000;2, CD000065.
72. Nyamtema AS, Urassa DP, Van Roosmalen J. Maternal health interventions in resource limited countries: a systematic review of packages, impacts and factors for change. BMC Pregnancy Childbirth. 2011;11:30.

2

A structural equation analysis on the relationship between maternal health services utilization and newborn health outcomes

Rornald Muhumuza Kananura[1,2,5*], Robert Wamala[2], Elizabeth Ekirapa-Kiracho[1], Moses Tetui[1,3], Suzanne N. Kiwanuka[1], Peter Waiswa[1,4,5] and Leonard K. Atuhaire[2]

Abstract

Background: Neonatal and maternal health services have a bearing on neonatal mortality. Direct and indirect factors affecting neonatal health outcomes therefore require understanding to enable well-targeted interventions. This study, therefore, assessed the interrelationship between newborn health outcomes and maternal service utilization factors.

Methods: We investigated maternal health utilization factors using health facility delivery and at least four Antenatal Care (ANC) visits; and newborn health outcomes using newborn death and low birth weight (LBW). We used data from a household cross-sectional survey that was conducted in 2015 in Kamuli, Pallisa and Kibuku districts. We interviewed 1946 women who had delivered in the last 12 months. The four interrelated (Endogenous) outcomes were ANC attendance, health facility delivery, newborn death, and LBW. We performed analysis using a structural equation modeling technique.

Results: A history of newborn death (aOR = 12.64, 95% CI 5.31–30.10) and birth of a LBW baby (aOR = 3.51, 95% CI 1.48–8.37) were directly related to increased odds of newborn death. Factors that reduced the odds of LBW as a mediating factor for newborn death were ANC fourth time attendance (aOR = 0.62, 95% CI 0.45–0.85), having post-primary level education (aOR = 0.68, 95% CI 0.46–0.98) compared to none and being gravida three (aOR = 0.49, 95% CI 0.26–0.94) compared to being gravida one. Mother's age group, 20–24 (aOR = 0.24, 95% CI 0.08–0.75) and 25–29 years (aOR = 0.20, 95% CI 0.05–0.86) compared to 15–19 years was also associated with reduced odds of LBW. Additionally, ANC visits during the first trimester (aOR = 2.04, 95% CI 1.79–2.34), and village health teams (VHTs) visits while pregnant (aOR = 1.14, 95% CI 1.01–1.30) were associated with increased odds of at least four ANC visits, which is a mediating factor for health facility delivery, LBW and newborn death. Surprisingly, newborn death was not significantly different between health facility and community deliveries.

(Continued on next page)

* Correspondence: mk.rornald@yahoo.com; mk.rornald@musph.ac.ug
[1]Makerere University School of Public Health (MakSPH), Makerere University College of Health Sciences, Kampala, Uganda
[2]Department of Planning and Applied Statistics, Makerere University School of Statistics and Planning, Kampala, Uganda
Full list of author information is available at the end of the article

(Continued from previous page)

Conclusions: Attending ANC at least four times was a mediating factor for reduced newborn death and low birth weight. Interventions in maternal health and newborn health should focus on factors that increase ANC fourth time attendance and those that reduce LBW especially in resource-limited settings. Targeting women with high-risk pregnancies is also crucial for reducing newborn deaths.

Keywords: Interrelationship, Structural equation modeling, Maternal health utilization, Newborn outcomes,

Background

Globally, at least four million newborns die within four weeks of life every year, of which 75% die within the first week [1]. The largest proportion of neonatal death occurs in low-and-middle-income countries (LMICs) where access to quality health care is low [1, 2]. Most of these newborns die without skilled care that could greatly increase their chances of survival [3]. Access to quality maternal and newborn health services in most of the LMCs is constrained due to various health systems, cultural, socioeconomic, and demographic factors [3]. Though the preventable causes of newborn death such as congenital malformations, tetanus, preterm delivery, diarrhea, pneumonia, intrapartum-related birth asphyxia, and consequences of LBW are well known [1, 4–7], addressing such causes becomes impossible in LMICs where health facilities always experience lack of skilled health workers and stock out of essential medicine and supplies [8, 9].

Uganda's neonatal death rate is estimated at 27 per 1000 live births, which is higher than that of her neighbors (Kenya at 23 and Tanzania at 21 per 1000 live births) [2]. A wider comparison with other African countries still finds Uganda's rate high; for example, Egypt has a rate of 11, South Africa, 15 and Morocco 17 deaths per 1000 live births according to a recent UNICEF report on child health outcomes [2]. Low birth weight (LBW) in Uganda is roughly estimated at 11% [10] given that almost a quarter of the newborns are not weighted [11]. LBW has been found to be significantly related to newborn deaths especially in resource-limited settings [4, 11, 12]; yet these could be saved with simple care such as warmth, feeding, hygiene and early treatment of infection [4, 6].

In addition, the utilization of maternal and newborn services such as ANC attendance, skilled delivery assistance, and postnatal care in Uganda is still below average. For example, ANC fourth time attendance, delivery under skilled assistance and postnatal care within 2 days are estimated at 48, 58, and 33% respectively [13]. Yet these services are cornerstones for assessing newborn and maternal danger signs during pregnancy, labor and after delivery [3, 6]. The utilization of these services is challenged by both demand and supply side constraints including; delays to seek care and system inefficiencies such as low staffing levels, poor care skills, frequent supplies and drugs stock outs and the lack of essential equipment [5]. On the demand side, access to finances has been indicated as the most important factor that affects the utilization of maternal and newborn services [14–16]. Studies done in Rwanda and Ghana have indicated the importance of insurance schemes in increasing the likelihood of maternal and newborn skilled service utilization [15, 16]. Women's access to and control over finances, not only guarantees timely access to services, but also to quality services [15, 16]. In Uganda, it is common for women to deliver at home or within the community because of inhibiting transport costs related to poor community transport systems [17, 18]. Increasing newborn survival, therefore, needs a continuum of care that addresses both the demand and supply side bottlenecks.

The predictors for newborn health outcomes (NHO) and maternal health care utilization (MHCU) are always determined based on approaches that assume direct associations rather than indirect factors [12, 19]. In this study, we considered newborn death (newborn died within 28 days after delivery) and LBW (newborn weight <2.5Kg) for NHOs, while for MHCU, we considered health facility delivery and ANC fourth time attendance. We sought therefore to breach this gap by exploring the interrelationship between factors for newborn outcomes and factors for health facility utilization in rural communities. We believe that health planners, policymakers, and other stakeholders especially from similar settings can use our findings to inform and guide policy formulation needed for the design of interventions aimed at achieving sustainable development goal three. In addition, our findings may contribute to the existing literature particularly on understanding the complexities around newborn death and its relations to low birth weight, health facility delivery, and ANC attendance.

Methods

Study design and population

Data for this study was from the end-line cross-sectional survey conducted by Makerere University School of Public Health in July/August 2015 for the evaluation of a Maternal and Neonatal Implementation for Equitable Systems (MANIFEST) project, which was a quasi-exprimental study implemented in the districts of Pallisa, Kibuku and Kamuli in Eastern Uganda from 2013–2015. The project aim was to improve maternal and neonatal health outcomes. The whole of Kibuku district was an intervention area because it only had one health sub-district. Kamuli and Pallisa had three health sub-districts (HSD), and so one HSD was selected as an intervention area and another as a comparison area in each of the district. The district team did the selection of the intervention and comparison area, which was purposively based on the district maternal and new-born service indicators. Data was collected from women who had delivered in the last 12 months irrespective of birth outcomes. The estimated population in the three districts is 1,106,100 [20].

Sample size and selection of study participants

The study sample size was determined using a two-sided Z-test of the difference between proportions with 80% statistical power, a 5% significance level and 1.5 design effect that resulted in a sample size of 2293 women. The assumption was that after three years (2013–2015) of implementation, skilled deliveries would have increased from 38 to 58%, 62 to 72% and 68 to 78% in the intervention area of Kibuku, Pallisa and Kamuli districts respectively. For the purpose of this study, the data sets for the two project study areas were pooled. However, to verify if the sample size was good enough to measure neonatal death risk factors, we re-estimated the sample size using openEpi [21] at 95% confidence interval with an expected newborn death rate of 27/1000, a precision of 9/1000 (27/1000 ± 9/1000) and a 1.5 design effect which gave us sample size 1867 women. The sample size was, therefore, sufficient to measure newborn death rate and its related predictors.

To select 2293 women, we created a sampling frame of all villages in each of the study areas and estimated 199 villages required to realize the calculated sample size based on an annual average of at least 12 newly delivered women in each village. The 199 villages were selected based on probability proportionate to size. Thereafter, we listed all households in order to identify women who had delivered in the last 12 months irrespective of the birth outcome. During listing, 1946 women were identified as eligible women and all considered for interviews since the estimated sample size was not realized. Trained research assistants made home visits and used a structured questionnaire to interview all eligible women (Additional file 1). The questionnaire was in local language. The principle investigators (RMK, SNK, EEK and MT) and supervisors checked the data collected each day while in the field for completeness. Women whose pregnancies were terminated before 20 weeks were not included. The questionnaires included items for socio-demographic characteristics, antenatal care, socio-economic factors, birth outcome, health system factors, and cultural factors. During analysis, we excluded 52 stillbirths since our focus was on the factors affecting the newborn deaths within 28 days after delivery.

Study variables

In this study, there were four simultaneous equations having at least one endogenous variable as independent variables in each of the equations. The four interrelated study outcomes (endogenous variables) were newborn death, LBW, at least four ANC visits, and health facility delivery. On the other hand, the exogenous factors were the history of newborn death, receiving VHT home visits, ANC first trimester attendance, gestational age, saving for maternal health, and other socio-demographic characteristics such as religion, occupation, marital status, education, age, gravida, and transport to the health facility.

Data analysis

We analyzed data using STATA 13.0 in three stages. Firstly, we did a descriptive summary of socio-demographic characteristics, health facility delivery, ANC attendance, newborn death, LBW, and other selected variables. Secondly, we performed a bivariate analysis using *ulogit* STATA command in order to attain the likelihood of the predictors of maternal health utilization and newborn outcomes. Thirdly, we used a generalized structural equation modeling multivariate approach with binomial logit link function since the study had more than one endogenous variable [22]. Only variables that were significant at bivariate analysis and those that were indicated by Marsh et al., 2002 as well as Mosley & Chen frameworks [6, 23] as potential determinants of maternal health utilization and newborn health outcomes were included in the multivariate analysis. We used pairwise correlation matrix to determine the correlation between the independent variables and likelihood ratio test to test for model goodness of fit.

Results

Description of study participants

Table 1 presents the description of 1894 mothers of newborns. The majority (92%) of participants were peasants, more than a half (62%) of the respondents had not attained any education and most (91%) were married. In addition, the motorcycle was the most common means of transport used to the health facility (66%) and followed by foot/bicycle (20%). Additionally, 15% were teenage mothers and 14% were of the age 35 and above. Furthermore, 33 per 1000 live births (63/1894) were newborns delivered at the gestational age of 5–7 months and almost two out of five (787/1894) respondents had at least five pregnancies. Fifty-seven per a thousand (109/1894) women had ever experienced a newborn death, 28% (530/1894) had ever received VHT visit after delivery and 35.7% (676/1894) had ever received VHT visit while pregnant. Additionally, 31% (596/1894)

Table 1 Distribution by socio-demographic/economic and health characteristics

Characteristics	$n = 1,894$	Percent (%)
Religion		
Catholic	423	22.3
Muslim	320	16.9
Protestant	823	43.5
Others	328	17.3
Marital status		
Not married	163	8.6
Married	1731	91.4
Education		
None	1177	62.1
Primary	549	29.0
Post-primary	168	8.9
Occupation		
Business	96	5.1
Peasant	1755	92.7
Salaried worker	43	2.3
Age group		
15–19	281	14.8
20–24	634	33.5
25–29	415	21.9
30–34	292	15.4
35–39	194	10.2
40+	78	4.1
Gestational age at birth		
5–6Months	21	1.1
7Months	42	2.2
8Months	271	14.3
9Months	1560	82.4
Gravida		
One	306	16.2
two	296	15.6
Three	284	15.0
Four	221	11.7
Five and above	787	41.6
Type of transport used to the facility		
Motorcycle	1,245	65.7
Vehicle	274	14.5
Others	375	19.8
Had a history of newborn death		
No	1,785	94.2
Yes	109	5.8
Attended ANC Early [a]		
No	1,298	68.5
Yes	596	31.5
Received VHT visits after delivery		
No	1,364	72.0
Yes	530	28.0
Received VHT visit while pregnant		
No	1,218	64.3
Yes	676	35.7
Saved money for maternal health services		
No	1,848	97.6
Yes	46	2.4
Newborn death[b]		
Alive	1843	97.3
Died	51	2.7
Delivered in the health facility		
No	563	29.7
Yes	1331	70.3
Attended at least 4 ANC visits		
No	724	38.2
Yes	1170	61.8
Low birth weight[c] $n = 1442$		
No	1249	86.6
Yes	193	13.4

[a] attended first ANC in first-trimester
[b] died within 28 days after birth

accessed ANC in their first trimester and only two percent (46/1894) had saved money for maternal health services.

Health facility utilization and newborn health outcomes

Seven out of ten (1331/1894) respondents delivered in the health facility and almost four out of ten (724/1894) did not attend all the four ANC visits. Low birth weight was found among 13.4% (193/1442) babies; however, 24% (452/1894) of the newborns were not weighed. Newborn death was estimated to be 27 per 1,000 (51/1894) live births with the majority (83%) dying within seven days after birth. In addition, 33 out of 51 newborn deaths (68%) happened within one day (24 h).

Maternal health utilization and newborn health predictors at bivariate level

Bivariate analysis was conducted for study variables that had the possibility of being predictors of health facility utilization in the multivariate analysis. Table 2 shows the variable relationships. Factors that significantly increased the odds of health facility delivery were being a salaried worker compared to those that had petty businesses, at

Table 2 Differentials in maternal health utilization by socio-demographic factors and health facility utilization

	Health facility delivery	ANC four-time attendance	Newborn death	Low birth weight
	Unadjusted OR (95%CI)	Unadjusted OR (95%CI)	Unadjusted OR (95% CI)	Unadjusted OR (95% CI)
Religion				
Catholic[a]	1.00	1.00	1.00	1.00
Muslim	0.80 (0.62–1.03)	0.87 (0.68–1.11)	1.44 (0.68–3.05)	1.04 (0.81–1.33)
Protestant	1.04 (0.86–1.27)	1.03 (0.85–1.24)	0.62 (0.32–1.21)	1.11 (0.92–1.34)
Others	1.10 (0.85–1.44)	0.88 (0.69–1.13)	1.86 (0.92–3.76)	0.91 (0.71–1.18)
Marital status				
No married[a]	1.00	1.00	1.00	1.00
Married	0.95 (0.67–1.36)	1.24 (0.90–1.72)	0.65 (0.25–1.69)	0.81 (0.58–1.12)
Education				
None[a]	1.00	1.00	1.00	1.00
Primary	1.25 (0.87–1.80)	1.34 (0.96–1.88)	1.48 (0.57–3.84)	0.63 (0.44–0.90)*
Post primary	1.22 (0.98–1.53)	1.15 (0.94–1.41)	0.34 (0.13–0.88)*	0.75 (0.61–0.93)*
Occupation				
Business[a]	1.00	1.00	1.00	1.00
Peasant	0.88 (0.60–1.30)	0.90 (0.63–1.29)	0.44 (0.18–1.06)	1.27 (0.88–1.85)
Salaried worker	2.65 (1.11–6.33)*	1.82 (0.91–3.64)	2.33 (0.54–9.97)	0.23 (0.09–0.59)*
Age group				
15–19[a]	1.00	1.00	1.00	1.00
20–24	0.94 (0.75–1.17)	1.21 (0.98–1.51)	0.61 (0.27–1.38)	0.98 (0.69–1.39)
25–29	0.91 (0.71–1.15)	1.21 (0.97–1.52)	0.62 (0.26–1.50)	0.40 (0.25–0.64)*
30–34	0.98 (0.74–1.28)	1.01 (0.78–1.31)	0.97 (0.40–2.33)	0.99 (0.65–1.50)
35–39	1.41 (0.99–1.99)	0.69 (0.51–0.93)*	1.26 (0.49–3.25)	1.04 (0.64–1.70)
40+	0.79 (0.49–1.27)	0.61 (0.38–0.95)*	0.59 (0.08–4.36)	1.04 (0.48–2.22)
Had a history of newborn death				
No[a]	1.00	1.00	1.00	1.00
Yes	1.02 (0.67–1.56)	0.81 (0.55–1.19)	12.62 (6.49–24.57)*	1.38 (0.93–2.04)
Attended at least 4 ANC visits				
No[a]	1.00	–	1.00	1.00
Yes	1.42 (1.17–1.75)*	–	0.83 (0.44–1.57)	0.62 (0.45–0.84)*
Attended ANC Early				
No[a]	1.00	1.00	1.00	1.00
Yes	0.95 (0.77–1.17)	3.27 (2.61–4.10)*	0.54 (0.25–1.18)	0.88 (0.64–1.24)
Received VHT visit while pregnant				
No[a]	1.00	1.00	–	1.00
Yes	1.31 (1.06–1.61)*	1.27 (1.05–1.55)*	–	1.03 (0.76–1.42)
Saved for money maternal health services				
No[a]	1.00	1.00	–	–
Yes	1.77 (1.18–2.64)*	1.04 (0.71–1.40)	–	–
Gravida				
One[a]	1.00	1.00	1.00	1.00
Two	0.86 (0.60–1.24)	0.98 (0.70–1.36)	1.15 (0.50–2.62)	1.1 (0.85–1.43)
Three	0.74 (0.51–1.06)	1.03 (0.74–1.44)	0.81 (0.31–2.08)	0.8 (0.61–1.05)
Four	0.84 (0.57–1.25)	1.31 (0.91–1.89)	0.84 (0.30–2.38)	1.06 (0.79–1.42)

Table 2 Differentials in maternal health utilization by socio-demographic factors and health facility utilization *(Continued)*

Five and above	0.72 (0.53–0.97)*	0.84 (0.64–1.11)	0.75 (0.39–1.45)	1.1 (0.91–1.33)
Gestational age at birth				
5–6Months	–	–	12.01 (3.85–37.47)*	–
7Months[a]	–	–	1.00	–
8Months	–	–	0.66 (0.23–1.87)	–
9Mmonths	–	–	0.43 (0.22–0.85)*	–
Type of Transport used to the health facility				
Motorcycle[a]	–	–	1.00	–
Vehicle	–	–	2.07 (1.09–3.94)*	–
foot/bicycle	–	–	1.25 (0.65–2.42)	–
Low birth weight				
No[a]			1.00	–
Yes			5.56 (2.70–11.44)	–
Delivered in the health facility				
No[a]	–	–	1.00	–
Yes	–	–	1.28 (0.62–2.63)	–
Received VHT visits after delivery				
No[a]	–	–	1.00	–
Yes	–	–	0.45 (0.2–1.07)	–
Baby experienced danger signs				
No[a]	–	–	1.00	
Yes	–	–	0.87 (0.45–1.68)	
Mother experienced danger signs				
No[a]	–	–	1.00	–
Yes	–	–	1.22 (0.65–2.29)	–

OR-Odds Ratio, * $p < 0.05$, [a]reference category, dash (–) denotes variables not considered for particular outcome

least four ANC visits, VHTs visits during pregnancy and saving money for maternal services ($p < 0.05$). The odds of health facility delivery was significantly reduced by being gravida 5+ compared to being gravida one ($p < 0.05$). Regarding the recommended ANC attendance, factors that significantly increased the probability of at least four ANC visits were attendance of ANC in the first trimester, and VHTs visits during pregnancy ($p < 0.05$). Furthermore, factors that significantly reduced the probability of having at least four ANC visits were belonging to the age group of 35+ years compared to the age group 14–19 years ($p < 0.05$).

Regarding newborn health outcomes, factors that significantly reduced the odds of neonatal death were post primary education completion compared to none and gestational age of eight months to nine months compared to the gestational age of 7 months ($p < 0.05$). In addition, factors that increased the odds of newborn death were the history of newborn death, LBW, gestational age at the time of birth of 5–6 months compared to the gestational age of 7 months and use of motor vehicle transport compared to the motorcycle ($p < 0.05$). Factors that significantly reduced the odds of LBW were at least four ANC visits, having at least primary education level compared to none and a salaried occupation compared to petty business.

The predictors of newborn death, LBW, health facility delivery and at least four ANC visits at bivariate level do not reveal causal linkages between the variables. Therefore, a structural equation modeling approach was used to understand the causal linkages as indicated in the next results-sub section. All significant variables identified in the bivariate analysis were considered for further analysis in the multivariate model. However, variables that were not significant such as age group, gravida, education, and occupation were controlled for in the multivariate analysis since available literature has indicated their contribution towards newborn death, low birth weight, and health facility utilization.

The interrelationship between health facility utilization and newborn health outcomes

Table 3 indicates the details of the interrelationship between health facility utilization and newborn health

Table 3 Analysis of interrelationship between maternal health utilization and newborn health outcomes using GSEM

	Newborn Outcome indicators		Facility utilization indicators	
	Newborn death (Y_1)	Low birth weight (Y_2)	Health facility delivery (Y_3)	ANC 4 time attendance (Y_4)
	Adjusted OR (95% CI)		Adjusted OR (95% CI)	
Delivered in the health facility				
No[a]	1.00	–	–	–
Yes	0.47 (0.19–1.26)	–	–	–
Attended at least 4 ANC visits				
No[a]	–	1.00	1.00	–
Yes	–	0.62 (0.45–0.85)**	1.43 (1.16–1.75)**	–
Age group				
15–19[a]		1.00	1.00	1.00
20–24		0.24 (0.08–0.73)*	1.04 (0.76–1.42)	1.17 (0.97–1.40)
25–29		0.20 (0.05–0.86)*	0.93 (0.66–1.30)	1.20 (0.98–1.47)
30–35		0.34 (0.10–1.17)	1.01 (0.70–1.45)	1.13 (0.91–1.41)
34–59		0.40 (0.11–1.42)	1.27 (0.86–1.86)	0.91 (0.73–1.13)
Attended ANC Early				
No[a]	–	–	–	1.00
Yes	–	–	–	2.04 (1.79–2.34)**
Received VHT visit while pregnant				
No[a]	–	–	–	1.00
Yes	–	–	–	1.14 (1.01–1.30)*
Marital status				
Not Married[a]	1.00	1.00	1.00	1.00
Married	0.77 (0.23–2.60)	0.90 (0.53–1.53)	0.94 [0.65,1.36]	1.15 [0.93–1.41]
Education Level				
None[a]	–	1.00	1.00	1.00
Primary	–	0.75 (0.38–1.45)	1.15 (0.76–1.72)	1.18 (0.92–1.50)
Post primary	–	0.68 (0.46–0.98)*	1.29 (1.02–1.63)*	1.11 (0.97–1.27)
Occupation				
Business[a]	1.00	1.00	1.00	1.00
Peasant	0.54 (0.11–2.65)	0.85 (0.40–1.79)	1.26 (0.80–1.97)	1.14 (0.87–1.49)
Salaried worker	0.42 (0.04–4.60)	1.07 (0.29–3.88)	2.84 (1.03–7.80)*	1.50 (0.88–2.53)
Had a history of newborn death				
No[a]	1.00	1.00	–	–
Yes	12.64 (5.31–30.10) **	1.33 (0.72–2.47)	–	–
Gravida				
One[a]	–	1.00	–	–
two	–	0.91 (0.53–1.54)	–	–
Three	–	0.49 (0.26–0.94)*	–	–
Four	–	0.65 (0.31–1.37)	–	–
Five and above	–	0.79 (0.39–1.60)	–	–
Type of Transport used to the facility				
Motorcycle[a]	1.00	–	–	–
Vehicle	0.79 (0.20–3.16)	–	–	–
Foot/bicycle	1.40 (0.49–3.93)	–	–	–

Table 3 Analysis of interrelationship between maternal health utilization and newborn health outcomes using GSEM *(Continued)*

Low Birth Weight				
No[a]	1.00	–	–	–
Yes	3.51 (1.48–8.37)**	–	–	–
Saved money for maternal health services				
No[a]	–	–	1.00	1.00
Yes	–	–	1.72 (1.14–2.58) **	0.92 (0.74–1.14)

OR-Odds Ratio, * $p< 0.05$, ** $p< 0.01$, *** $p< 0.001$, [a]reference category, dash (–) denotes variables not considered for particular outcome

outcomes. The direct predictors of newborn death were LBW and history of newborn death, while the indirect factors were at least four ANC visits, education, gravida, ANC first attendance in the first trimester of pregnancy, VHTs visits during pregnancy, and religion. Newborns with low birth weight and those born to mothers with a history of newborn death were more likely to die within 28 days after birth (aOR = 3.51, 95% CI 1.48–8.37) and (aOR = 12.64, 95% CI 5.31–30.10) respectively). The odds of the newborn death was not significantly different between those delivered within and outside of the health facilities.

The factors for LBW as a mediating variable for newborn death were at least four ANC visits, education, gravida, and age. Women who attended ANC at least four times had 38% reduced odds of delivering low birth weight babies compared to those who attended ANC less than four times (aOR = 0.62, 95% CI 0.45–0.85). Mothers who had post-primary education had 32% reduced odds of delivering low birth weight babies compared to those who had no education at all (aOR = 0.68, 95%CI 0.46–0.98). Mothers who were gravida three had 51% reduced odds of delivering low birth weight babies compared to those who were gravida one (aOR = 0.49, 95% CI = 0.26–0.94). LBW was less likely among children born to mothers aged 20–24 (aOR = 0.24, 95% CI 0.07–0.73) and 25–29 (aOR = 0.20, 95% CI 0.05–0.86) years compared to those aged 15–19 years. No significant associations identified among women aged above 29 years.

The factors for attending ANC at least four times as a mediating variable for newborn death and LBW were ANC first attendance in the first trimester of pregnancy, VHTs visits during pregnancy and religion (Table 3). Women who attended ANC in the first trimester were

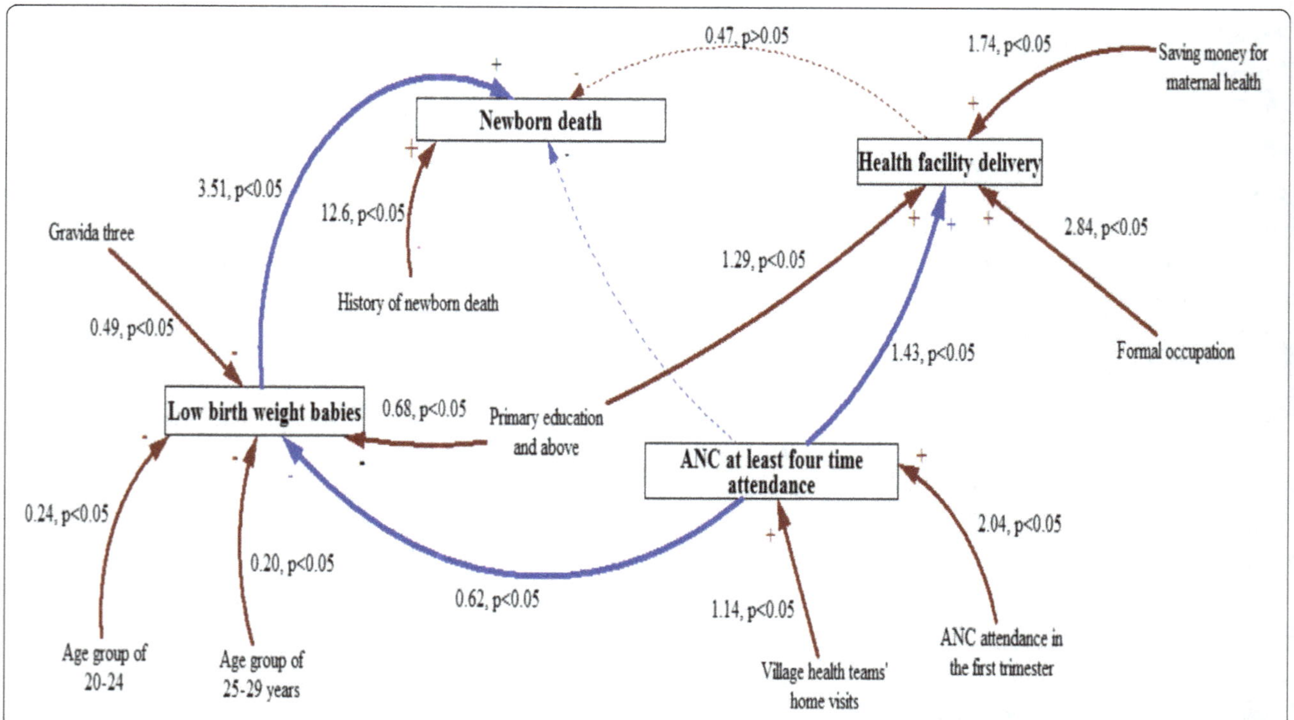

Fig. 1 Causal loop for maternal health utilization and newborn health outcome. Note: – negative effect, + positive effect, Negative effect though not significant. Negative effect but dropped because of multicollinearity

two times more likely to attend ANC at least four times relative to those who attended ANC in the second trimester or later (aOR = 2.04, 95% CI 1.79–2.34). Women who were visited by the VHTs while pregnant had 14% increased odds of attending ANC at least four times (aOR = 1.14, 95% CI 1.01–1.30).

Figure 1 is a causal loop diagram that summarizes the interconnectedness between the maternal health care utilization and newborn health outcome factors.

Discussion

This study has indicated a high proportion of LBW babies in these rural communities and this might be underestimated since almost a quarter of the newborns were not weighed as found in a similar study [11]. Newborn mortality rate was 27 per 1,000 live births, similar to the national average [24]. As noted in similar studies, the newborn mortality rate was high within seven days after delivery (83%) with the majority (68%) of newborns dying within one day [1, 25]. This is an indication of the critical care needed at the time of birth and the immediate period thereafter for newborns to survive [1]. Newborn deaths in the first seven days are mainly attributed to maternal pregnancy and childbirth related complications and infections [12, 26]. Death occurring within one day might be closely related to community and health facility challenges that include delays in seeking care, poor community transport systems, lack of skilled health workers, lack of equipment and drugs at the health facilities and poor referral networks from the lower level to the higher levels [5].

Interrelationship between newborn outcomes and health utilization factors

The direct determinants of newborn death were LBW, history of newborn death and mother's age. Since LBW is an endogenous variable, LBW and any other endogenous variable that affect LBW are mediating variables for newborn death. The odds of dying among children born to mothers who had a history of losing newborns was 12 times higher compared to those born by mothers who had no history of newborn death. This was found to be consistent with other studies [24, 27–31]. Other studies have also indicated that women who experienced a pregnancy loss or stillbirth or lost a baby within 28 days in the past are more likely to lose a baby in the subsequent pregnancy [24, 30, 31]. There is, therefore, a need for an examination of historical cohorts of newborns and immediate family members with respect to genetic, chromosomal and congenital predispositions in order to elicit more precise conclusions [32].

The likelihood of increased deaths among LBW newborns was not surprising, since this has been reported in a number of studies done in similar settings [11, 12, 33]. These studies have shown that LBW babies are at a higher risk of a number of health complications, which increase their chances of death if appropriate care is not given. Moreover, the low capacity of health facilities in LMICs to prevent, screen and manage the LBW babies' complications makes it hard for newborns to survive. Therefore, interventions aimed at building the capacity of health workers on how to screen and care for LBW babies at health facilities are vital.

The factors associated with the odds of LBW as a mediating factor for newborn death were education, at least four ANC visits, mother's age, and religion. Post-primary level education of mothers was positively related to the birth weight of newborns; a finding that is consistent with existing studies undertaken in other LMICs [34–36]. Lower education levels have been associated with lower health awareness and health seeking behavior as well as low dietary literacy among mothers, which have been found to have a bearing on LBW [35]. Additionally, LBW among babies born to mothers who were gravida three was found to be lower compared to those whose mothers who were gravida one. Similar studies indicated that mothers who are pregnant for the first time are more likely to deliver LBW than mothers with two to four pregnancies [13, 34, 37]. Furthermore, women aged 20–29 years were less likely to deliver LBW babies compared to women aged 15–19 years and there was no significant association established among mothers aged above 29 years. The increased LBW among children born to mothers aged 15–19 years has been associated with the problems faced by such adolescent mothers, who are often women from vulnerable populations, which predisposes them to less access to care [13, 34, 37, 38]. Poor knowledge levels and nutrition status coupled with underdeveloped reproductive organs further increase the chances of adolescents to deliver LBW babies [36]. Additionally, the increased odds of LBW among elderly mothers might be related to poor child spacing [36].

Regarding attending ANC at least four times as a mediating factor for LBW and newborn death, newborns whose mothers attended ANC at least four times were less likely to be LBW babies compared to those who attended for less times, which was consistent with other studies [12, 34, 37]. The World Health Organization (WHO) recommends a minimum of four antenatal visits during pregnancy since this is a period when newborns are affected by problems such as preterm birth, restricted fetal growth and congenital infections that might increase the chances of newborn death [39]. Furthermore, attending ANC has been indicated as a potential avenue for women and their families to receive information and advice on obstetric care as well as identification and management of infections such as Malaria, HIV/AIDS, Syphilis, and other sexually transmitted diseases

[39] that have an effect on the fetus. This confirms the importance of conducting population-oriented programs that encourage early ANC attendance [37].

In this study, women who attended ANC in the first trimester had two times the odds of attending ANC at least four times relative to those who attended ANC in the second trimester and above, which was in agreement with a study done in Malawi and Ghana [40]. In addition, the odds of at least four ANC visits was higher among women visited by VHTs while pregnant. This confirms the importance of community health workers in promoting maternal service utilization particularly in rural communities as reported in other studies done in Sub-Saharan Africa [5, 39, 41–45]. These studies have highlighted the importance of community health workers in identifying pregnant women in the community, sensitizing, encouraging and empowering them to seek maternal health services from a qualified health worker. Home visits by VHTs encourages women to attend ANC early (in the first trimester), which helps them benefit fully from preventive strategies, such as iron and folic acid supplementation, treatment of helminthic infections, and intermittent preventive treatment with sulfadoxine-pyrimethamine for malaria in pregnancy among other interventions [39, 46].

Surprisingly, the proportion of newborn deaths for women who delivered in the health facility was not statistically different from those who delivered in the community, which is consistent with recent studies in similar settings [11, 12]. This indifference has been linked to the poor quality of care in the health facilities as well as the possibility of births happening in health facilities but without skilled personnel assistance [33, 47]. This is made worse by system-wide challenges such as drugs and supplies shortages, the lack of essential equipment and shortage of health workers exemplified by a similar study done in Eastern Uganda [48]. This therefore indicates that increasing health facility deliveries without addressing supply side constraints is unlikely to reduce the newborn mortality. In fact, poor quality services at the health facilities reduce utilization of maternal and newborn services. Interventions seeking to improve neonatal health outcomes, therefore, need to consider tackling both demand and supply side constraints.

Limitations of the study

The analysis was limited to the available information on variables given the nature of the dataset. In addition, the results are generalizable to communities in rural Eastern Uganda but can also be generalized to areas that have a similar context. Additionally, recall bias might have affected the study results but we minimized this by including only women who had delivered in the last 12 months. In addition, excluding 52 records of stillbirth might have had an effect on the health facility and ANC four-time attendance outcomes, however, the records were less than 3% of the total number of participants. The study also did not assess causes of death by timing.

Conclusions

The interdependence between the predictors of maternal health care utilization and newborn health outcomes highlight important areas of focus for interventions aimed at reducing neonatal mortality. Community health interventions such as home visits by village health teams should be strengthened in order to improve early ANC attendance and recommended ANC visits. There is a need to target women with high risk pregnancies in particular those with a previous history of neonatal mortality and teenage pregnancy. In addition, low cost interventions that improve identification and survival of low birth weight babies in low resource settings should be strengthened.

Abbreviations

ANC: Antenatal Care; IRB: Institutional Review Board; LBW: Low birth weight; MakSph: Makerere University School of Public Health; MCHCU: Maternal Health Care Utilization; UDHS: Uganda Demographic Health Survey; UNCST: Uganda National Council for Science and Technology; VHTs: Village Health Teams; WHO: World Health Organization

Acknowledgements

We are thankful to the study participants and the district health office from the districts of Kamuli, Kibuku and Pallisa for their time during data collection. We are grateful to Future Health System and Makerere University School of Public Health for their technical support during the design and the implementation of this study.

Funding

The MANIFEST study was funded by Comic Relief grant code 112483. The funding body did not play any direct role in the study data collection, analysis and writing of the manuscript. The content is solely the responsibility of the authors and does not necessarily represent the official views of Comic Relief.

Authors' contributions

RMK carried out data collection, analysis and led the writing of the manuscript with the contribution from all authors. RW participated in conceiving and reviewing the study, EE-K provided general guidance and participated in drafting and reviewing the manuscript, MT, SNK and PW participated in reviewing the study, and LKA provided guidance in data analysis and presentation.

Competing interests

The authors declare that they have no competing interests.

Author details

[1]Makerere University School of Public Health (MakSPH), Makerere University College of Health Sciences, Kampala, Uganda. [2]Department of Planning and Applied Statistics, Makerere University School of Statistics and Planning, Kampala, Uganda. [3]Epidemiology and Global Health Unit, Department of Public Health and Clinical Medicine, Umeå University, Umeå, Sweden. [4]Global Health Division, Department of Public Health Sciences, Karolinska Institutet, Stockholm, Sweden. [5]Maternal and Newborn Centre of Excellence, Makerere University School of Public Health, Kampala, Uganda.

References

1. Lawn JE, Cousens S, Zupan J. 4 Million neonatal deaths: When? Where? Why? Lancet. 2005;365:891–900.
2. UNICEF. The State of the World's Children 2014 -Every Child Counts. New York; 2014. http://www.unicef.org/sowc2014/numbers/documents/english/SOWC2014_In Numbers_28 Jan.pdf.
3. Ayele DZ, Belayihun B, Teji K, Ayana DA. Factors affecting utilization of maternal health care services in Kombolcha District, Eastern Hararghe Zone, Oromia Regional State, Eastern Ethiopia. Int Sch Res Not. 2014;2014:7.
4. Kinney MV, Kerber KJ, Black RE, Cohen B, Nkrumah F, Coovadia H, et al. Sub-Saharan Africa's mothers, newborns, and children: Where and why do they die? PLoS Med. 2010;7:1–9.
5. Waiswa P, Kallander K, Peterson S, Tomson G, Pariyo GW. Using the three delays model to understand why newborn babies die in eastern Uganda. Trop Med Int Heal. 2010;15:964–72. doi:10.1111/j.1365-3156.2010.02557.x.
6. Marsh DR, Darmstadt GL, Moore J, Daly P, Oot D, Tinker A. Advancing newborn health and survival in developing countries: a conceptual framework. J Perinatol. 2002;22:572–6.
7. Chou D, Daelmans B, Jolivet RR, Kinney M, Say L. Ending preventable maternal and newborn mortality and stillbirths. Bmj. 2015; h4255. doi:10.1136/bmj.h4255.
8. Penfold S, Shamba D, Hanson C, Jaribu J, Manzi F, Marchant T, et al. Staff experiences of providing maternity services in rural southern Tanzania - a focus on equipment, drug and supply issues. BMC Health Serv Res. 2013;13:61. doi:10.1186/1472-6963-13-61.
9. Dogba M, Fournier P. Human resources and the quality of emergency obstetric care in developing countries: a systematic review of the literature. Hum Resour Health. 2009;7:7. doi:10.1186/1478-4491-7-7.
10. Namiiro FB, Mugalu J, McAdams RM, Ndeezi G. Poor birth weight recovery among low birth weight/preterm infants following hospital discharge in Kampala, Uganda. BMC Pregnancy Childbirth. 2012;12:1.
11. Kananura RM, Tetui M, Mutebi A, Bua JN, Waiswa P, Kiwanuka SN, et al. The neonatal mortality and its determinants in rural communities of Eastern Uganda. Reprod Health. 2016;1–9. doi:10.1186/s12978-016-0119-y.
12. Kassar SB, Melo AMC, Coutinho SB, Lima MC, Lira PIC. Determinants of neonatal death with emphasis on health care during pregnancy, childbirth and reproductive history. J Pediatr (Rio J). 2013;89:269–77.
13. Ministry of Health Uganda and ORC Macro. Uganda Demographic and Health Survey 2011. 2011. http://ubos.org/onlinefiles/uploads/ubos/pdf documents/Uganda DHS 1988–89 Final Report.pdf.
14. Chi PC, Bulage P, Urdal H, Sundby J. A qualitative study exploring the determinants of maternal health service uptake in post-conflict Burundi and Northern Uganda. BMC Pregnancy Childbirth. 2015;15:18. doi:10.1186/s12884-015-0449-8.
15. Amoakoh-Coleman M, Ansah EK, Agyepong IA, Grobbee DE, Kayode GA, Klipstein-Grobusch K. Predictors of skilled attendance at delivery among antenatal clinic attendants in Ghana: a cross-sectional study of population data. BMJ Open. 2015;5:e007810. doi:10.1136/bmjopen-2015-007810.
16. Joharifard S, Rulisa S, Niyonkuru F, Weinhold A, Sayinzoga F, Wilkinson J, et al. Prevalence and predictors of giving birth in health facilities in Bugesera District, Rwanda. BMC Public Health. 2012;12:1049. doi:10.1186/1471-2458-12-1049.
17. Anyait A, Mukanga D, Oundo GB, Nuwaha F. Predictors for health facility delivery in Busia district of Uganda: a cross sectional study. BMC Pregnancy Childbirth. 2012;12:132. doi:10.1186/1471-2393-12-132.
18. Kiwanuka SN, Ekirapa EK, Peterson S, Okui O, Rahman MH, Peters D, et al. Access to and utilisation of health services for the poor in Uganda: a systematic review of available evidence. Trans R Soc Trop Med Hyg. 2008;102:1067–74. doi:10.1016/j.trstmh.2008.04.023.
19. Christiana RT, Michael JD, Kingsley A, Christine LR, Hall J. Determinants of neonatal mortality in Indonesia. BMC Public Health. 2008;8:232.
20. UBOS. Uganda Bureau of Statistics; 2014 Statistical Abstract. 2014.
21. Dean A, Sullivan K, Soe M. OpenEpi: Open Source Epidemiologic Statistics for Public Health. Updat 2011/23/06. 2011;:Version 2.3.1. www.OpenEpi.com.
22. Huber C. Generalized Structural Equation Modeling Using Stata. 2013.
23. Mosley WH, Chen LC. An analytical framework for the study of child survival in developing countries. 1984. Bull World Health Organ. 2003;81:140–5. http://www.pubmedcentral.nih.gov/articlerender.fcgi?artid=2572391&tool=pmcentrez&rendertype=abstract.
24. Getahun D, Lawrence JM, Fassett MJ, Strickland D, Koebnick C, Chen W, et al. The association between stillbirth in the first pregnancy and subsequent adverse perinatal outcomes. Am J Obstet Gynecol. 2009;201:378–80. doi:10.1016/j.ajog.2009.06.071.
25. Rammohan A, Iqbal K, Awofeso N. Reducing Neonatal Mortality in India: Critical Role of Access to Emergency Obstetric Care. PLoS One. 2013;8:3.
26. Pedrosa LDCO, Sarinho SW, Ordonha MR. Quality of information analysis on basic causes of neonatal deaths recorded in the Mortality Information System: a study in Maceió, Alagoas State, Brazil, 2001–2002. Cad Saude Publica. 2007;23:2385–95.
27. van Dinter MC, Graves L. Managing adverse birth outcomes: helping parents and families cope. Am Fam Physician. 2012;85:900–4.
28. Turton P, Hughes P, Evans CD, Fainman D. Incidence, correlates and predictors of post-traumatic stress disorder in the pregnancy after stillbirth. Br J Psychiatry. 2001;178:556–60. doi:10.1192/bjp.178.6.556.
29. August EM, Salihu HM, Weldeselasse H, Biroscak BJ, Mbah AK, Alio AP. Infant mortality and subsequent risk of stillbirth: a retrospective cohort study. BJOG. 2011;118:1636–45.
30. Mahande MJ, Daltveit AK, Mmbaga BT, Obure J, Masenga G, Manongi R, et al. Recurrence of perinatal death in Northern Tanzania: a registry based cohort study. BMC Pregnancy Childbirth. 2013;13:166. doi:10.1186/1471-2393-13-166.
31. Reddy Uma M, Katherine Laughon S, Liping S, James T, Willinger M, Jun Z. Prepregnancy risk factors for Antepartum stillbirth in the United States. Obstet Gynecol. 2010;116:1119–26.
32. Williams B, Datta S. Previous fetal death. In: A Textbook of Preconceptional Medicine and Management. 2012. p. 241–50. https://www.glowm.com/resources/glowm/preconception_pdf/old/Preconceptional%20MedicineFull.pdf#page=149.
33. Ogi S, Odimegwu C. Perinatal mortality in Nigeria: Do place of delivery and delivery assistants matter? Open Demogr J. 2011;4:1–10. https://benthamopen.com/contents/pdf/TODEMOJ/TODEMOJ-4-1.pdf.
34. Khatun S, Rahman M. Socio-economic determinants of low birth weight in Bangladesh: a multivariate approach. Bangladesh Med Res Counc Bull. 2008;34:81–6.
35. Muula AS, Siziya S, Rudatsikira E. Parity and maternal education are associated with low birth weight in Malawi. Afr Health Sci. 2011;11:65–71.
36. Manna N, Sarkar J, Baur B, Basu G, Bandyopadhyay L. Socio-biological determinants of Low birth weight: a community based study from rural field practice area of medical college, Kolkata, West Bengal (India). Iosr J Drg. 2013;4:33–9. http://www.iosrjournals.org/iosr-jdms/papers/Vol4-issue4/H0443339.pdf.
37. Alemseged A, Mektie W, Semarya B. Maternal risk factors associated with low birth weight. J Coll Physicians Surg Pak. 2003;13:25–8.
38. Ydav D, Chaudhray U, Shrestha N. Maternal risk factors associated with low birth weight. J Nepal Heal Res Counc. 2011;9:159–64.
39. Lincetto O, Mothebesoane-anoh S, Gomez P, Munjanja S. Antenatal Care: Opprotunities for Africa's Newborns. Int J Sci Technol Res. 2013;2:51–62.
40. Pell C, Meñaca A, Were F, Afrah NA, Chatio S, Manda-Taylor L, et al. Factors affecting antenatal care attendance: results from qualitative studies in Ghana, Kenya and Malawi. PLoS One. 2013;8:e53747. doi:10.1371/journal.pone.0053747.
41. Ediau M, Wanyenze RK, Machingaidze S, Otim G, Olwedo A, Iriso R, et al. Trends in antenatal care attendance and health facility delivery following community and health facility systems strengthening interventions in Northern Uganda. BMC Pregnancy Childbirth. 2013;13:189. doi:10.1186/1471-2393-13-189.
42. Lema IA, Sando D, Magesa L, Machumi L, Mungure E, Mwanyika Sando M, et al. Community health workers to improve antenatal care and PMTCT uptake in Dar es Salaam, Tanzania: a quantitative performance evaluation.

J Acquir Immune Defic Syndr. 2014;67 Suppl 4:S195–201. doi:10.1097/QAI.0000000000000371.
43. Gogia S, Sachdev HS. Home visits by community health workers to prevent neonatal deaths in developing countries: a systematic review. Bull World Health Organ. 2010;88:658–666B.
44. Gilmore B, McAuliffe E. Effectiveness of community health workers delivering preventive interventions for maternal and child health in low- and middle-income countries: a systematic review. BMC Public Health. 2013;13:847. doi:10.1186/1471-2458-13-847.
45. Aboubaker S, Qazi S, Wolfheim C, Oyegoke A, Bahl R. Community health workers: a crucial role in newborn health care and survival. J Glob Health. 2014;4:1–5. www.ncbi.nlm.nih.gov/pmc/articles/PMC4267086/.
46. van Eijk AM, Bles HM, Odhiambo F, Ayisi JG, Blokland IE, Rosen DH, et al. Use of antenatal services and delivery care among women in rural western Kenya: a community based survey. Reprod Health. 2006;3:2.
47. Nathan R, Mwanyangala M. Survival of neonates in rural Southern Tanzania: does place of delivery or continuum of care matter? BMC Pregnancy Childbirth. 2012;12:18. doi:10.1186/1471-2393-12-18.
48. Tetui M, Ekirapa E, Bua J, Mutebi A, Tweheyo R, Waiswa P. Qaulity of Antenatal care services in eastern Uganda: implications for interventions. Pan Afr Med J. 2012;13:1–15. http://www.panafrican-med-journal.com/content/article/13/27/full/.

3

Factors affecting effective community participation in maternal and newborn health programme planning, implementation and quality of care interventions

Lisa Howard-Grabman[1*], Andrea Solnes Miltenburg[2], Cicely Marston[3] and Anayda Portela[4]

Abstract

Background: Community participation in in health programme planning, implementation and quality improvement was recently recommended in guidelines to improve use of skilled care during pregnancy, childbirth and the postnatal period for women and newborns. How to impement community participation effectively remains unclear. In this article we explore different factors.

Methods: We conducted a secondary analysis, using the Supporting the Use of Research Evidence framework, of effectiveness studies identified through systematic literature reviews of two community participation interventions; quality improvement of maternity care services; and maternal and newborn health programme planning and implementation.

Results: Community participation ranged from outreach educational activities to communities being full partners in decision-making. In general, implementation considerations were underreported. Key facilitators of community participation included supportive policy and funding environments where communities see women's health as a collective responsibility; linkages with a functioning health system e.g. via stakeholder committees; intercultural sensitivity; and a focus on interventions to strengthen community capacity to support health. Levels of participation and participatory approaches often changed over the life of programmes as community and health services capacity to interact developed.

Conclusion: Implementation requires careful consideration of the context: previous experience with participation, who will be involved, gender norms, and the timeframe for implementation. Relevant stakeholders must be actively involved, particularly those often excluded from decision making. Current limited evidence suggests that the vision of community participation as a process and the presence of a focus to strengthen community capacity to participate and to improve health may be a key factor for long term success;

Keywords: Community participation, Maternal and newborn health, Quality improvement, Health programme planning and implementation

* Correspondence: lhowardg@trg-inc.com
[1]Training Resources Group, Inc., 4301 Wilson Boulevard, Suite 400, Arlington, VA 22203, USA
Full list of author information is available at the end of the article

Background

Community participation in health is: 'a process whereby people, both individually and in groups, exercise their right to play an active and direct role in the development of appropriate health services, in ensuring the conditions for sustained better health and in supporting the empowerment of community to help development' p.10 [1]. Involving communities in assessing their own needs and in developing strategies to meet those needs can increase intervention ownership and sustainability, while responsiveness to community needs in planning and implementation of health programmes can help improve health equity, service delivery, and uptake of care [2–4]. Various reviews and World Health Organization (WHO) Guidelines have highlighted the importance of community participation for improved health [5–9].

The WHO commissioned systematic reviews of health promotion interventions involving community participation. We performed a secondary analysis on two of them here [10]: 1) quality improvement of maternity care services where community members participate in processes to review the quality of health services either as informants or as partners with health providers in planning and implementation to improve quality; and 2) maternal and newborn health programme planning and implementation, where community members are involved in planning, designing, implementing and monitoring strategies and interventions. Based on these reviews, community participation in quality improvement and in health programme planning and implementation is now recommended by WHO to improve use of skilled care during pregnancy, childbirth and the postnatal period for women and newborns, increase the timely use of facility care for obstetric and newborn complications and improve maternal and newborn health [10]. In addition to the available evidence on the impact of participation, it is also important to understand which factors influence implementation of community participation interventions for maternal and newborn health. This article addresses this question, exploring stakeholder perspectives and experiences of the two community participation interventions, and identifying barriers and facilitators to successful implementation.

Methods

We analysed the studies included in systematic reviews of published and unpublished grey literature used to inform WHO health promotion guidelines for maternal and newborn health [10]. The methods for the review are described in the WHO document.

The systematic reviews included articles published between 2000 and 2012 initially identified from a systematic mapping of maternal health research in low- and middle-income countries [11]. Studies included RCTs as well as any other study design that included at least one data collection point prior to the intervention and one during or after the intervention. Studies reporting qualitative data were included. The systematic reviews themselves are not the topic of this paper.

We extracted data from 16 studies that could shed light on factors influencing implementation using an adapted 'SURE (Supporting the Use of Research Evidence) framework' [12]. The framework includes a comprehensive list of barriers and facilitators to implementing health systems interventions including stakeholder knowledge and attitudes, health service delivery factors, and social and political considerations. Starting from the categories within the broad SURE framework the authors identified further, specific themes of interest from the primary empirical data presented in the included articles and from the author discussion and conclusions from those articles.

Results

Description of included studies

Table 1 shows characteristics of included studies. 16 papers reported on 13 separate programmes: seven in Asia (India $N = 1$; Bangladesh $N = 1$; Pakistan $N = 2$; Nepal $N = 1$; China $N = 1$, Indonesia $N = 1$), three in East Africa (Tanzania $N = 1$; Uganda $N = 1$; Kenya $N = 1$) and three in Latin America (Peru $N = 2$; Honduras $N = 1$). Implementation approaches for community participation varied. They included forming stakeholder committees [13–21], mobilizing communities to take action [14, 22–25], community based monitoring of health outcomes or services [17–19, 25, 26], community outreach activities to increase awareness of health issues [13, 16, 27] and facilitating stakeholder dialogues [19, 28]. Many of the studies were complex, multiple intervention programmes that combined community participation with health system strengthening and some also combined multiple approaches to participation. There was no consistent definition of 'community' and some studies did not define 'community' at all.

Community participation did not always fit neatly into one category, ranging from communities being the recipients of health messages to high level engagement where community members and groups played active roles in decision-making, planning and implementation [29]. In six programmes, community members participated at different levels at different points during the intervention [17, 18, 22, 23, 25, 26, 28]. Communities were involved in designing programmes from the beginning in only two cases [19–21]; in four programmes, communities provided input on interventions [25–28]; and in seven, programme teams designed the programme and chose the interventions. The communities were then asked to adapt and implement them [13–18, 22–24]. Women participated at

Table 1 Characteristics of studies and description of interventions

No	Study	Setting	CP[a]	Time frame	Approach	Level	General description of intervention or aim of the study
1	Purdin S, et al. (2009). Reducing maternal mortality among Afghan refugees in Pakistan	Pakistan: Hangu district of Khyber Pakhtunkhwa Province (rural refugee settlements)	P&I	1980–2007`	Community outreach and stakeholder committee	Outreach	Provision of reproductive health services for Afghan refugees through establishment of Basic Health Units and Basic Emergency Obstetric Care facilities. Camp-based health committees included community representatives who attended bi-monthly meetings with health staff to discuss project activities and provide feedback to providers on services provided. The Basic Health Unit staff trained Community Health Workers and committee members including men on safe motherhood and reproductive health topics to educate others in the refugee community.
2	Ahluwalia I, et al. (2003). An evaluation of a community-based approach to safe motherhood in northwestern Tanzania (See also Ahluwalia, 2003)	Tanzania: Kwimba Missungwi districts (rural)	P&I	1998–2000	Community mobilizing	Outreach, Consult, Involve	As part of a Community Based Reproductive Health Project (CBRHP) strengthening of community level services was done through a special activity called the Community Capacity Building and Empowerment Project. The project aimed for local problem solving through 1) training, technical assistance, and support for (village health workers) VHWs who provided educational house visits on topics such as recognition of danger signs and birth preparedness; [2] developing community-based plans for transportation to health facilities and [3] increasing participation by community members in planning and decision-making through community meetings, aiming to identify and solve local health problems.
3	Ahluwalia I, et al. (2010). Sustainability of community-capacity to promote safer motherhood in northwestern Tanzania: what remains? (See also Ahluwalia, 2010)	Tanzania: Kwimba Missungwi districts (rural)	P&I	2006	Community mobilizing	Outreach, Consult, Involve	This study reports on a follow-up study of Ahluwalia (2003) with the aim to examine the remains of the CBRHP as described above. Activities continued from 2001 to 2006 without project support. A post project assessment was conducted with focus on the CBRHP components, including community supported transport systems; village health workers; and changes in selected maternal health service use indicators at the district level.
4	Bhutta Z, et al. (2011)	Pakistan: 2 towns in Sindh with 1400 villages (rural)	P&I	2006–2008	Stakeholder committee and Community mobilizing	Outreach	Community-based intervention package principally delivered through training of Lady Health Worker (LHW) and *Dais* (traditional health workers) and promotion of liaison between them together with facilitation of the creation of voluntary community health committees (CHC). In addition to advocacy work with community elders and local

Table 1 Characteristics of studies and description of interventions *(Continued)*

							political leaders, the CHCs were encouraged to organize an emergency transport fund and the use of vehicles using local resources. The CHCs facilitated the LHWs in accessing women and in conducting group education sessions in the intervention villages.
5	Paxman J, et al. (2005). The India Local Initiatives Program: A Model for Expanding Reproductive and Child Health Services	India: 4 northern states in Kolkata, the hills of the Himalayas, Punjab plains, and mountains of Himachal Pradesh (urban & rural)	P&I	1999–2003	Stakeholder committee	Involve	NGOs help to organize or strengthen a reproductive and child health committee composed of influential community members. The committees recruit, train and oversee the work of community health volunteers (CHVs), raise money for health activities and support, and enlist support of local government, social and religious leaders. CHVs provided health information to households and kept track of their health status, provided some basic health services including some family planning methods, organized educational activities and referred clients to additional services outside their communities. CHVs tracked health status making use of a pictorial map to facilitate use by people with limited literacy skills, which helped project staff to monitor performance.
6	Kaufman J, et al. (2012). Improving reproductive health in rural China through participatory planning	China: Dafang and Zhenning counties in Guizhou Province, Luoping County in Yunnan Province (rural)	P&I	2002–2006	Community outreach	Involve	The Gender and Health Equity Network (GHEN) project aimed to improve health further for poor rural women by increasing women' s participation in planning and resource allocation through capacity building through training of township women's representatives and local officials in gender and health. Women's health promotion groups and demonstration households were established. Demonstration households collected information on local health service needs and shared this with the health promotion team who communicated to higher-level health authorities. Women and their families were taught how to prevent and treat common health problems and were motivated to use services. Health education activities were organized at least once per month. County and township supervision meetings were held once every two months to provide direction, identify and solve problems.
7	Harkins T, et al. (2008). The health benefits of social mobilization: experiences with community-based Integrated Management of Childhood	Peru: Chao district (peri-urban) and Honduras: San Luis district (rural)	P&I	2004–2005	Stakeholder committee, community outreach	Involve	Multiple government agencies, private sector and non-governmental organizations along with representatives of community-based organizations established or strengthened existing committees that were tasked by the

Table 1 Characteristics of studies and description of interventions *(Continued)*

	Illness in Chao, Peru and San Luis, Honduras						project with disseminating key Integrated Management of Childhood Illness health messages to their various constituencies through their networks with the aim of involving families and communities in maternal and child health approaches. Members of the committee were trained and they in turn capacitated community members. The committees could be creative about how they disseminated the messages. The committee was responsible for organizing the training and events and the supporting logistics for their activities.
8	Sood S, et al. (2004). Measuring the effects of the SIAGA behavior change campaign in Indonesia with population-based survey results	Indonesia, West-Java	P&I	1999–2004	Community mobilizing	Involve	Social mobilization campaign consisted of a mass media component that targeted husbands (Suami SIAGA), birth attendants (Bidan SIAGA), and communities (Warga SIAGA) and villages (Desa SIAGA) with radio and television spots and shows that modeled the desired attitudes and behaviors of "alert" husbands, midwives and communities that support the health of their mothers and babies. There was also a community participation component for the "alert village" that built on a traditional concept of the value of community help. This component aimed at motivating people to establish life-saving systems in their villages (transport, emergency funds, blood)
9	Mathur, et al. (2004). Youth Reproductive Health in Nepal – is participation the answer? (See also Malhotra, 2005)	Nepal: Nawalparasi and Kawasoti Districts (rural Terai) & two urban suburbs of Kathmandu	P&I	1998–2004	Stakeholder committee	Shared Leadership	A youth centered participation project was initiated through a formative research process, which included a needs assessment on how issues of youth reproductive health were relevant in the communities of interest. The project staff facilitated an action planning process through which results of the needs assessment were shared with community members. The project established two community-based advisory groups, the Adolescent Coordination Team (ACT) and the Project Advisory Committee (PAC) consisting of adults. This was followed by formation of separate task forces consisting of youth representatives to develop interventions and an intervention plan. The task forces then came together to integrate their plans after seeking advice from resource people in the community. This was followed by implementation of the interventions. This study documents the process and results of the project.

Table 1 Characteristics of studies and description of interventions *(Continued)*

10	Malhotra, et al. (2005). Nepal: The Distributional Impact of Participatory Approaches on Reproductive Health for Disadvantaged Youth (See also Mathur, 2004)	Nepal: Nawalparasi and Kawasoti Districts (rural Terai) & two urban suburbs of Kathmandu	P&I	1998–2004	Implementation planning through youth involvement taskforces	Shared Leadership	This study reports on the impact of participatory approaches in improving youth reproductive health as reported by Mathur (2004). The authors examine whether the participatory or the non-participatory intervention approach is more successful in reducing the gaps between the disadvantaged and the advantaged in access to youth reproductive health services and in outcomes.
11	Kaseje D, et al. (2010). Evidence-based dialogue with communities for district health systems' performance improvement	Kenya: 6 districts in Nyanza Province: Nyando, Siaya, Kisumu, Rachuonyo, Suba, Bondo (urban & rural)	P&I, QI	2005–2007	Stakeholder committees, facilitation of dialogue, community based monitoring	Collaborate	An evidence-based dialogue model was introduced to community members, district health management teams, and service providers through a series of three, three-day workshops. The intervention package included the development of committees at the village, community and health facility levels; identify, train and deploy Community Health Extension Workers (CHEWs) as facilitators of dialogue at the community level, supporters of CHWs, and maintainers of a community-based information system; identify and train CHWs to support households in health improvement activities, maintain village register and facilitate dialogue at household level; establishment of village registers of all households; improvement and timeliness of analysis, dissemination and utilization of health management information system data; analyze suggestions collected from suggestion boxes on a monthly basis; and, hold dialogue sessions based on data from the community and health facilities every month at household and community levels and every four months at health facility and sub-district levels. In dialogue sessions, data were displayed, discussed and consensus was built on what was acceptable and what needed to be improved.
12	Bjorkman M, and Svensson J (2009). Power to the People: Evidence from a randomized field experiment on community-based monitoring in Uganda	Uganda: 50 communities from 9 districts in all four regions of Uganda (rural)	P&I, QI	2004–2006	Community-based monitoring	Collaborate (most villages), Shared Leadership (some villages)	With the aim to strengthen providers' accountability to citizen-clients an NGO-facilitated approach was implemented. First community members were presented with baseline information (a "report card") which was a summary of information gathered from both community members and service providers as well as data collected from service registers to reflect the status of health service delivery relative to other providers and the government standards. During community meetings community members developed a shared view on how to improve service delivery

Table 1 Characteristics of studies and description of interventions *(Continued)*

							and monitor the providers. A facility meeting was held with health facility staff to present the results of the household survey and contrast the results to the results of the information provided by services providers. An interface meeting between community representatives elected at the earlier community meeting and health service providers discussed proposed suggestions for improvement and came to agreement on an action plan and a plan for how the community would monitor progress. After six months, health facility staff and community members jointly assessed and analyzed progress.
13	Sinha D (2008). Empowering communities to make pregnancy safer: an intervention in rural Andrha Pradesh.	India: Mominpet in Rangareddy District in Andhra Pradesh (rural)	QI	2004–2006	Community mobilizing and community based monitoring	Shared Leadership (some villages)	Community organizers raised awareness of village councils and youth organizations about the powerful role they could play in ensuring that public health facilities provide the services they are required to deliver and instructed them on how to use a monitoring tool to compare actual performance with expected service delivery. Village councils then held regular monthly meetings to which they invited representatives of local organizations, youth groups, schools, mother's committees, and community level health workers. Participants in the meetings reviewed service performance, health data and service utilization statistics, identified problems and worked to solve them. When solutions did not work, they initiated action with higher authorities. Meetings were also held at the lower levels. Youth leaders, initially young men but later joined by young women, organized meetings in the villages to raise awareness of young people to hold providers accountable for good service. Eventually, the young people formed a "Youth Committee for Right to Health" that met monthly.
14	Gabrysch S, et al. (2009). Cultural adaptation of birthing services in rural Ayacucho, Peru.	Peru: All 17 villages in the Santillana district, Ayacucho region (rural)	QI	1997–2001	Facilitation of dialogue	Consult, Collaborate	Program cycle approach to engaging pregnant women and health providers in the development of maternity services that met both service provider and community expectations for quality care. Phase 1: detailed formative research by project team to understand perceptions and practices related to reproductive health and health services. Phase 2: 3 facilitated meetings of pregnant women, TBAs, CHWs and health providers to design a birthing service that was ` to all

Table 1 Characteristics of studies and description of interventions *(Continued)*

							parties. Phase 3: Implementation of newly designed birthing service through capacity building workshops for health providers and TBAs to teach each other; sharing of evidence-based practices; informing of the population about the new service. Phase 4: Project evaluation followed by minor adaptation to the model. Phase 5: Routine monitoring and assessment of sustainability until 2007.
15	Barbey A, et al. (2001). Dinajpur SafeMother Initiative Final Evaluation Report (see also Hossain & Ross, 2006)	Bangladesh: Dinajpur & Panchagarh in northwestern Bangladesh (rural)	QI	1998–2001	Stakeholder committees and community based monitoring	Involve	This study reports on an evaluation of the Dinajpur Safe motherhood Initiative (DSI) to examine and validate the achievements, and explain the attribution of the specific project interventions. The DSI had the primary aim of testing the impact of a defined package of interventions. Facility interventions included facility upgrades to provide basic Emergency Obstetric Care (EmOC) and improvements of quality of care through the creation of Stakeholder Committees, with representation of health providers and 11 community members (leaders, active TBAs, CBOs) to build rapport between the community and the health care system and through the enhancement of health service provider capacity. The stakeholder committee met regularly and monitored service cleanliness and client perceptions of services, as well as reviewed maternal death or near-miss cases. Community interventions included: birth planning education through home visits and group discussions at clinic and village meetings by SBAs, fieldworkers and village doctors who were trained to disseminate BP messages that were also incorporated into a variety of visual aids; the establishment of Community Support System (CmSS) including emergency funds for EmOC, emergency transportation for referral to another health facility, identification of volunteers to accompany women to facilities or to provide financial support and a list of volunteers who are available to donate blood in case of emergency. DSI specifically aimed to ensure quality services for all women subjected to violence, particular during pregnancy.

Table 1 Characteristics of studies and description of interventions *(Continued)*

16	Hossain & Ross (2006). The effect of addressing demand as well as supply of emergency obstetric care in Dinajpur, Bangladesh (see, also Barbey et al., 2001)	Bangladesh: Dinajpur & Panchagarh in northwestern Bangladesh (rural)	QI	1998–2001	Stakeholder committees and community based monitoring	Involve	This study reports on the impact of the Dinjpur Safe motherhood Initiative (DSI) as reported by Barbey (2001) on utilization of EmOC services.

[a]CP – Community Participation in P&I (Programme planning and implementation), QI (Quality Improvement) and/or MDSR (Maternal Death Surveillance and Response)

lower levels than men in many of the studies, [13, 14, 17, 18], however, one study focused exclusively on women's participation [27].

Implementation barriers and facilitators

Tables 2 and 3 present barriers and facilitators to successful implementation across the two distinct interventions.

We identified five categories of implementation barriers and facilitators reported by the studies: 1) the extent to which there was an enabling and supportive environment or not; 2) the nature of community capacity; 3) health system factors; 4) features of the interface between community and health services; and, 5) intercultural competence and sensitivity of the programmes.

The findings across the two interventions were very similar so in this analysis we discuss them together. However, Tables 2 and 3 provide the reader with specific details about which factors were reported in each study.

Enabling and not-so-enabling environments

The Millennium Development Goals triggered supportive maternal and newborn health policies and political commitment at the highest levels of government in many countries which changed the overall context for these programmes. Community participation interventions in Bangladesh, India, Peru, China, and Indonesia were implemented in the context of new government schemes and approaches to upgrade services and make them more accessible and affordable [16–18, 24, 25, 27]. For example, through the National Rural Health Mission, the Indian government introduced subsidies and incentives to make services more accessible and affordable for pregnant women and their families [25]. In China, a rural health insurance scheme was introduced which allowed local officials to decide on which services would be covered. This, in turn, created opportunities for programme participants to advocate for more accessible services for women [27]. At the district and village levels, NGOs involved in establishing health committees with the India Local Initiatives Programme characterised the urban environment as highly politicized with disputes that interrupted progress. The study also reported that politicians did not collaborate with the programme when they saw no benefit for themselves [15].

Cultural norms of collective responsibility helped communities to plan and work together to address barriers to accessing quality care. In Indonesia, the SIAGA social mobilization project intentionally built on the traditional value of collective help (*gotong royong*) as the foundation for their "alert community" campaign. This aimed at motivating people to establish life-saving systems in their villages (transport, emergency funds, blood) [24]. In Tanzania, one study showed how community members initially perceived women's health as the responsibility of individuals and were not inclined to work together to address barriers to service use [22, 23]. As the programme evolved, however, the study authors report that community awareness grew: both about the nature of the challenges and how they could help by working together. Over time, the members of the community began to value collective responsibility and action [22, 23]. The communities where this shift in norms occurred were also reportedly more likely to sustain their efforts to improve health and maintain mechanisms such as transport systems compared with those that remained focused on individual responsibility [23].

Community capacity

Studies reported many facilitating and inhibiting factors related to community capacity development, both generally in terms of community leadership, governance and management, and more specifically in relation to health knowledge, skills and abilities. Many programmes worked with committees and stakeholder groups that helped facilitate the participation process. In Bangladesh and Kenya, lack of transparency in decision-making and management of resources led to the committees dissolving and compromised the trust necessary for villagers to work together successfully [17–19]. Bhutta, et al. (2011) observed that leadership transitions were a challenge to implementation; trust and relationship building had to begin again with each new leader [14]. Eight of the studies noted the value of multiple organizations at multiple levels working in partnership, recognizing that improving maternal and child health would require participation and support of many stakeholders [15–18, 22–24, 27]. The majority of studies reviewed that worked with committees reported that committees were most successful when their purpose and individual roles and responsibilities within the committees were clear [13]. Strong and stable community leadership was highlighted as a key facilitator to effective implementation in six studies [15, 17, 18, 22, 23, 26]. While many of the studies opted to involve leaders and influential people in quality improvement stakeholder committees and groups, some authors emphasized the importance of ensuring representation for those who often did not have a voice in community planning and implementation. They underscored the importance of providing opportunities for women and young people to develop and exercise leadership skills and have a forum for their participation on issues that clearly and directly affect and interest them [16, 17, 19, 25, 26]. In general, studies reported value in having regular meetings to monitor progress, adapt strategies as necessary and solve problems [17–19, 25, 26].

Table 2 Facilitators of implementation cited in studies included in the systematic review for each research question

Facilitators of implementation	Community participation in quality improvement	Community participation in MNH programme planning & implementation
ENABLING/SUPPORTIVE ENVIRONMENT		
A supportive political environment with supportive policies makes it easier to implement programmes.	18, 19	28
Community awareness of and interest in MNH are high.		
• When mortality is high, it is more likely that community members will see the problem and perceive the need for change. • Use mass media campaigns (radio/TV) and other outreach methods to increase awareness of the issue.	18, 19	17, 25
Reinforce or nurture cultural norm of collective responsibility for better maternal & newborn health.		23, 24
Build on and/or develop more cohesive populations with tighter social networks. Rural programme sites had an easier time implementing than those in urban sites in part due to more cohesive populations, tighter social networks.		16, 21, 22
COMMUNITY CAPACITY		
Community leadership		
Having strong and stable community leadership facilitates implementation.	18, 19, 27	16, 18, 23, 24, 27
Improve community leadership, ownership & governance of programme	18, 20, 26, 27	16, 18, 20
Provide women/young people with opportunities for leadership, forum for participation	18, 20, 26	16, 18, 20, 21, 22, 28
Increase focus and attention to health in local council meetings	26, 27	25, 27
COMMUNITY PARTICIPATION & GOVERNANCE		
Ensure representation of the voices and perspectives of different groups	20, 26, 27	17, 20
Increase participation of marginalized, disadvantaged, less powerful groups	26, 27, 29	21,22, 27
Increase women's participation in decision-making		23, 24, 28
Work with existing structures when they are functional or have flexibility to form new structures/mechanisms when they don't exist or are dysfunctional (need to understand their purpose, roles and responsibilities). Establish and/or strengthen committees or other planning & coordination structures.	18, 19, 20, 26, 27	14, 15, 16, 17, 18, 21, 22, 23, 24, 25, 27, 28
COLLABORATION & PARTNERSHIP		
Establish and/or strengthen multi-organization partnership including public sector/local government at multiple levels.	18, 19	16, 17, 23, 24, 25, 28
Improve community - health services interaction/relations.	18, 19, 20, 29	15, 18, 20, 21, 22, 27
Increase awareness and support of community health workers.		14, 15, 23, 24
Strengthen social networks for information exchange/support.		21, 22, 25
• Violence against women advocacy support network established, action taken to address this issue	18, 19	18, 19
COMMUNITY MANAGEMENT CAPACITY		
Strengthen community ability to use data for decision-making, monitoring, accountability & advocacy.		
• Communities, households, services with more complete data; using data	20, 26	14, 20
• Use of data for decision-making, advocacy	20, 26, 27	
• Improved community monitoring and accountability of health services	18, 19, 26, 27	21, 22, 27
Strengthen community ability to leverage and manage resources.		
• Transparency in decision-making and management of resources	18, 19, 20	18, 20, 23, 24
• Community capacity to leverage and manage resources	18, 20	16, 20, 23, 24, 25
Strengthen community ability to plan; development of written action plan, "community contract" that guided implementation.	18, 19, 20, 27	20, 21, 22, 23, 24, 27
Strengthen community ability to problem-solve.	18, 19	18
Community capacity: health related technical knowledge, skills & abilities		

Table 2 Facilitators of implementation cited in studies included in the systematic review for each research question *(Continued)*

Train village health workers/community volunteers to be able to provide health education and services.	19, 20, 26	14, 16, 17, 23, 24
Develop blood donor lists to identify potential donors, if needed.	18, 19	18, 19, 25
Improve knowledge of danger signs.	18, 19	17,18, 19
HEALTH SYSTEM		
Sufficient number of trained staff in health facilities		14, 15
Improve quality of care/upgrade services	[aim of all studies for this intervention]	14, 15, 18
Availability of accurate data on health situation, health services	19, 20, 27	16, 20, 27
Leadership at district and health facility levels	18, 19	
COMMUNITY & HEALTH SYSTEM INTERACTION		
Community health workers play a vital role linking communities and health services	18, 19, 20, 26, 29	14, 15, 16, 20, 23, 24
NGOs can facilitate the process, provide technical support to communities to help them develop capacity to plan and implement. Existing relationships of NGOs with communities and health services facilitate implementation. NGOs can support inter-cultural interaction.	18, 19, 27, 29	14, 16, 17, 18, 23, 24, 27
Bring communities and health service providers together to participate in joint assessment and dialogue before planning.	20, 29	20, 28
Use key questions to drive planning process dialogue.	20, 29	20
Schedule regular meetings (monthly, bimonthly, quarterly) to monitor, adjust strategies, problem-solve.	18, 19, 20, 26, 27	
INTERCULTURAL SENSITIVITY /COMPETENCE		
Acknowledge and build on existing traditional/local beliefs and practices.	29	25
Develop/use culturally appropriate materials in local languages that are suitable for the range of literacy/numeracy skills in the programme context.	18, 19, 27, 29	15, 16, 18, 25, 27
Understand social networks and focus on changing social norms.	26	21, 22, 25
Maintain a gender rights focus and consider gender roles.	18, 19	16, 18, 25, 28
OTHER PROGRAMME CONDITIONS		
Use participatory methodology and techniques		21, 22, 25
Use a synergistic package of complementary interventions		18
Provide funding support for a longer period of time (this study was funded for 4 years)		28
Train programme facilitators (in MNH topics, data interpretation, dissemination, conflict resolution, management)		14, 15, 17, 18, 23, 24, 27

Note: see numbered list of references at the end of the article to interpret the numbers presented in the columns below. This is a descriptive, qualitative analysis based on what the reviewed studies reported. The number of studies reporting each facilitating factor is not intended to be an indicator of the level of importance of the factor.

A key factor influencing implementation in most studies included whether interventions helped communities address the issues that affected them. Some programmes were designed with this aim in mind; for example, the youth participation programme in Nepal and the Gender and Health Equity Network in China helped groups of socially marginalised people learn how to influence decision-making on health policy making and practice [20, 21, 27]. In Uganda, the programme "encouraged communities to be more involved with the state of health service provision and strengthened their capacity to hold their local health providers to account for performance" [26]. In other studies this type of process occurred not by design, but serendipity: the community mobilization study in India, for instance, relied on the programme's community organizers to act as intermediaries between communities and health services as part of the intervention which in turn increased community willingness and ability to hold health workers accountable for services [25]. Studies that did not include elements of community capacity development ran into implementation challenges. For example, several studies describe how community, facility and government stakeholders needed time to develop ways of planning and working together which did not always fit programme timelines [15, 19–23, 27]. Sometimes communities had limited understanding of how to interpret and manage health data, which hindered effectiveness of community based monitoring [17–19].

Table 3 Implementation barriers and challenges cited in studies included in the systematic review for each research question

Implementation barriers & challenges	Community participation in quality improvement	Community participation in MNH programme planning & implementation
Not-so-enabling environment		
Need more supportive maternal health policies		1, 2
Low status of women, gender inequity	18, 19, 26	14, 28
Discrimination against indigenous people, ethnic groups, poor people	29	
Conflict, insecurity and violence against women	18, 19, 29	14
Politicians do not collaborate when they see no benefit for themselves		16
Urban environment highly politicized		16
Urban setting negatively affects time available to participate, especially for men; recruitment and retention of community health volunteers is also more challenging.		16, 21, 22
Community capacity		
Community leadership		
Changes in leadership		15
Community leadership doesn't prioritize maternal health or health more generally.	19	
COMMUNITY GOVERNANCE & MANAGEMENT		
Community capacity to plan and work together is limited. Takes time to develop.	20	16, 20, 21, 22, 23, 24, 28
Trust issues exist among different groups.	18, 19	16, 18, 22
• Lack of transparency in management of community funds.	18, 19	18
Ineffective structures		
• Existing structures are dysfunctional	27	27
• At sub-district level, organizational structures are less defined and many different local groups exist. (Dinajpur Safe Motherhood Initiative chose to develop a Community Support System structure to address this challenge.)		18, 19
Health system		
Managing resources & resource constraints		
• Human resource constraints of public health system		15
• Health services supervision system weak, irregular	27	27
• Services lack "modern equipment and advanced technology"	18, 19	18, 21, 22
Health facility data inconsistent and incomplete – difficult to plan effectively and difficult to assess attribution of programme outcomes; limited capacity for data management	18, 20, 29	18, 20
Service provider attitudes are resistance to change	29	21, 22
Wider health system issues such as ineffective referral system (outside of local control)	29	
Community -health system interaction		
MANAGEMENT OF RESOURCES & RESOURCE CONSTRAINTS		
• Limited access to facilities (distance, difficult terrain)	20	17, 20
• Lack of funds (for transport)	20	20
• Lack of financial and technical resources (MOH, community)	20	20, 23, 24
• Rotation of health personnel doesn't allow time to develop trusting relationships with community	29	
• Expectations of community health workers are unrealistic; too many tasks		15
Poor communication	20	20
Need to improve linking/interface of communities with services	18, 19	18, 23, 24
Intercultural sensitivity/competence		
Cultural traditions of women delivering and residing in other homes outside of study area for postnatal period affects birth preparedness plans and postnatal follow-up care.		15

Table 3 Implementation barriers and challenges cited in studies included in the systematic review for each research question *(Continued)*

Reluctance of families to travel long distances for neonatal care (cultural practice and security issues underlie this reluctance)		15
Increasing empowerment of youth led to conflict at times		21, 22
Reaching and including people with low literacy and numeracy skills	29	17
May not be reaching the poorest and most vulnerable with the strategies used, strategies may not be effective for these groups	18, 19	18
General programme design/implementation challenges		
Proxy indicators have some limitations (e.g., utilization of EmOC for "met need")	18, 19	18
Expansion and scaling up	20, 26, 29	
Low coverage and high complexity of the intervention		15
Volunteers taking on too many tasks		15

Note: see numbered list of references at the end of this article to interpret the numbers presented in the columns below. This is a descriptive, qualitative analysis based on what the reviewed studies reported. The number of studies reporting each barrier or challenge is not intended to be an indicator of the level of importance of the factor.

Health system factors

Limitations within health systems were highlighted in many studies. For instance, five studies highlighted the importance to health facilities of having accurate data on population health, health services and case studies of maternal deaths and "near-misses" to improve quality and planning within services, as well as to share with the broader community to raise awareness about health priorities and to monitor progress over time [15, 17–19, 25, 26]. Yet, incomplete and inconsistent data at health facilities made it difficult to plan effectively, and also made it hard for programmes to assess the effects of changes they had made [17, 19, 28]. Resource constraints also presented challenges to effective implementation [14, 14, 17, 18, 20, 21]. Two studies reported that having trained staff in health facilities and upgrading the quality of care helped facilitate work with communities [13, 14]. A persistent challenge in many health programmes that was also evident in the studies reviewed here was a weak, irregular and ineffective supervision system for healthcare staff [26]. Barbey (2001) indicates that health system leadership at the district and facility levels is key to quality improvement efforts [17].

Interface between community and health services

Communities and health services may face challenges in coming together to plan and implement programmes. Some communities had limited access to facilities because of distance, difficult terrain and lack of funds for transport, while health service providers may face problems trying to reach communities and supervise community health workers [16, 18, 19]. Poor communication and lack of financial and technical resources on both sides (public health sector and community) can limit communities' and service providers' ability to meet, which can limit the effectiveness of such partnerships in improving healthcare [19, 22, 23].

Several studies reported that joint assessments between healthcare providers and members of the community helped improve quality by providing valuable information to feed into priority setting and identify opportunities and challenges [19, 27, 28]. Community health workers, volunteers, and NGOs play important roles in linking communities with health systems by facilitating dialogue, providing health education and services through community outreach, collecting health and community data, and by drawing on existing relationships which help them understand the local context and priorities [13–15, 17–19, 22, 23, 25, 28]. Sometimes, however, volunteers were expected to take on too many tasks and thus could not complete all of them well [14]. Barbey et al. (2001) advise that facilitators be well-trained in facilitation, coaching and training skills [17].

Intercultural competence and sensitivity of the programmes

Culturally-appropriate materials in local languages are needed that are suitable for a range of literacy and numeracy skills for programmes where community members participate in analysis of health data as a basis for decision-making and action [14, 15, 17, 18, 24, 28]. Programmes in Indonesia, India and Nepal highlighted the importance of programme personnel understanding and working to mobilize social networks in culturally-sensitive ways to bring about changes in social norms [20, 21, 24, 25]. A gender roles analysis study in China advocated a gender rights focus as a way to help raise community awareness about inequities in women's access to services and other opportunities, making the case for women's participation in bottom up planning processes in resource-poor settings where women's status is low to better inform decision-makers about women's needs and views [27].

Women's low status appears to have influenced how community priorities were set, how decisions were made at the household level, and also influenced women's level of participation. Gender inequity manifested in different ways in different places. For instance, in Peru, Quechua women were discriminated against and treated poorly by health services staff. Ongoing local conflict also affected their sense of security and limited access to health facilities [16]. Similarly, in India husbands were reluctant to participate in maternal health interventions, describing maternal health as a "women's issue." Study authors reported, "It was clear that efforts to make husbands more supportive questioned deep-rooted norms and beliefs, and met with considerable resistance; consequently, husbands were slow to change their views." [27]. The studies in Bangladesh showed how women suffered from violence in multiple settings: at home, in communities and in health services [17, 18].

Benefits and harms

Reported benefits of community involvement in monitoring health data and quality included increased accountability of the health system to the community. Studies also reported reduced absenteeism [25, 26], reduced drug stock-outs [19, 26], reduced waiting time [26], better examination procedures [26], improved facility infrastructure and equipment [19, 25, 27] and reduced use of untrained providers [25] as well as generally improved quality of care [17, 18]. Other cited benefits included policies and actions that reflected and addressed women's needs [27].

At community level reported benefits included improved abilities of individuals, groups and communities in governance of programmes [15, 17, 19, 25, 26], management, planning and using data for group decision-making [13, 19–23, 25, 26], obtaining and managing resources [15, 17, 19–24], facilitating group processes to include new voices [20–23, 25–28], monitoring and evaluation, conflict management, and problem-solving [17, 18, 20, 21, 24–26]. In addition, participation interventions helped community members improve their knowledge and skills about maternal and newborn health, which enabled them to carry out specific health related tasks or functions [13, 14, 17, 18, 22, 23]. Two studies suggested that community capacity development can also help sustain improvements in health [20, 23].

Most studies did not report on specific harms. In a study from Peru, the authors noted that it was important to attend to both the personal needs of community members as well as ensure adequate medical quality [28]. In addition, increased empowerment of young people in Nepal sometimes led to conflict when it challenged existing social norms [20, 21].

Stakeholder perspectives and experiences

The quality improvement studies provided very limited information on stakeholder perspectives. Stakeholder dialogue in developing culturally-acceptable childbirth services in Peru was reported to have helped create mutual understanding between communities and service providers and the new services developed as a result were hailed as a success locally [28]. A study in India [25] using community mobilization and monitoring noted: "Community leaders reported that as a result of direct interaction with government officials on problems faced by health providers and the women themselves, there was more openness among officials to resolving issues and a greater willingness to accept feedback from the community" p14 [25]. Women in the same study said there was more community support for pregnancy-related care. Interventions at family level found approaching mothers-in-law helpful, as they were more receptive to community organizers than husbands [25].

Studies on community participation in planning and implementation of health programmes reported positive experiences of programme participants, although they reported few details. Stakeholder committees in Bangladesh were reported to be generally acceptable, with the strongest committees recognizing they could apply their strengthened problem-solving skills to other issues beyond health, and saying that they appreciated programme staff assistance in how they motivated committees to come up with their own solutions [18]. Members of committees in India and Kenya were reported to appreciate having a better understanding of their own roles and responsibilities, for instance in the decision making process for resource allocation and financial management [15, 19]. In Nepal, where young people participated to try to improve reproductive health, 'community members and, in particular, young people, felt a strong enough sense of ownership over the project to demand accountability from the implementation team. By the end of the project, young people were leading many of the intervention activities, with the implementation team acting only as facilitators' [20, 21]. Study authors reported that community outreach through dissemination of health messages by health promotion groups or committees was widely accepted in Peru and China [18, 27]. Health providers in Peru reportedly said that families became more knowledgeable about maternal and child health danger signs, and of how to care for children with diarrhoea [16]. Four studies [14, 24–26] did not report any stakeholder perspectives or experiences, including whether or not the intervention was acceptable to them.

Discussion

Linking implementation factors to health outcomes

The designs of the original studies, along with the complexity of the integrated multi-component interventions and the different approaches to community participation, make it difficult to link specific implementation strategies to specific outcomes [7, 8]. The studies themselves attribute the following positive outcomes to participation strategies: increased community awareness of danger signs and complications [15, 16, 24]; an increase in appropriate care-seeking [12, 14–23, 25, 26, 30]; improved transport to services, either through financial support being made available after community meetings, or because of increased awareness through educational materials, or broader programme activities [15, 16, 20–24]; and creating a process for community members to use health data to identify and address barriers to survival [15–19, 23, 25].

Rifkin argues that approaching community participation as a process rather than an intervention influences how the effect of community participation should be evaluated [7]. Process evaluations were not usually documented in the studies included here, a finding which is in line with previous reviews [8, 9]. For studies where communities played more active roles, particularly in planning and implementing health programmes [19–21, 25–27], rather than more passive roles as recipients of community outreach [13, 14, 16], development of community capacity to address programme challenges and barriers and increase programme ownership was a key factor, whether or not this was an intended programme goal. Strengthened abilities of community members and groups to plan and implement programme-related activities acquired through experience and training can be applied beyond the programme, enhancing community participation in broader civil society in the immediate and longer term [22, 23, 25, 26]. However, the Nepal youth study suggests that strengthening a community's capacity to work together effectively without paying careful attention to developing specific health-related knowledge and skills may not result in the desired improvement of specific health outcomes, at least in the short term (presumably in a context in which community level health related knowledge and skills are not well developed) [26, 27]. Strengthened capacity can lead to shifts in the balance of power through partnerships or coalitions between different groups (for example through stakeholder committees) or increased skills, education and confidence of members who become empowered to tackle their own problems (for example through community-based monitoring and increased accountability) [5, 31–34].

Limitations

Our findings are limited by the following: a relatively small number of studies met the inclusion criteria for the original WHO reviews of effectiveness; there is little detail in these studies about stakeholder perspectives and the context and conditions in which programmes were implemented. Most studies did not report on their definition of 'community' and it is unclear whether they had operational definitions or were working with implicit understandings such as a rough geographical definition. The way community is defined has programmatic implications in terms of organization, leadership, representation, governance and decision-making processes, particularly when programme implementers choose to work with existing structures and organizations and so clearly influences the process of community participation. Lack of clear definitions of who comprises 'community' suggests a lack of focus in the implementation, which could be problematic – for instance if the intervention amplifies already-heard voices at the expense of marginalised groups.

Across studies there was limited discussion about why the programmes chose the approaches they implemented and the extent to which these approaches seemed to work, or needed to be adjusted during the programme. Authors provided very little information on the process of participation, what motivated different community members to participate, and how their participation contributed to successful outcomes. They also did not discuss certain key details that could inform implementation of programmes in the future, for instance, which theoretical or pedagogical approach(es) they used, the particular roles that community and programme team members played in the learning process or how these roles may or may not have changed over time as community capacity grew and environmental conditions changed. Most authors did not report on how programme team members developed their own capacity to design, facilitate and support these processes and how relationships and personalities influenced effectiveness during implementation.

There is an urgent need for better qualitative data to be collected in future studies to ensure that dynamics and processes are captured to inform future participation programs [4, 7]. Documenting, evaluating and reporting on highly complex and dynamic community participation approaches using conventional evaluation methods and designs with the rigor required to establish a strong evidence base may be difficult for implementers who may lack relevant resources and expertise. Conventional quantitative and qualitative evaluation methods supplemented by systems thinking [35, 36], complexity aware monitoring [37], realist evaluation and other methods [38] may provide greater insight into how these processes work in different contexts and conditions, but such evaluation methods require adequate resources and staff to be done thoroughly.

Conclusion

While the conclusions from the secondary analysis presented here are necessarily tentative, a key element of successful health programme interventions through community participation appears to be the extent to which community, facility and government stakeholders develop their capacity to work effectively together to design, manage, and monitor health programmes as well as their health-related knowledge and skills. We identified the following factors to consider when supporting community participation programmes:

- *Enabling or not-so-enabling environment* – the extent to which political will, community awareness and sentiment, policies and available resources are supportive of maternal and newborn health and community participation;
- *Community leadership and governance* characterized by stability and strength of local leadership, the extent to which marginalized voices are represented in decision-making and whether and how to work with existing structures;
- *Community management capacity* to leverage and manage resources, use data for decision-making and for planning, monitoring, and accountability;
- *Community and health system capacity to interact* including the roles and relationships that community health workers, NGOs and others can play to link communities and health systems, and the use of regularly scheduled effective processes that use key questions to drive constructive dialogue; and,
- *Intercultural sensitivity/competence* that acknowledges, respects and builds on existing local beliefs and practices, considers gender rights and roles, understands social networks and norms, uses local languages and materials accessible to the range of literacy and numeracy skills within the programme context.

While some facilitating and inhibiting factors identified in this secondary analysis may be beyond the control or influence of a particular programme, it may be helpful for programme designers and implementers to be aware of them and the possible implications they may have for implementation and results. For example, working in a setting in which there is a very low level of trust among members of the community is likely to require a great deal more time and effort spent on building trust before meaningful engagement in joint programme planning can take place.

Better understanding of how best to support community participation processes to improve maternal and newborn health is essential, particularly methods of investigating adequately the effects of different programmes in what are inevitably complex and dynamic social settings.

Abbreviations

ANC: Antenatal care; MDSR: Maternal death surveillance and response; MNH: Maternal and newborn health; SURE : Supporting the Use of Research Evidence; WHO: World Health Organization

Acknowledgements

This paper draws from an initial report produced by Lisa Howard-Grabman for the World Health Organization. We would like to gratefully acknowledge the contributions of the participants of the WHO Technical Consultation on Health Promotion Interventions for Maternal and Newborn Health that took place between 15 and 17 of July 2014 at WHO headquarters in Geneva, for discussing the preliminary outcomes of the systematic reviews and for their contributions to the first version of the report.

Funding

The study was funded by the WHO Department of Maternal, Newborn, Child, and Adolescent Health through a grant received from the Norwegian Agency for Development Cooperation.

Authors' contributions

LHG performed the analysis and developed the initial reports. LHG, ASM, CM and AF drafted the article. All authors approved the final version. Anayda Portela is a staff member of the World Health Organization and is responsible for the views expressed in this article which do not necessarily represent the decisions, policy or views of the World Health Organization.

Competing interests

The authors declare that they have no competing interests.

Author details

[1]Training Resources Group, Inc., 4301 Wilson Boulevard, Suite 400, Arlington, VA 22203, USA. [2]Institute of Health and Society, Department of Community Medicine and Global Health, Faculty of Medicine, University of Oslo, P.O. Box 1072 Elindern, 0316 Oslo, Norway. [3]Faculty of Public Health and Policy, London School of Hygiene & Tropical Medicine, 15-17 Tavistock Place, London WC1H 9SH, UK. [4]World Health Organization Department of Maternal, Newborn, Child and Adolescent Health, 20 Avenue Appia, 1211 Geneva, Switzerland.

References

1. Oakley P, Kahssay H. Community involvement in health development: an overview. In: Kahssay H, Oakley P, editors. Community involvement in health development: a review of the concept and practice. Geneva: WHO; 1999. p. 3–19.
2. Draper AK, Hewitt G, Rifkin S. Chasing the dragon: developing indicators for the assessment of community participation in health programmes. Soc Sci Med. 2010;71(6):1102–9.
3. Zakus JD, Lysack CL. Revisiting community participation. Health Policy Plan. 1998;13(1):1–12.
4. Marston C, Renedo A, McGowan CR, Portela A. Effects of community participation on improving uptake of skilled care for maternal and newborn health: a systematic review. PLoS One. 2013;8(2):e55012.
5. Rosato M, Laverack G, Grabman LH, Tripathy P, Nair N, Mwansambo C, et al. Community participation: lessons for maternal, newborn, and child health. Lancet. 2008;372(9642):962–71.

6. Rifkin SB. Lessons from community participation in health programmes: a review of the post Alma-Ata experience. Int Health. 2009;1(1):31–6.
7. Rifkin SB. Examining the links between community participation and health outcomes: a review of the literature. Health Policy Plan. 2014; 29:ii98-ii106.
8. George AS, Mehra V, Scott K, Sriram V. Community participation in health systems research: a systematic review assessing the state of research, the nature of interventions involved and the features of engagement with communities. PLoS One. 2015;10(10):1–25.
9. O'Mara-Eves A, Brunton G, McDaid D, Oliver S, Kavanagh J, Jamal F, et al. Community engagement to reduce inequalities in health: a systematic review, meta-analysis and economic analysis. Public Heal Res. 2013;1(4):1–526.
10. World Health Organization. WHO recommendations on health promotion interventions for maternal and newborn health. Geneva: WHO. 2015:2015.
11. MASCOT. Study group. Systematic review draft protocol: Health system and community-based interventions for improving maternal health and for reducing maternal health inequalities in low- and middle-income countries: a two-stage mixed-methods research synthesis. 2014.
12. The SURE Collaboration. SURE Guides for Preparing and Using Evidence-Based Policy Briefs: identifying and addressing barriers to implementing policy options. [Internet]. 2011. Available from: epoc.cochrane.org/sites/epoc.cochrane.org/files/public/uploads/SUREGuides-v2.1/Collectedfiles/sure_guides.html.
13. Purdin S, Khan T, Saucier R. Reducing maternal mortality among afghan refugees in Pakistan. Int J Gynaecol Obstet. 2009;105(1):82–5.
14. Bhutta ZA, Soofi S, Cousens S, Mohammad S, Memon ZA, Ali I, et al. Improvement of perinatal and newborn care in rural Pakistan through community-based strategies: a cluster-randomised effectiveness trial. Lancet. 2011;377(9763):403–12.
15. Paxman JM, Sayeed A, Buxbaum A, Huber SC, Stover C. The India local initiatives program: a model for expanding reproductive and child health services. Stud Fam Plan. 2005;36(3):203–20.
16. Harkins T, Drasbek C, Arroyo J, McQuestion M. The health benefits of social mobilization: experiences with community-based integrated Management of Childhood Illness in Chao, Peru and San Luis. Honduras Promot Educ. 2008;15(2):15–20.
17. Barbey A, Faisel AJ. Myeya J. Stavrou V, Psych MC, et al. Dinajpur SafeMother Initiative Final Evaluation Report. CARE: Mh ADD; 2001.
18. Hossain J, Ross SR. The effect of addressing demand for as well as supply of emergency obstetric care in Dinajpur. Bangladesh IJOG. 2006;92(3):320–8.
19. Kaseje D, Olayo R, Musita C, Oindo CO, Wafula C, Muga R. Evidence-based dialogue with communities for district health systems' performance improvement. Glob Public Health. 2010;5(6):595–610.
20. Malhotra A, Mathur S, Pande R, Roca E. Nepal: the distributional impact of participatory approaches on reproductive health for disadvantaged groups. In: Gwatkin DR, Wagstaff A, Yazbeck AS, editors. Reaching the poor with health, nutrition, and population services: what works, what doesn't, and why. Washington: The World Bank; 2005.
21. Mathur S, Mehta M, Malhotra A. Youth reproductive health in Nepal. 2004. International Center for Research on Woman.
22. Ahluwalia IB, Schmid T, Kouletio M, Kanenda O. An evaluation of a community-based approach to safe motherhood in northwestern Tanzania. Int J Gynecol Obstet. 2003;82(2):231–40.
23. Ahluwalia IB, Robinson D, Vallely L, Gieseker KE, Kabakama A. Sustainability of community-capacity to promote safer motherhood in northwestern Tanzania: what remains? Glob Health Promot. 2010;17(1):39–49.
24. Sood S, Chandra U, Palmer A, Molyneux I. SIAGA behavior change campaign in Indonesia SIAGA behavior change campaign in Indonesia. Matern Neonatal Heal. 2004;
25. Sinha D. Empowering communities to make pregnancy safer: an intervention in rural Andhra Pradesh. Population Council: New Delhi; 2008.
26. Bjorkman M, Svendsson J. Power to the people: evidence from a randomized field experiment on community based monitoring in Uganda. Q J Econ. 2009;124(2):735–69.
27. Kaufman J, Liu Y, Fang J. Improving reproductive health in rural China through participatory planning. Glob Public Health. 2012;7(8):856–68.
28. Gabrysch S, Lema C, Bedriñana E, Bautista MA, Malca R, Campbell OMR. Cultural adaptation of birthing services in rural Ayacucho, Peru. Bull World Health Organ. 2009;87(9):724–9.
29. WHO. Working with individuals, families and communities to improve maternal and newborn health. Geneva: WHO; 2010.
30. World Health Organization. WHO recommendation on community mobilization through facilitated participatory learning and action cycles with women's groups for maternal and newborn health. WHO. 2014:2014.
31. Laverack G, Labonte R. A planning framework for community empowerment goals within health promotion. Health Policy Plan. 2000; 15(3):255–62.
32. Gibbon M, Labonte R, Laverack G. Evaluating community capacity. Heal Soc Care Community. 2002;10(6):485–91.
33. Crisp. Four approaches to capacity building in health: consequences for measurement and accountability. Health Promot Int 2000;15(2):99–107.
34. Hawe P. Working invisibly: health workers talk about capacity-building in health promotion. Health Promot Int. 1998;13(4):285–95.
35. De Savigny D, Adam T, WHO. Systems Thinking for Health Systems Strengthening. Geneva: WHO; 2009.
36. Dooris. Healthy settings: challenges to generating evidence of effectiveness. Health Promot Int 2005; 21(1):55–65.
37. Britt H. Patsalidis M. Complexity-Aware Monitoring. USAID: Discusion Note; 2013.
38. Butterfoss FD. Process evaluation for community participation. Annu Rev Public Health. 2006;27:323–40.

4

Establishing partnership with traditional birth attendants for improved maternal and newborn health: a review of factors influencing implementation

Tina Miller[1*] and Helen Smith[2]

Abstract

Background: Recent World Health Organization recommendations recognize the important role Traditional Birth Attendants (TBAs) can play in supporting the health of women and newborns. This paper provides an analysis of key factors that affect the implementation of interventions to develop partnerships with TBAs to promote improved access to skilled care at birth.

Methods: We conducted a secondary analysis of 20 papers identified through two systematic reviews that examined the effectiveness of interventions to find new roles for TBAs on maternal and newborn health outcomes, as well as papers identified through a systematic mapping of the maternal health literature. The Supporting the Use of Research Evidence framework (SURE) guided the thematic analysis to explore the perceptions of various stakeholders and implementation barriers and facilitators, as well as other contextual issues.

Results: This analysis identified countries that have implemented interventions to support the transition from birth with a TBA to birth with a skilled birth attendant. Drawing on the experiences of these countries, the analysis highlights factors that are important to consider when designing and implementing such interventions. Barriers to implementation included resistance to change in more traditional communities, negative attitudes between TBAs and skilled attendants and TBAs concerns about the financial implications of assuming new roles. Facilitating factors included stakeholder involvement in devising and implementing interventions, knowledge sharing between TBAs and skilled birth attendants, and formalised roles and responsibilities and remuneration for TBAs.

Conclusions: The implementation barriers identified in this analysis could, if not addressed, prevent or discourage TBAs from carrying out newly defined roles supporting women in pregnancy and childbirth and linking them to the formal health system. This paper also identifies the factors that seem critical to success, which new programmes could consider adopting from the outset. In most cases a multi-faceted approach is needed to prepare TBAs and others for new roles, including the training of TBAs to strengthen their knowledge and skills to enable them to be able to assume new roles, alongside the sensitization of healthcare providers, communities, women and their families. Further research is required to map the transition process and stakeholder experiences in more detailed ways and to provide longer-term monitoring of existing interventions.

Keywords: Traditional birth attendant (TBA), New roles, Partnership, Maternal health, Newborn health, Implementation

* Correspondence: tamiller@brookes.ac.uk
[1]Department of Social Sciences, Oxford Brookes University, Oxford OX3 0BP, UK
Full list of author information is available at the end of the article

Background

Improving access to skilled care during pregnancy, childbirth, and postpartum remains a priority strategy for improving maternal health and is key to achieving one of the many indicators specified in sustainable development goal (SDG) 3, reducing the global maternal mortality ratio. In 2004 the World Health Organization (WHO), the International Confederation of Midwives (ICM) and the International Federation of Gynaecology and Obstetrics (FIGO) issued a joint statement defining 'skilled birth attendants' and their role. Although the statement did not include traditional birth attendants (TBAs), countries were encouraged to work with TBAs to define new roles for them and ensure cooperation between TBAs, skilled attendants, and staff in referral facilities [1]. Subsequent recommendations on optimising lay health worker roles [2], and WHO's framework for working with individuals, families and communities [3] both identify a need to specify the responsibilities of TBAs for maternal and newborn health (MNH) in countries where they are an important source of childbirth care.

Specifying roles for TBAs acknowledges their cultural and social acceptability and the important role that they play in supporting the health of women and newborns and linking women, families and communities to the formal health system [3]. Strategies to increase use of Skilled Birth Attendants (SBAs) where TBAs are providers of childbirth care have generally involved linking TBAs with formal health services, increasing partnerships or teamwork with TBAs, or finding new roles. New roles for TBAs in the formal health system include encouraging and accompanying women to attend antenatal and postnatal care and have skilled care during birth, providing companionship to women during and after childbirth, as well as broader roles that they can play in community-level health education and community mobilization strategies to improve MNH. Strategies to increase partnerships with TBAs include developing collaborative relationships through opportunities for reciprocal sharing of traditional and professional knowledge between TBAs and SBAs, emphasising such collaboration in in-service midwifery training [4, 5], as well as including TBAs in community level networks and as links in referral chains for skilled care [6, 7].

Recent WHO guidance on health promotion interventions for maternal and newborn health endorses previous statements and recommends dialogue with TBAs, women, families, communities and service providers in order to define and agree alternative roles for TBAs in contexts where TBAs remain the main providers of care at birth [8]. The expert group reviewed the available evidence on the effect of establishing partnerships and new roles for TBAs on facility birth and birth with a SBA [8]. Overall, the evidence suggests improvements in use of SBAs, some increase in facility births, as well as some improvements in antenatal care (ANC) use and postpartum visits to women following the implementation of TBA interventions [8].

In the last 15 years countries have started to implement alternative roles and partnerships with TBAs, typically as part of complex and multifaceted interventions to increase skilled care which are difficult to evaluate. This makes it challenging to measure the contribution of TBA interventions, and to determine which strategies or which combination of strategies for TBA partnership are most effective [9, 10]. Nonetheless the recent WHO guidance recommends alternative roles for TBAs, and in this paper we turn attention towards understanding how best to implement these interventions. We summarise the available evidence and information on stakeholder perspectives and experiences in these interventions and the factors influencing implementation in different countries and contexts. This secondary analysis draws on studies from recent systematic reviews together with country experiences captured in descriptive accounts in order to synthesise: stakeholder experiences of partnerships and new roles for TBAs; the barriers and facilitators to implementation of partnerships and new roles; and how implementation factors relate to care seeking outcomes [8–10].

It is important to note the diversity in the country contexts in this paper and their stage of transition from TBA to skilled attendance. TBAs constitute a diverse group and may have had some basic training, for example when to refer a woman to a facility [4, 5] or be unskilled. They may also be described in different ways, for examples as 'Traditional Midwives' in Mexico and Nigeria [11, 12] and as 'Dayas' in Pakistan [13]. Detailed definitions of types of TBAs were not reported in the studies, but descriptions provided in the studies enabled a generic definition to be determined of a TBA as a non-professional, who has conducted home births, but lacks technical skills and training to manage obstetric complications. The TBA may have received training for the management of referrals [4–6].

Methods

We conducted a secondary analysis of implementation factors identified in studies included in a systematic review of the effects of new roles and partnership with TBAs on MNH outcomes [8]. Our secondary analysis aimed to examine the included studies further to identify ideas about implementation that were not necessarily the central focus of the original research [14]. We considered the re-use of existing data an efficient way of generating new insights into implementing new roles for TBAs and extending the contexts in which the original qualitative research data could be interpreted [15]. The systematic review identified two existing reviews [9, 10] and included six studies identified through a mapping of maternal health literature published from 2000 to 2012 (focused on health system and community-based interventions for improving maternal health)[16]. For the analysis reported in this paper we include these six studies, which contained information about implementation, and they were quality assessed as part of the systematic review process. A further 14 sources were also identified, containing descriptions of implementation efforts to partner with or find new roles for TBAs; 13 of these from the inventory compiled in one of the abovementioned systematic reviews [8–10], and another paper was identified during the more recent systematic mapping process reported above. These 14 sources contain useful information on countries' experiences of implementing new roles or partnerships with TBAs; they mostly comprise review articles and grey literature without empirical data and so were not quality assessed.

The SURE (Supporting the Use of Research Evidence) framework was used to guide the extraction of information from papers and synthesis of factors influencing implementation presented in this article [17]. Dominant factors and recurrent themes were identified across the included studies and used to organise the data. These are reported below in relation to stakeholder perspectives and experiences as well as barriers and facilitators to implementation of new roles and partnership with TBAs.

Results

A total of 20 papers comprising six studies identified through the systematic review process, and 14 additional sources, were included in this secondary analysis. The six research studies involved complex interventions, evaluated the use of different study designs and focused to varying degrees on improving MNH outcomes through interventions which included new roles for TBAs and TBA partnership [18]. Table 1 summarises the characteristics of these studies and the 14 additional sources. The countries represented in the six studies were: Bangladesh [6], Indonesia [4, 5], Myanmar [7], Peru [19] and Pakistan [13]. These studies report on various interventions to link TBAs with health services, increase partnerships with or find new roles for TBAs. Four studies evaluated community-based partnership interventions where midwives were trained and posted to work in poor, remote, or vulnerable communities and encouraged to work in collaboration with TBAs [4–7]. The other two studies evaluated new roles for TBAs within broader safe motherhood programmes; one culturally appropriate childbirth care model with TBAs and family members to encourage women to deliver in facilities [19] and the other multifaceted programme involved TBAs in raising awareness of services and reproductive health issues at community level [13]. The additional sources provided information on implementation of new roles or partnerships with TBAs in: East Africa (n = 3); West Africa (n = 1); South Asia (n = 1); South East Asia (n = 4); Central America (n = 3); South America (n = 1); and multiple countries (n = 1). The interventions described include: promoting partnerships between midwives, doctors, or health services and TBAs [11, 12, 20–24]; and creating new roles for TBAs including accompanying women to services [25, 26], supporting women during labour or childbirth [27, 28], and offering financial incentives to TBAs to refer women [12, 28].

Stakeholder experiences of partnerships and new roles for TBAs

The stakeholders most often identified in the interventions are TBAs, community-based SBAs (trained midwives), facility-based SBAs, women service users, family members and local communities including men and religious leaders. The perspectives of each of these groups on partnership and new roles for TBAs are not detailed in depth in any of the included sources, but our analysis identified some insights into how these interventions are received and experienced.

TBA, community-based SBAs, and facility-based staff experiences

Interventions to develop collaborative partnerships between TBAs, SBAs and facility-based staff have involved relationship-building integrated into midwifery training in Indonesia [4], and integration of TBAs into a 'referral chain' with nurse midwives in Bangladesh [6]. TBA-facilitated sessions on traditional birth and medications and village midwives working 'side-by-side' with TBAs have been used to promote partnership in Peru [19] and Indonesia [4, 5] respectively, and in Sudan incentive schemes to motivate TBAs to work collaboratively have been introduced [24]. In Myanmar links with TBAs have been strengthened through a network of community-based provision in which maternal health workers have responsibility for overseeing the work of TBAs [7].

Reports suggest that TBA experiences of new partnership working with SBAs and facility-based staff are varied. In Guatemala, TBAs describe their increased confidence, for example when giving information to families and persuading husbands to support use of facility care [27]. But others in the same programme report suspicion of their new roles by some members of their communities and a lack of consideration for their personal needs when accompanying women to a hospital facility (e.g. food and accommodation) [27]. Further

Table 1 Characteristics of included studies and additional sources

Author	Study design	Setting	Description of intervention
Fauveau et al., 1991 [6]	Pre and post intervention study	BANGLADESH, rural Matlab	Nurse-midwives posted in outposts of programme area. The nurse-midwives' duties included working with CHWs and TBAs to ensure that they were called during labour.
Frankenberg et al., 2009 [4]	Longitudinal panel survey	INDONESIA	A village midwife programme where midwives were trained and placed in poor communities far from health centres. Responsibilities included developing collaborative relationships with traditional village midwives.
Gabrysch et al., 2009 [19]	Pre and post comparative study	PERU, Ayacucho rural Santillana district	A culturally appropriate childbirth care model developed with Quechua communities and health professionals. Key features included a rope and bench for vertical delivery position, inclusion of family and TBAs, use of the Quechua language and health professionals that were respectful of culture.
Mullany et al., 2010 [7]	A pre and post intervention study (2-stage cluster-sampling surveys before and after programme implementation)	MYANMAR, Shan, Mon, Karen, and Karenni regions	A community-based project, collaboration to improve coverage of maternal health services in vulnerable communities. Strategy of a 3-tiered network of community-based providers: TBAs created links between community member and senior workers, HWs strengthened links between TBAs and lead health workers, and MHWs, who oversaw the work of TBAs and other HWs.
Purdin et al., 2009 [13]	Programme evaluation using health information system/ retrospective pre-post analysis	PAKISTAN, Hangu district, Afghan refugee camp	Male involvement interventions relating to safe motherhood, services established, and training provided to different community actors including TBAs to raise awareness of services and reproductive health issues. Outreach and community input. Each refugee camp has a health committee with community representatives and health service staff that meet bi-monthly to discuss project activities and provide feedback to health workers on health services provided. Basic emergency obstetric care facilities, community-based education provided to key community representatives including CHWs, female health workers, women of reproductive age, men, health committee members (all men), teachers, religious l eaders and private practitioners.
Ronsmans et al., 2001 [5]	A pre and post intervention study, including mixed methods	INDONESIA, three districts in South Kalimantan	A midwife placed in each village and at least one doctor with obstetric skills in each district. Financial access was facilitated for the poor. Village midwives were encouraged to work side by side with TBAs. TBAs supported to refer women with a complication and to work in collaboration with village midwives.
Additional sources			
Andemichael et al., 2009 [25]	Published article – rapid assessment	ERITREA	Improve access to services: addressing geographical barriers. New role for TBA: accompanying women to health services.
Braine, T. 2008 [11]	Published article - opinion	MEXICO	New role for TBA: Doctor + TBA partnership. Cultural adaptation of institutional childbirth.
Davis-Floyd, R. 2001 [30]	Published article – qualitative research	MEXICO	Improve access to services: addressing geographical barriers. New role for TBA: midwife + TBA partnership.
Fonseca-Becker et al., 2004 [27]	Published (online) report	GUATEMALA	New roles for TBA as a key component of newly established health committee. Recognises TBAs importance as a (culturally acceptable) bridge between pregnant women and the health system. TBAs incorporated into activities in health facilities as part of MNH. TBA giving emotional support and coaching during

Table 1 Characteristics of included studies and additional sources *(Continued)*

Author	Study design	Setting	Description of intervention
			labour, passing instruments to SBA and acting as interpreter.
Koblinsky et al., 1999 [28]	Published article – review paper	MULTIPLE COUNTRIES	Improve access to services: addressing geographical and financial barriers. New role for TBA: support at childbirth with health workers.
Murigi, S.F. 2010 [26]	Newspaper article	UGANDA	TBAs prohibited for childbirth. New role for TBA: community advocacy and accompanying women to health services
Onuki, D. 2002 [29]	Published article - opinion	BOLIVIA	New role for TBA: paid to refer pregnant women to health services. Cultural adaptation of institutional childbirth.
Ministry of Health, Myanmar 2010	Personal communication	MYANMAR	Improve access to services: addressing geographical barriers. New roles for TBA: community advocacy; health services + TBA partnership.
Ministry of Health, Nigeria, 2010	Unpublished concept note	NIGERIA	New role for TBA: community advocacy, accompanying women to services, support for women during labour and childbirth, paid to refer or accompany women to health services, provide a link between women and families and health services.
Ministry of Health, Southern Sudan, 2009	Unpublished report	SOUTH SUDAN	New role for TBA: accompany women to health services, financial incentives to TBAs, midwife + TBA partnership.
Save the Children, 2008	Unpublished report	AFGHANISTAN	Human resources development and deployment Policies to increase access to services, quality of the services, community participation and midwife + TBA partnership
UNICEF Indonesia, 2010 [21]	Published (online) report	INDONESIA	New role for TBA: midwife + TBA partnership.
Weber, M. 2010	Innovation 'letter to a friend' ('surat dari sahabat'). Also described in reference [21]	INDONESIA	New role for TBA: midwife + TBA partnership. Community advocacy.
World Bank, 2010 [22]	Published (online) report	INDONESIA	Human resources development and deployment Improve access to services: addressing geographical and financial barriers. New role for TBA: midwife + TBA partnership.

evidence from the Guatemala case study suggests that TBAs collaborate with the facility and accompany women as an 'obligation' to women who need help, and because it helps give the hospital a 'good image' with the population [27]. In Malaysia collaborative working between TBAs and SBAs was reported to have improved previously poor relations as TBAs had been gradually shifted to 'a more exclusively family supportive role' since 1973 [28].

There are also reports of facility staff having a low opinion of TBAs, and thereby making them feel unwelcome [27]. But improved relationships between TBAs and facility personnel were reported in Mexico and Peru [11, 19] following a broad participatory approach, and the design of a culturally appropriate model of care which included TBAs in Peru [19]. Integrating TBAs as birth companions (to give traditional massage and drinks) [11, 19] and as interpreters [19, 28] was accepted positively by facility staff and TBAs.

Women service users, family members and wider community experiences

Few papers report directly or in detail on women's experiences of new roles or interventions to promote partnerships with TBAs. The need to include 'key decision-makers' from communities including men (who are often household decision-makers) and religious leaders in TBA partnership interventions was noted in some papers [5, 6, 13], but only scant reporting of their experiences was included in the analysed papers. Involving household stakeholders (women, mothers-in-laws and husbands) and TBAs in assessing reproductive health information materials was a strategy used in Indonesia to foster collaboration [5]. Community empowerment and an increase in men's awareness of maternal and neonatal health was also reported following partnership working in Indonesia [21]. The need to establish 'strong links with the community' when implementing changes to models of care was reported more generally [28] and in particular the importance of community 'consideration', 'consultation', 'mobilisation' and 'inclusion' noted in relation to TBA partnership in Peru [19], Nigeria [12], Guatemala [27] Myanmar [7] and Indonesia [4, 5], even though detailed reporting of community stakeholder experiences was limited, with the exception of a case study conducted in Guatemala [27]. Some studies emphasised the value of 'intercultural adaptation' [29] and 'culturally appropriate' skilled care provision which retained TBAs as companions and interpreters [11, 19, 27, 30]. For example, in Guatemala, hospital workers were observed to show more patience, consideration, and respect to the women using their services, and for women, having access at the facility to an interpreter who spoke their language was 'deemed extremely positive' [27]. Trust between the hospital staff and local women was reported to have increased as a result of the changes to the organisation of care including recognising TBAs as a culturally acceptable bridge between women and the health system [28]. In Peru, family members being allowed to stay at the facility was also regarded positively by the families [19]. But in Myanmar concern was expressed by some family members about the financial costs (including loss of work time) and disruption to family life associated with childbirth at a facility and the need to leave the family home [23].

Barriers and facilitators to implementation of new roles for TBAs

Implementation challenges exist at the individual, community, facility and wider health system levels. The factors identified in the papers broadly focus on the importance of sensitising key stakeholders in order to change traditional TBA practices and achieve partnership with health service personnel, shifting attitudes and strengthening working relationships between TBAs and other health workers, and finding ways to adequately reward and incentivise TBAs in their new roles. It was also recognised that it could take time for new ways of working to become accepted and for behaviours to change.

Changing traditional TBA roles and practices

The continued adherence to traditional practices and a 'greater degree of traditionalism' in some communities [4] and countries [6, 23] have been identified as barriers to change and reasons why TBA partnership and anticipated shifts to SBA have not occurred in ways, or at a pace, anticipated [4, 28]. A continued preference for TBAs and traditional birth practices was noted in Eritrea [25] and Myanmar [23] and cultural practices in some regions [11, 19, 20, 23, 27, 28, 30] have been recognised as a barrier to skilled care use as women and community members still trust and prefer to use TBAs. A lack of available or accessible skilled care in some remote communities is also a reason given for continued use of TBAs [21–23, 26].

In contrast, several countries have experienced gradual shifts in traditional practices and cultural beliefs towards acceptance of new roles for TBAs and greater trust in midwives for technical aspects of childbirth [21]. This has been achieved through sharing of knowledge between TBAs, community-based SBAs, and facility-based staff and through community involvement especially in relation to designing culturally-appropriate facility care in Peru [19], Guatemala [27], Mexico [11, 30] and Bolivia [29]. This has led to improved relationships between multiple stakeholders [19]. But changing traditional practices in some communities has been slow [4, 26, 28] and community involvement was widely identified as essential in changing behaviours towards skilled care at birth [11, 19, 27]. The inclusion of key decision makers, including men, in information campaigns to increase demand for skilled care at birth and raise awareness of new roles for TBAs was also noted in Pakistan [13] and in Indonesia [5]. In Peru using an inclusive, 'participatory approach' to identify local needs facilitated the introduction of culturally-appropriate skilled care, and ensured that service use was sustained [19]. Involving TBAs and community members in the assessment of information materials as a means to facilitate partnership and community support was reported in Indonesia, where local radio was also used as a community information tool [5].

Working relationships between TBAs and other health workers

As new roles for TBAs lead to closer working with SBAs and facility-based staff, rivalry and negative attitudes among the different cadres have been reported [5]. A review paper summarising different models of childbirth care highlights that in countries where home birth is predominant and the government attempts to link with TBAs, they are likely to view government staff as competitors for the same clients; government health workers on the other hand may have a low opinion of TBAs [28]. There are however examples in the included studies of how TBAs and other health workers have developed mutually respectful working relationships. For example, in Brazil TBAs were made to feel part of the formal health system by being granted access to a telephone for arranging transport to a facility and (in some cases) provision of a uniform, and this reportedly helped to overcome negative attitudes towards TBAs among skilled birth attendants [28]. In Myanmar integrating TBAs into a three-tiered network of care providers [7] and allocating them specific roles in providing antenatal care, conducting uncomplicated births, and creating links with upper-tier workers helped to promote good partnership working within the context of camps for internally displaced populations in the eastern border. The supervision of partnership working together with strong referral mechanisms was acknowledged more generally as a way to facilitate good working relations [28]. As part of the TBA-midwife partnership project in Indonesia, TBAs no longer help women give birth but their 'social status' has been retained helped by the formal acknowledgement of the TBA in the health system [21]. In many countries identifying new roles for TBAs (for example adapting facility care to include TBAs as birth companions) involved consultation with all stakeholders, which was found to facilitate better partnership working and helped to overcome rivalry between TBAs and skilled attendants [7, 11, 19, 27, 28, 30]. Many reports emphasised the importance of defining new roles for TBAs (for example, ANC, family health, postpartum care, breastfeeding and weaning, as advocates for MNH needs) and committing to these at the policy level [12]. The introduction of formal agreements ('contracts') between TBAs, SBAs and health services was reported to facilitate implementation in Brazil [28] and Indonesia [21].

Rewards and incentives for TBAs in new roles

As TBAs take up new roles and transition to partnership working they can experience an erosion of income and payment-in-kind previously received for conducting childbirth in the community. Performing new roles such as referring and accompanying women to facilities [25–27] and acting as a birth companion also involves new costs (e.g. transport and food) which some TBAs expressed concern about [27]. The need to ensure financial remuneration for TBAs was noted in several countries [4, 12, 28] and addressed through a formal signed agreement in Indonesia [21]. In Bolivia [29], Sudan [24], Indonesia [4] and Nigeria [12] payment for TBA referral or post-partum care [4] was introduced or recommended. Paid referral included encouraging TBAs to provide lists of pregnant women and referring women for skilled care in Indonesia [4], Peru [19] and Sudan [24]. In Indonesia, TBAs were encouraged to work collaboratively with midwives and report pregnancies to the health centre so that midwives could invite the woman for antenatal care by personal letter [21], and in Guatemala TBAs agreed to prepare lists of pregnant women for the health committee [27]. In Bolivia TBAs received payment for referral of pregnant women to a medical institution [29]. TBAs were also encouraged to refer women to Maternity Waiting Homes in Eritrea [25]. The introduction of performance based incentives for TBAs was recommended in Nigeria as a means to build capacity in their new social support role [12].

Discussion

Our analysis has identified that in countries where TBAs have been encouraged to work in more collaborative ways with formal health systems, TBAs, community-based SBAs, and facility-based staff had mixed experiences of the interventions. As old practices change and new ways of working in partnership are introduced this can affect working relationships between TBAs and SBAs. For example, our analysis highlights rivalry and competition for the same clients and implies unequal power relations between TBAs and formal health workers who may have a low opinion of TBAs. Community suspicion of new roles, poor working relationships with SBAs, and not being made welcome at facilities are some of the challenges TBAs face in their new roles and working alongside skilled birth attendants. However, when programmes used broad participatory approaches to design new models of care which included TBAs, and where TBAs were given clearly defined roles (such as birth companions or interpreters for women during labour and birth) they were more readily accepted by facility staff and TBAs. The included studies contained little information about the experiences of women service users, families, and communities of alternative roles for TBAs. However, when programmes placed emphasis on culturally appropriate skilled care and included roles for TBAs, this was regarded positively by women and families who may previously have felt emotionally unsupported by SBAs [19, 27, 31]. In services that included TBAs as a bridge to women and communities trust between women and facility staff increased. Barriers and facilitators to changing traditional TBA practices and achieving partnership with SBAs and facilities were also identified in the literature [4, 6, 8–10, 23, 28]. These included strengthening working relationships and reducing suspicion between TBAs and other health workers, and adequately rewarding and incentivising TBAs in their new roles.

What factors are critical to the success of TBA interventions?

To better understand the factors critical to the success of interventions to introduce new roles for TBAs, we considered the perspectives and implementation factors identified in this analysis in relation to the care seeking outcomes (birth with a skilled birth attendant or facility birth; ANC use (one to four visits) and postnatal visits for the woman) reported in the original systematic review. Table 2 lists the perspectives and implementation factors that made a difference in contexts where care seeking outcomes improved, together with key barriers to success. Of the six studies included in the original systematic review, three studies [4, 7, 13] reported improvements in number of ANC visits and coverage

Table 2 Implementation factors linked to systematic review outcomes

Studies from systematic review that report overall improvement in care seeking outcomes		Findings from synthesis of factors influencing implementation	
Author, year	Country, setting	Facilitating factors critical to successful outcomes	Barriers to successful outcomes
Fauveau et al., 1991 [6]	BANGLADESH, rural Matlab	Collaborative working between trained midwives, nurse-midwives, CHW's and TBAs - Integration of TBAs into a 'referral chain' working with skilled personnel	- Continued adherence to traditionalism and traditional practices - Men as main decision-makers in the family may be unwilling to seek external assistance
Frankenberg et al., 2009 [4]	INDONESIA	- Collaborative relationships with TBAs identified as a duty of trained midwives posted in villages	- Greater degree of traditionalism in some villages where trained midwife posted
Gabrysch et al., 2009 [19]	PERU, Ayacucho rural Santillana district	- Adopting a participatory approach including TBAs and family members to design culturally appropriate childbirth services - TBAs accommodated as birth companions to help with pushing and giving drinks and to provide a culturally appropriate facility birth - TBAs involved in capacity building workshops with other health workers	- Providers continuing to ascribe high levels of home births as due to 'cultural preference' or 'ignorance' rather than offering culturally accessible services
Mullany et al., 2010 [7]	MYANMAR, Shan, Mon, Karen, and Karenni regions	- Integration of TBA into a 3 tiered network of community based providers - Training of HWs and TBAs to strengthen their working relationship - TBAs used to create links between community members and senior health workers - TBAs used to provide improved ANC - Supervision of TBA role a responsibility of MHWs	
Purdin et al., 2009 [13]	PAKISTAN, Hangu district, Afghan refugee camp	- TBAs provided with reproductive health (RH) training along with other community members - TBAs active in awareness raising, including RH	
Ronsmans et al., 2001 [5]	INDONESIA, three districts in South Kalimantan	- Village midwives encouraged to strengthen their relationships with TBAs - TBAs identified as one of several 'key decision-makers' - TBAs involved in accessing information, education and communication (IEC) materials for community use	

following the implementation of a TBA intervention and four of the six studies [5–7, 13] showed that postpartum visits to women increased over time following the implementation of a TBA intervention. Where TBA partnership interventions were reported to improve care-seeking outcomes, the interventions included community involvement, both to ensure culturally appropriate service provision, and community acceptance of new roles for TBAs. Within this dialogue, the involvement of men as key decision-makers in households was important to help change traditional care seeking behaviours. Bringing TBAs and skilled birth attendants together to work in partnership is best achieved where individual roles are clearly defined and supervised. Formal recognition of new roles for TBAs within health service systems also helps community acceptance of new responsibilities for example a broader, more family supportive role in the community. Formal recognition will also maintain the social status of the TBA.

Limitations

Owing to the comprehensive search strategies employed in the systematic reviews and systematic mapping exercise, we are confident we have located the available literature, published and unpublished, on implementation of TBA partnerships and new roles, albeit limited to publications written in English. There is a possibility we may have missed reports or evaluations from projects or programmes in South or Central America or West Africa. Our findings indicate important implementation considerations common across different contexts, but our understanding of how these factors change over time or how they interrelate to prevent or promote skilled care at birth is limited. None of the studies reporting evaluations of TBA interventions explicitly collected data on stakeholder preferences or attitudes towards the interventions, nor did they provide detailed descriptions of the TBA interventions such as how partnerships were built or strengthened and how new roles were identified and by whom. This could be because the TBA interventions were implemented as part of larger community or facility based programmes to increase skilled attendance and facility birth, and the evaluations focused on the programmes overall and not the contribution of the component parts. The additional and largely unpublished sources included in this analysis describe to some extent the nature of partnerships between SBAs, facilities and TBAs, but very little is revealed about how to nurture and sustain collaborative working, or the views of women service users, TBAs, and health workers about acceptability and appropriateness of the new roles and partnerships. Although there is an obvious value and efficiency in using already collected data to answer additional research questions, secondary analysis can pose a threat to fidelity in interpretation of findings beyond those presumed in the original research [ref Thorne 1998]. The themes identified in this paper reflect our critical analysis of data already interpreted and contextualised by authors of the primary studies. However we feel the threat is minimal as we did not set out to build theory or develop a higher order analysis, we simply extracted information on themes that primary authors had identified themselves.

Research implications

Longer-term monitoring of TBA interventions, as new roles and partnership working become established, could help programme planners and policy makers identify what works and direct resources towards improvements or modifications. Better reporting of intervention characteristics including details of the type of TBA could help other programmes or countries decide what aspects to replicate or implement. There is also a need for more in-depth qualitative research and case studies, focusing on multi- stakeholder perspectives, to better understand what aspects of interventions (in different country settings and populations) facilitate acceptance of new roles for TBAs and lead to improvements in use of skilled childbirth care. Future evaluations could usefully explore and record the preferences articulated by those providing and receiving care in more detailed and rigorous ways. We would encourage publication of case studies from countries that have implemented policies to ban TBAs and the effect of these policies, as well as those countries with experience in changing the role of TBAs but which may not yet be documented in the literature, such as in Latin America. Future studies should include an estimation of costs, since exact costs were not reported in the literature we reviewed. We could infer from the different studies only limited information about costs incurred. These were dependent on the intervention type, including provision of payments to TBAs to take on new roles such as referring pregnant women, accompanying them to the facility, reimbursing transport costs or other costs associated with assuming a new role. It is also important to consider any additional cost burden to women and families, especially if there is an expectation that they should pay or compensate TBAs for helping them to access services for example. This is particularly relevant in countries where maternity care is not provided for free.

Conclusion

Interventions to support countries to transition from birth with a TBA to birth with a SBA are important and timely in light of priority strategies to increase skilled care at birth and the human resource challenges in achieving this goal. The implementation barriers identified in this analysis could, if not addressed, prevent or discourage TBAs from carrying out newly defined roles supporting women in pregnancy and childbirth and linking them to the formal health system. This paper also identifies the factors that seem critical to success, which new programmes could consider adopting from the outset. In most cases a multi-faceted approach is needed to prepare TBAs and others for new roles, including the training of TBAs to strengthen their knowledge and skills to enable them to be able to assume new roles, alongside the sensitization of healthcare providers, communities, women and their families. The integration of other stakeholders to contribute to a support and monitoring system for the transition period is also recommended. As with many other interventions for improving maternal and newborn health, the availability and accessibility of skilled care and other health systems challenges remain important barriers; not least identifying a sustainable source of funding to compensate and incentivise TBAs in their new roles.

Acknowledgements
The authors wish to thank Annie Portela of the Department of Maternal, Newborn, Child and Adolescent Health, WHO, for her helpful feedback on earlier drafts of the paper and for editing the series of which this paper is part.

Funding
The authors did not receive any funding for the production of this article.

Authors' contributions
TM produced the first complete draft of the manuscript. HS revised the manuscript and both authors edited, read and approved the final version.

Competing interests
The authors declare that they have no competing interests.

Author details
[1]Department of Social Sciences, Oxford Brookes University, Oxford OX3 0BP, UK. [2]Centre for Maternal and Newborn Health, Liverpool School of Tropical Medicine, L3 5QA, Liverpool, UK.

References

1. World Health Organization. Making pregnancy safer: the critical role of the skilled attendant: a joint statement by WHO, ICM and FIGO. Geneva: World Health Organization; 2004.
2. World Health Organization. WHO Recommendations – Optimize MNH: optimizing health worker roles for maternal and newborn health interventions through task shifting. Geneva: World Health Organization; 2012. Available from: http://apps.who.int/iris/bitstream/10665/77764/1/9789241504843_eng.pdf. Accessed 25 May 2015.
3. World Health Organization. Working with individuals, families and communities to improve maternal and newborn health. Geneva: Department of Making Pregnancy Safer; 2010. p. 2010.
4. Frankenberg E, Buttenheim A, Sikoki B, Suriastini W. Do women increase their use of reproductive health care when it becomes more available? Evidence from Indonesia. Stud Family Plann. 2009;40(1):27–38.
5. Ronsmans C, Endang A, Gunawan S, et al. Evaluation of a comprehensive home-based midwifery programme in South Kalimantan, Indonesia. Trop Med Int Health. 2001;6(10):799–810.
6. Fauveau V, Stewart K, Khan SA, Chakraborty J. Effect on mortality of community-based maternity-care programme in rural Bangladesh. Lancet. 1991;338(8776):1183–6.
7. Mullany LC, Lee TJ, Yone L, et al. Impact of Community-Based Maternal Health Workers on Coverage of Essential Maternal Health Interventions among Internally Displaced Communities in Eastern Burma: The MOM Project. PLoS Med. 2010;7(8):e1000316. https://doi.org/10.1371/journal.pmed.1000316.
8. World Health Organization. WHO recommendations on health promotion interventions for maternal and newborn health. Geneva: World Health Organization; 2015. Available from: http://www.who.int/maternal_child_adolescent/documents/health-promotion-interventions/en/. Accessed 20 Apr 2017.
9. Byrne A, Morgan A. How the integration of traditional birth attendants with formal health systems can increase skilled birth attendance. Int J Gynaecol Obstet. 2011;115:127–34. https://doi.org/10.1016/j.ijgo.2011.06.018.
10. Vieira C, Portela A, Miller T, Coast E, Leone T, Marston C. Increasing the use of skilled health personnel where traditional birth attendants were providers of childbirth care: a systematic review. PLoS One. 2012;7(10):e47946. https://doi.org/10.1371/journal.pone.0047946.
11. Braine T. Mexico's midwives enter the mainstream. B World Health Organ. 2008;86(4):244–5.
12. Federal Government of Nigeria. Changing roles – refocusing traditional birth Attendant towards accelerated reduction of Maternal and newborn mortality in Nigeria: concept note. Abuja: Federal Ministry of Health; 2010.
13. Purdin S, Khan T, Saucier R. Reducing maternal mortaility among Afghan refugees in Pakistan. Int J Gynecol Obstet. 2009;105:82–5.
14. Heaton J. Secondary analysis of qualitative data. Social Research Update. 1998; issue 22. Available from: http://sru.soc.surrey.ac.uk/SRU22.html
15. Thorne S. Ethical and representational issues in qualitative secondary analysis. Qual Health Res. 1998;8(4):547–55.
16. World Health Organisation, Department for Maternal, Newborn, Child and Adolescent health (WHO/MCA) MASCOT/Wotro Map of Maternal Health Research (database). Hosted by EPPI Centre, UCL Institute of Education, London, UK.
17. The SURE Collaboration. SURE Guides for Preparing and Using Evidence-Based Policy Briefs: identifying and addressing barriers to implementing policy options. Geneva: World Health Organization; 2011.
18. WHO recommendations on health promotion interventions for maternal and newborn health: evidence base. Geneva: World Health Organization; 2015. Available from: http://www.who.int/maternal_child_adolescent/documents/health-promotion-interventions/en/. Accessed 29 Oct 2015.
19. Gabrysch S, Lema C, Bedrinana E, Bautista MA, Malca R, Campbell OM, Miranda JJ. Cultural adaptation of birthing services in rural Ayacucho, Peru. BWorld Health Organ. 2009;87(9):724–9.
20. Save the Children. Saving the Lives of Mothers and Newborns in Afghanistan: Afghanistan Newborn Health Situation Analysis. Washington DC: Save the Children; 2008
21. UNICEF Indonesia. Programme experiences in Indonesia: documentation collection. Jakarta: UNICEF Indonesia; 2010. Available from: https://www.unicef.org/indonesia/Programme_Experiences-UNICEF_Indonesia_2010.pdf. Accessed 13 Nov 2015.
22. World Bank. "...and then she died": Indonesia Maternal Health Assessment. Washington DC: World Bank; 2010. Available from: http://documents.worldbank.org/curated/en/718951468040488082/pdf/533270ESW0Whit10Box345625B01PUBLIC1.pdf. Accessed 29 Oct 2015.
23. Win LL, Sein TT, Tin N, Win SS. Utilization of antenatal care and birth delivery services in rural areas of Kyauk-padaung township, Myanmar. Unpublished report, Department of Medical Research (Lower Myanmar), Yangon, May 2006.
24. Government of Southern Sudan. Maternal, Neonatal and Reproductive Health strategy 2009–2012. Southern Sudan: Ministry of Health; 2009.
25. Andemichael G, Haile B, Kosia A, Mufunda J. Maternity waiting homes: a panacea for maternal/neonatal conundrums in Eritrea. J Eritrean Med Assoc. 2009;4(1):18–21.
26. Murigi SF. Should Uganda ban traditional birth attendants? Guardian. 2010.27. https://www.theguardian.com/katine/katine-chronicles-blog/2010/mar/30/traditional-birth-attendants-ban. Accessed 30 Mar 2010.
27. Fonseca-Becker F, Cordon O et al. Impact Evaluation: Community Mobilization and Behavior Change, Maternal and Neonatal Health Component, Ministry of Health and Public Assistance. Baltimore: Johns Hopkins Bloomberg School of Public Health Center for Communication Programs; 2004. Available from: http://www.jhuccp.org. Accessed 29 Oct 2015.
28. Koblinsky MA, Campbell O, Heichelheim J. Organizing delivery care: What works for safe motherhood? B World Health Organ. 1999;77(5):399–406.
29. Onuki D. Humanization of childbirth in Bolivia. Midwifery Today-International Midwife. 2002;64:54–5.
30. Davis-Floyd R. La partera profesional: articulating identity and cultural space for a new kind of midwife in Mexico. Med Anthropol. 2001;20(2–3):185–243.
31. van Roosmalen J, Walraven G, Stekelenburg J, Massawe S. (2005) Editorial: integrating continuous support of the traditional birth attendant into obstetric care by skilled midwives and doctors: a cost-effective strategy to reduce perinatal mortality and unnecessary obstetric interventions. Trop Med Int Health. 2005;10(5):393–4.

5

Measurement properties of comorbidity indices in maternal health research

Kazuyoshi Aoyama[1,2,4,5,7,8*], Rohan D'Souza[6,7], Eiichi Inada[5], Stephen E. Lapinsky[2,4] and Robert A. Fowler[3,4,7]

Abstract

Background: Maternal critical illness occurs in 1.2 to 4.7 of every 1000 live births in the United States and approximately 1 in 100 women who become critically ill will die. Patient characteristics and comorbid conditions are commonly summarized as an index or score for the purpose of predicting the likelihood of dying; however, most such indices have arisen from non-pregnant patient populations. We sought to systematically review comorbidity indices used in health administrative datasets of pregnant women, in order to critically appraise their measurement properties and recommend optimal tools for clinicians and maternal health researchers.

Methods: We conducted a systematic search of MEDLINE and EMBASE to identify studies published from 1946 and 1947, respectively, to May 2017 that describe predictive validity of comorbidity indices using health administrative datasets in the field of maternal health research. We applied a methodological PubMed search filter to identify all studies of measurement properties for each index.

Results: Our initial search retrieved 8944 citations. The full text of 61 articles were identified and assessed for final eligibility. Finally, two eligible articles, describing three comorbidity indices appropriate for health administrative data remained: The Maternal comorbidity index, the Charlson comorbidity index and the Elixhauser Comorbidity Index. These studies of identified indices had a low risk of bias. The lack of an established consensus-building methodology in generating each index resulted in marginal sensibility for all indices. Only the Maternal Comorbidity Index was derived and validated specifically from a cohort of pregnant and postpartum women, using an administrative dataset, and had an associated c-statistic of 0.675 (95% Confidence Interval 0.647–0.666) in predicting mortality.

Conclusions: Only the Maternal Comorbidity Index directly evaluated measurement properties relevant to pregnant women in health administrative datasets; however, it has only modest predictive ability for mortality among development and validation studies. Further research to investigate the feasibility of applying this index in clinical research, and its reliability across a variety of health administrative datasets would be incrementally helpful. Evolution of this and other tools for risk prediction and risk adjustment in pregnant and post-partum patients is an important area for ongoing study.

Keywords: Systematic review, Comorbidity index, Maternal Health Research, Measurement properties, Charlson comorbidity index, Maternal comorbidity index, Elixhauser comorbidity index

* Correspondence: kazu.aoyama@utoronto.ca
[1]Department of Anesthesia and Pain Medicine, The Hospital for Sick Children, University of Toronto, Toronto, Canada
[2]Intensive Care Unit, Mount Sinai Hospital and University Health Network, University of Toronto, Toronto, Canada
Full list of author information is available at the end of the article

Background

Maternal critical illness is a medical condition of pregnant and postpartum women which may result in end-organ injury, morbidity or death; and, generally requires treatment with organ supporting care – mechanical ventilation for respiratory failure, intravenous vasoactive medications for septic shock, or transfusions for peripartum haemorrhage [1]. Maternal critical illness occurs in 1.2 to 4.7 of every 1000 live births in the United States and is associated with a fetal loss rate of 30% [2–4].

Within developed countries, for every 100 episodes of maternal critical illness [5], one woman will die. While approximately 30–40% of maternal critical illness is preventable [6], the events leading to deterioration and risk of death can be rapid and insidious. Effective monitoring and early intervention for those at risk are not always planned or available. Clinicians, patients and families would therefore benefit from a tool that could predict the risk of maternal mortality from commonly available data, across a range of gestational age in order to assist with decision-making on an appropriate level of monitoring and care. Maternal health research would also be assisted by a tool to help risk-adjust in observational studies among patients with different probabilities of death.

Kirshner and Guyatt [7] suggest a methodological framework for the development of predictive measurement tools for clinical and health services research that considers all potential predictive factors of outcomes and include patient-related and health-system domains. In maternal critical care, maternal age, comorbidities, features of the present illness, physiological status and biological profiles have individually been shown to influence the risk of maternal mortality and morbidity [8, 9]. An ideal predictive tool for maternal mortality would therefore incorporate all these domains, and guide management by indicating which patients require an increased level of observation or care in order to prevent critical illness or death.

Patient characteristics and comorbid conditions are commonly used to describe patient populations and are often summarized as an index or score for the purpose of predicting the likelihood of dying. Such an index can also assist in adjusting potential confounding factors in clinical and health services research when attempting to quantify the association of a particular factor with an outcome such as death. Prior studies have shown inconsistent performance (with respect to discrimination and calibration) of common physiology-based indices for pregnant and post-partum women (e.g. Acute Physiology And Chronic Health Evaluation (APACHE) score, the Simplified Acute Physiology Score (SAPS), the Mortality Prediction Model (MPM) and their adaptations) [10–12]. An increasing volume of maternal health research uses administrative datasets; however, there is no existing systematic review and appraisal of comorbidity indices appropriate for health administrative datasets in maternal health research.

Objective

The objective was to conduct a systematic review to identify and critically appraise measurement properties of comorbidity indices predicting mortality among pregnant and post-partum women.

Methods

Criteria for considering studies for review:

Type of studies

Studies eligible for inclusion included prospective and retrospective cohort studies, excluding case-reports, case-series and case-control studies.

Participants

Participants were pregnant and postpartum women in general wards and ICUs at acute care hospitals. The postpartum period was defined as within 6 weeks from the date of delivery or fetal demise. Patients in outpatient clinics or emergency rooms, not admitted to hospital, were excluded.

Index models (prediction models for clinical outcomes being evaluated in this review) [13]

We focused on comorbidity indices. We exclude models based upon physiology-based indices with vital signs and laboratory results because health administrative data sets rarely have this level of granular detail.

Target conditions for predicting mortality

The target conditions were comorbidities of hospitalized pregnant and postpartum women.

Reference standards to confirm mortality

Clinical follow-up in hospital, or up to 30 days following discharge to determine survival or death during the index hospital stay in each study. Studies that reported on mortality as a composite outcome with other outcomes (e.g. organ dysfunction) were eligible.

Data sources and search strategy

We performed a literature search using MEDLINE and EMBASE (1946 to May 2017 in MEDLINE, 1947 to May 2017 in EMBASE) for all publications on comorbidity indices, not including vital signs and laboratory results, in the context of maternal health research, using the search terms associated with "pregnant women" as study participants, terms identifying comorbidity indices ("health status indicators") and index models of interest and "mortality" as the outcome of index models. The detailed search strategy is provided in Additional file 1: Appendix A. The reference lists of identified relevant articles and also the references that cited identified articles were reviewed through Web of Science. In addition, narrative review articles and book chapters were examined. No language restriction was applied for the literature search.

Data collection

Selection of studies

The two independent reviewers (KA, RD) scanned the titles and abstracts of every record retrieved to determine the studies to be assessed further. If it was clear from the title and abstract that the article was not relevant, according to the above eligibility criteria, the reviewers rejected the record. The full texts of the remaining articles were retrieved. Two reviewers (KA, RD) independently assessed and determined the eligibility of studies. Disagreements were resolved by discussion and, when necessary, a third reviewer (RF) was consulted to assist in adjudicating a final decision.

Data extraction

Each study was described by general information (title, journal, year of publication status and study design [prospective or retrospective]), study descriptors (number of included patients, age, subgroups, type of comorbidity index, and stated purpose of the model), follow-up information (outcome including mortality rate) and predictive validity (calibration and discrimination).

Assessment of methodological quality

The quality of studies was assessed using Hayden's six-domain risk of bias tool for prognostic studies [14] that has been used widely for methodological quality in systematic reviews of risk prediction models [15–17]. The Hayden guidelines address 6 components: 1) Study participation (definition and description of the study subjects); 2) Study attrition (study loss to follow-up); 3) Prognostic factor measurement (quantitatively measured predictors of interest); 4) Outcome measurement (quantitatively measured outcome of interest); 5) Confounding measurement and adjustment; and, 6) Analysis (calibration and discrimination). Each component comprises items that are scored and summed to measure bias within a particular study [14]. Two reviewers (KA, RF) independently assessed the risk of bias for identified studies.

Search for measurement properties of identified comorbidity indices

A highly sensitive methodological PubMed search filter was applied for each identified comorbidity index [18]. The title and abstract of all search results were then screened, to ensure each study included pregnant or post-partum women. A full literature review was conducted for all remaining articles after the screening of titles and abstracts.

We organized findings according to De Vet measurement tool [19] *development, sensibility, reliability* and criterion *validity*. Development: The 'clinimetric' properties of the indices were evaluated on the domains of item generation, item reduction and item weighting, as suggested by Feinstein [20]. Sensibility in general refers to the "usefulness" of an instrument; for example, describing the tool's comprehensiveness, clarity and face validity. A common sensibility assessment framework consists of *purpose, population and setting, face* and *content validity,* and *feasibility* [21]. Face validity is the extent to which a test is subjectively viewed as covering the concept it purports to measure. Content validity refers to the extent to which a measure represents all facets of a given construct (e.g. whether items sufficiently address construct domains of the comorbid conditions). That is to say, content validity refers to what the test actually measures, while face validity refers to what it appears to measure. Feasibility addresses features such as simplicity, training requirements and time for administration or completion. Reliability is defined as consistency or stability of measurement [22]. Criterion validity can be assessed by comparing the performance of an index with another measurement in the same clinical situation [19], ideally with the currently accepted gold standard.

Results

Our initial search retrieved 8944 citations, 8295 of which remained after removal of duplications. Figure 1 represents the study selection process. Screening of the titles and abstracts resulted in 61 relevant articles for which the manuscript full text was assessed for eligibility. From these, 59 studies were excluded, for the following reasons: 10 because there was insufficient information provided in the conference abstract and there was no subsequent full-text article, 6 that did not focus on mortality prediction, 13 that did not report upon model performance, 24 that explored physiology based indices initially developed for non-pregnant populations, in ICU settings, and which employed vital signs and laboratory results in addition to comorbidities (i.e. APACHE, SAPS, the MPM, Sepsis-related Organ Failure Assessment [23–26]), and 6 studies that did not focus on comorbidities. Finally, two eligible articles were identified. One described three comorbidity indices appropriate for health administrative data: the Maternal comorbidity index, the Charlson comorbidity index and the Elixhauser Comorbidity Index [27]. The other article was an external validation of the Maternal Comorbidity Index using Canadian health administrative datasets [28].

Description of included study and indices

Characteristics of included articles and the three indices are described in Table 1. Bateman and colleagues have recently developed a new measurement tool – the maternal

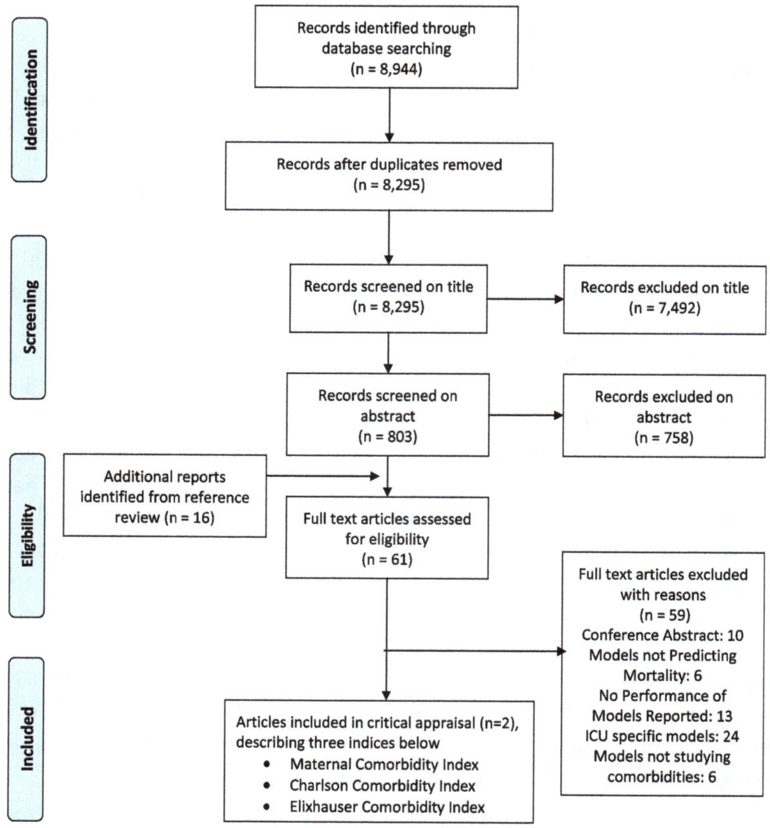

Fig. 1 PRISMA flow diagram for MEDLINE, EMBASE

comorbidity index, which predicts an occurrence of maternal end-organ injury or death during the delivery hospitalization through 30 days postpartum, and then validated the index in comparison to the Charlson comorbidity index and the Elixhauser Comorbidity Index [27]. The cohort was derived from the Medicaid Analytic eXtract (a United States-based health administrative dataset). The data set contained 854,823 completed pregnancies and then was separated into a two-thirds development cohort and a one-third validation cohort. The derived index included 20 maternal conditions and maternal age (Additional file 1: Appendix B) [27]. Each condition has a weighted score and the final score is a summation of all conditions.

In the validation cohort, the Maternal Comorbidity Index was assessed for calibration and discrimination properties and was also compared with the Charlson comorbidity index and the Elixhauser Comorbidity Index, using c-statistics and reclassification measure. C-statistics were 0.657 (95% CI 0.647–0.666) in the Maternal Comorbidity Index, 0.578 (95% CI 0.570–0.585) in the Charlson comorbidity index and 0.586 (95% CI 0.575–0.597) in the Elixhauser Comorbidity Index, respectively. The net reclassification improvement (a mechanism to evaluate correct or incorrect classification of risk groups in comparison to the actual outcome group or other indices) for the Maternal Comorbidity Index was 0.118 ($p < 0.001$) when comparing with the Charlson comorbidity

Table 1 Measurement properties of included indices

Study	Year	Design	n	Comorbidity Index	Outcome	C-statistic (95% CI)
Bateman et al. [27]	2013	Retrospective Cohort	854,823	The maternal comorbidity index	Organ injury or death	0.657 (0.647–0.666)
				The Charlson comorbidity index	Organ injury or death	0.578 (0.570–0.585)
				The Elixhauser comorbidity Index	Organ injury or death	0.586 (0.575–0.597)
Metcalfe et al. [28]	2015	Retrospective Cohort	5995	The maternal comorbidity index	Organ injury	0.67 (0.58–0.76)

CI Confidence Interval

index. This means, in comparison with the Charlson comorbidity index, the maternal comorbidity index correctly reclassified 20.8% of women while incorrectly reclassifying only 9.0%, demonstrating improvement in classification for 11.8% of the validation cohort [27, 29, 30].

Thereafter, Metcalfe validated discrimination and calibration properties of the Maternal Comorbidity Index within Canadian health administrative datasets [28]. The main outcome of this validation study was end-organ injury rather than original composite outcome of end-organ injury or death by Bateman. C-statistics for predicting the outcome in hospitalization data was 0.67 (95% Confidence Interval 0.58–0.76). The calibration was high with the Brier score of 0.01 which quantifies the difference between the predicted probability and the actual probability of the outcome, ranging from 0 to 1 (a number closer to 0 has better calibration).

Methodological quality

The risk of bias of these two articles was assessed according to the Hayden's guidelines [14], and summarized in Table 2. While the retrospective nature of the identified studies precludes assessment of study attrition, and there remains the potential for unmeasured and unaccounted for confounding variables, overall, the studies have a low risk of bias.

Studies for measurement properties

All three comorbidity indices were searched in PubMed, using a methodological PubMed search filter [18], leading to 42, 599 and 34 results for the Maternal, the Charlson and the Elixhauser Comorbidity Indices respectively. Development and sensibility of all three comorbidity indices were assessed on the basis of their original articles [27, 31, 32]. With regard to reliability and validity, we conducted a manual screening of titles and abstracts on the search results in each index. There were no existing studies regarding reliability of all three comorbidity indices in maternal health research. Predictive validity (i.e. discrimination and calibration) of the maternal comorbidity index was investigated in the original article and externally [27, 28].

Discussion

Our systematic literature search identified only three comorbidity indices that have been directly compared in maternal health research: The Maternal Comorbidity Index, the Charlson Comorbidity Index and the Elixhauser Comorbidity Index. Additional literature search with a methodological PubMed search filter revealed two studies that explored the *validity* of these indices in maternal health research [27, 28]. There is no study assessing *reliability* of these indices in maternal health research. The measurement properties of all three indices are summarized in Table 3 and detailed below.

The maternal Comorbidity index

The Maternal Comorbidity Index was developed from an existing United States database, the Medicaid Analytic eXtract, to predict end-organ injury and 30 day mortality of hospitalized pregnant woman [27]. The included comorbidities are available in Additional file 1: Appendix B. Although potential items in the index were based on clinical relevance and existing literature, no consensus method (e.g. Delphi technique) was used in generating potential items for evaluation and inclusion. Item reduction and weighting were derived on the basis of an odds ratio and coefficients of variables from previously published models predicting outcomes. As a part of a sensibility evaluation, the face validity and content validity was reasonable. Yet, no study has investigated feasibility of applying and incorporating the index into clinical research. C-statistics were near 0.7, indicating acceptable applicability. Although the external validity of the Maternal Comorbidity Index has been investigated [28], subsequent studies investigating reliability have not yet been reported.

The Charlson Comorbidity index

The Charlson Comorbidity Index was developed on the basis of one-year mortality from a cohort study of 604 patients admitted to an internal medicine service at a New York Hospital during 1 month in 1984 [31]. In the item generation phase, the initial list of 29 potential items was developed based on all comorbidities present in that the cohort. In the item reduction phase, all potential 29 comorbid diseases were investigated in a multi-variable backward proportional hazard model to calculate the adjusted relative risk of one-year mortality using all potential prognostic determinants. The authors excluded determinants with a p-value above 0.1 or with an adjusted relative risk below 1.2. Finally, 19 predictors remained in the Charlson Comorbidity Index. The Charlson Comorbidity

Table 2 Risk of Bias in Methodological qualities of identified articles

Study	Study Participation	Study Attrition	Prognostic Factor Measurement	Outcome Measurement	Confounding Measurement and Account	Analysis
Bateman et al. [27]	Low	NA	Low	Low	Moderate	Low
Metcalfe et al. [28]	Low	NA	Low	Moderate	Moderate	Low

NA Not Applicable

Table 3 Key features of Maternal, Charlson and Elixhauser comorbidity indices

	Maternal Comorbidity Index	Charlson Comorbidity Index	Elixhauser Comorbidity Index
Development			
Item generation	Based on clinical relevance and literature, but no consensus method applied	No input from previous index, and no consensus method applied	Based on review of published studies, but no consensus method applied
Item reduction	Odds ratio and p-value from statistical model applied	Adjusted relative risk from statistical model applied, but no clinical relevance for pregnant population	A series of univariable and multivariable regression models
Item weighting	Weights of coefficients from statistical model used	Weights of coefficients from statistical model used	No weighting
Sensibility			
Purpose	Predict end-organ injury or death during the delivery hospitalization to 30 days	Predict 1-year mortality	In-hospital mortality
Population	Women who delivered in hospital	General medical patients	Adult, non-maternal inpatients
Setting	Hospitals in U.S.	Medical ward in a hospital	Hospitals in California
Face validity	Exists	Exists	Exists
Content validity	Reasonable	Challenging	Reasonable
Feasibility	No study	Marked training required	No study
Reliability	Not studied	Excellent in general No maternal studies	Not studied
Criterion validity			
Concurrent validity	Not studied	No maternal studies	No maternal studies

Index was formulated on the basis of item weighting according to weights of coefficients derived from the mathematical models predicting outcome in nearly exclusively, non-pregnant patients. The components of the weighted index are shown in Additional file 1: Appendix C [31]. The main challenge in the item reduction of the Charlson Comorbidity Index is that it lacks clinical relevance for pregnant patients – the co-morbid conditions common to patients admitted to an internal medicine ward have minimal to modest overlap with pregnant or post-partum patients. Also, the development of the Charlson Comorbidity Index did not include quantitative input from experts and clinicians, which has a significant impact on content validity as a part of sensibility evaluation. In addition, there have been no prior studies to investigate the reliability of the Charlson Comorbidity Index among pregnant patients. Finally, the index showed poor discriminative ability with c-statistics less than 0.6 among pregnant women [27].

The Elixhauser Comorbidity index

The Elixhauser Comorbidity Index was developed using a California-based population dataset of adult, non-maternal inpatients from 438 acute care hospitals in 1992 [32]. The dataset included 1,779,167 patients and 41 comorbidities were listed. No consensus method was employed for making a list of potential candidates for the comorbidity index. Outcomes were defined as length of stay, charges and in-hospital mortality. Statistically unrelated comorbidities to the outcomes were excluded after a series of univariable and multivariable analyses, leading to a final set of 30 comorbidities (Additional file 1: Appendix D) [32]. The authors did not employ item weighting in the phases of development. The Elixhauser Comorbidity Index was developed mainly for use with administrative data. The index has good face validity as well as content validity as the items are mutually exclusive. Feasibility of using the index was not examined in maternal or related research. In the context of maternal health research, the reliability and criterion validity of the Elixhauser Comorbidity Index have not been elucidated. Lastly, discriminative ability of the index among pregnant women was poor (c-statistic <0.6) [27].

There have been an increasing number of 'big data' studies using health administrative datasets in medicine. However, there are many pitfalls in undertaking such studies, most commonly related to unmeasured or unaccounted for confounding in the relationship between exposures and outcomes. Because the severity of patients' medical conditions is a very common source of potential confounding, risk adjustment among patients with different severity of illness is essential within health administrative datasets in order to more validly estimate the true association of exposures and outcomes. Despite its modest discriminative performance, the Maternal Comorbidity Index is currently the most reasonable comorbidity index for maternal health research using health administrative datasets.

Overall, no comorbidity indices used in maternal health research employed a consensus method to identify or refine variable choices and this limits the sensibility of all indices. Reliability of these indices has not been investigated in maternal health research. Only two articles have explored predictive validity of the indices among pregnant women, showing that the Maternal Comorbidity Index appears better able to predict maternal mortality in comparison with the Charlson and Elixahuser Comorbidity Index [27, 28].

Our review has limitations. First, we did not determine how often these comorbidity indices are used in daily clinical practice, or in maternal health research. Instead, we have identified all available indices in the field and their related measurement properties with a methodological PubMed search filter. Second, there is no standard method to report risk of bias in studies of prediction models. We employed the Hayden's framework for our study, but the Prediction model study Risk Of Bias Assessment Tool (PROBAST) [33] could be an alternative to assess risk of bias in these studies that will soon be available and may provide an improved approach to bias description.

Conclusion

Based on this systematic review of the existing literature, the Maternal Comorbidity Index appears to be the most appropriate comorbidity index for use with health administrative datasets of pregnant or post-partum women; however, it requires further appraisal of feasibility and reliability, in order to better appreciate its ability to perform outcome prediction and risk adjustment. Also, given the modest discrimination of the Maternal Comorbidity Index, evolution of this and other tools for risk-adjustment in pregnant and post-partum patients will be an important area for ongoing study.

Abbreviations

CI: Confidence Interval; ICU: Intensive Care Unit

Acknowledgements

KA receives Fellowship funding from the Canadian Institutes of Health Research, to pursue the PhD stream of Clinical Epidemiology & Health Care Research at Institute of Health Policy, Management and Evaluation, University of Toronto.

Funding

CIHR Transitional Open Operating Grant (#342397).

Authors' contributions

KA conceived this paper. KA, RD and RAF performed the systematic review. KA performed the analysis on the result of the literature search, and RD, SEL, EI and RAF provided input on the interpretation. KA wrote the initial draft of the manuscript, and RD, SEL, EI and RAF helped draft the final version, which was approved by all authors.

Competing interests

The authors declare that they have no competing interests.

Author details

[1]Department of Anesthesia and Pain Medicine, The Hospital for Sick Children, University of Toronto, Toronto, Canada. [2]Intensive Care Unit, Mount Sinai Hospital and University Health Network, University of Toronto, Toronto, Canada. [3]Department of Critical Care Medicine, Sunnybrook Health Science Centre, University of Toronto, Toronto, Canada. [4]Interdepartmental Division of Critical Care Medicine, University of Toronto, Toronto, Canada. [5]Department of Anesthesiology and Pain Medicine, School of Medicine, Juntendo University, Tokyo, Japan. [6]Department of Obstetrics and Gynaecology, Division of Maternal-Fetal Medicine, Mount Sinai Hospital, University of Toronto, Toronto, Canada. [7]Institute of Health Policy, Management and Evaluation, University of Toronto, Toronto, Canada. [8]555 University Ave, Room 2211, Toronto, ON M5G 1X8, Canada.

References

1. Einav S, Bromiker R, Sela HY. Maternal Critical Illness. Curr Anesthesiol Rep. 2017;7:55–66.
2. Pollock W, Rose L, Dennis C. Pregnant and postpartum admissions to the intensive care unit: a systematic review. Intensive Care Med. 2010;36:1465–74.
3. Aoyama K, Seaward P, Lapinsky SE. Fetal outcome in the critically ill pregnant woman. Crit Care. 2014;18:307.
4. Say L, Pattinson RC, Gülmezoglu a M. WHO systematic review of maternal morbidity and mortality: the prevalence of severe acute maternal morbidity (near miss). Reprod Health. 2004;1:3.
5. Waterstone M, Bewley S, Wolfe C. Incidence and predictors of severe obstetric morbidity: case-control study. BMJ. 2001;322:1089-93–4.
6. Geller SE, Adams MG, Kominiarek M a, Hibbard JU, Endres LK, Cox SM, Kilpatrick SJ. Reliability of a preventability model in maternal death and morbidity. Am J Obstet Gynecol. 2007;196:57.e1–6.
7. Kirshner B, Guyatt G. A methodological framework for assessing health indices. J Chronic Dis. 1985;38:27–36.
8. Senanayake H, Dias T, Jayawardena a. Maternal mortality and morbidity: epidemiology of intensive care admissions in pregnancy. Best Pract Res Clin Obstet Gynaecol. 2013;27:811–20.
9. Zeeman GG. Obstetric critical care: a blueprint for improved outcomes. Crit Care Med. 2006;34(9 Suppl):S208–14.
10. el-Solh AA, Grant BJ. A comparison of severity of illness scoring systems for critically ill obstetric patients. Chest. 1996;110:1299–304.
11. Hazelgrove JF, Price C, Pappachan VJ, Smith GB. Multicenter study of obstetric admissions to 14 intensive care units in southern England. Crit Care Med. 2001;29:770–5.
12. Rojas-Suarez J, Paternina-Caicedo AJ, Miranda J, Mendoza R, Dueñas-Castel C, Bourjeily G. Comparison of severity-of-illness scores in critically ill obstetric patients: a 6-year retrospective cohort. Crit Care Med. 2014;42:1047–54.
13. Deeks J, Wisniewski S, Davenport C. Guide to the contents of a Cochrane diagnostic test accuracy protocol. Cochrane Handb Syst Rev Diagnostic Test Accuracy Version. 2013;100:1–15.
14. Hayden JA, Côté P, Bombardier C. Evaluation of the quality of prognosis studies in systematic reviews. Ann Intern Med. 2006;144:427–37.
15. Kansagara D, Englander H, Salanitro A, Kagen D, Theobald C, Freeman M, Kripalani S. Risk prediction models for hospital readmission: a systematic review. JAMA. 2011;306:1688–98.
16. Minne L, Ludikhuize J, de Jonge E, de Rooij S, Abu-Hanna A. Prognostic models for predicting mortality in elderly ICU patients: a systematic review. Intensive Care Med. 2011;37:1258–68.
17. Nassar AP, Malbouisson LMS, Moreno R. Evaluation of simplified acute physiology score 3 performance: a systematic review of external validation studies. Crit Care. 2014;18:R117.
18. Terwee CB, Jansma EP, Riphagen II, De Vet HCW. Development of a methodological PubMed search filter for finding studies on measurement properties of measurement instruments. Qual Life Res. 2009;18:1115–23.

19. de Vet HCW, Terwee CB, Mokkink LB, Knol DL. Measurement in Medicine: a Practical Guide. First. Cambridge: Cambridge University Press; 2011.
20. Feinstein AR. Clinimetrics. New Haven, MA: Yale University Press; 1987.
21. Bombardier C. Sensibility assessment worksheet. Toronto; 2014.
22. Mokkink LB, Terwee CB, Patrick DL, Alonso J, Stratford PW, Knol DL, Bouter LM, de Vet HCW. The COSMIN study reached international consensus on taxonomy, terminology, and definitions of measurement properties for health-related patient-reported outcomes. J Clin Epidemiol. 2010;63:737–45.
23. Knaus WA, Draper EA, Wagner DP, Zimmerman JE. APACHE II: a severity of disease classification system. Crit Care Med. 1985;13:818–29.
24. Le Gall J-R, Lemeshow S, Saulnier F. Simplified acute physiology score (SAPS II) based on a European / north American multicenter study. JAMA. 1993;270:2957–63.
25. Lemeshow S, Teres D, Klar J, Avrunin JS, Gehlbach SH, Rapoport J. Mortality probability models (MPM II) based on an international cohort of intensive care unit patients. JAMA. 1993;270:2478–86.
26. Vincent JL, Moreno R, Takala J, Willatts S, De Mendonça A, Bruining H, Reinhart CK, Suter PM, Thijs LG. The SOFA (sepsis-related organ failure assessment) score to describe organ dysfunction/failure. On behalf of the working group on sepsis-related problems of the European Society of Intensive Care Medicine. Intensive Care Med. 1996;22:707–10.
27. Bateman BT, Mhyre JM, Hernandez-Diaz S, Huybrechts KF, Fischer M a, Creanga A a, Callaghan WM, Gagne JJ: Development of a comorbidity index for use in obstetric patients. Obstet Gynecol 2013, 122:957–965.
28. Metcalfe A, Lix LM, Johnson J, Currie G, Lyon AW, Bernier F, Tough SC. Validation of an obstetric comorbidity index in an external population. BJOG. 2015;122:1748–55.
29. Cook NR, Ridker PM. Advances in measuring the effect of individual predictors of cardiovascular risk: the role of reclassification measures. Ann Intern Med. 2009;150:795–802.
30. Pencina MJ, D'Agostino RB, Vasan RS. Evaluating the added predictive ability of a new marker: from area under the ROC curve to reclassification and beyond. Stat Med. 2008;27:157-72–12.
31. Charlson ME, Pompei P, Ales KL, MacKenzie CR. A new method of classifying prognostic comorbidity in longitudinal studies: development and validation. J Chronic Dis. 1987;40:373–83.
32. Elixhauser a, Steiner C, Harris DR, Coffey RM. Comorbidity measures for use with administrative data. Med Care. 1998;36:8–27.
33. PROBAST steering committee. Prediction risk of bias assessment tool (PROBAST) [Internet]. Kleijnen Syst Rev Ltd, 2013 [accessed 22/07/2015] .

6

Handheld ultrasound to avert maternal and neonatal deaths in 2 regions of the Philippines: an iBuntis® intervention study

Godofreda V. Dalmacion[1,2,3*], Ramon T. Reyles[4], Antonia E. Habana[5], Lalaine Mae V. Cruz[3], Maricelle C. Chua[4], Analyn T. Ngo[6], Milagros J. Tia-Jocson[7] and Emmanuel S. Baja[2,3]

Abstract

Background: The major causes of maternal and neonatal mortality in the Philippines are hemorrhages and obstructed labor due to placental implantation abnormalities (PIAs), twin pregnancies and fetal malpresentations. All of which are all easily detected by ultrasound. However, women in rural areas and low-income groups do not have access to ultrasound during their prenatal care. We aimed to provide additional evidence on the benefits of handheld ultrasound (HU) for screening pregnancy related abnormalities in order to avert maternal and neonatal deaths.

Methods: Using a HU, we trained community healthcare workers (CHWs) to identify 5 obstetrical conditions: fetal viability and number, placental localization, amniotic fluid volume (AFV) and fetal presentation. Women, between 20th and 24th weeks age of gestation from 2 regions of the Philippines, were scanned using the HU and the GE Logic 5 Premium ultrasound machine for validation. Maternal and neonatal deaths averted were estimated as health outcome measures of the study.

Results: Four hundred sixty women were scanned of which 146 (31.7%) showed abnormal ultrasound readings consisting of 17 PIAs, 123 fetal malpresentation, 3 twins and 3 AFV abnormalities. The use of HU could have possibly averted 29 (6.3%) maternal deaths and 14.6% neonatal deaths at the time of delivery. Thirty-two out of the 460 women (~7%) delivered at home and 93% in hospitals or birthing facilities/lying–in centers. We observed approximately 95% agreement between the ultrasound readings of the trainees and the trainers, and 99% agreement between the readings made from the HU with the validation machine.

Conclusion: CHWs could be trained in the use of HU for scanning 5 obstetrical parameters. Early detection of abnormalities in these 5 obstetrical parameters can lead to early referral to facilities that are better equipped to manage obstetrical emergencies. Prenatal ultrasound can be an excellent point of care test for screening pregnant women at risk for possible complications and even death during labor and delivery.

Keywords: Handheld ultrasound, Screening, Access to prenatal care, Maternal and neonatal mortality

* Correspondence: jody.dalmacion@gmail.com
[1]Department of Pharmacology and Toxicology, College of Medicine, University of the Philippines-Manila, Manila, Philippines
[2]Department of Clinical Epidemiology, College of Medicine, University of the Philippines- Manila, Manila, Philippines
Full list of author information is available at the end of the article

Background

Based on a 2013 UNICEF Philippine Report, 13 mothers die every day in the country from pregnancy-related complications [1]. It reported a high maternal death rate of 162 per 100,000 livebirths in 2000 escalating further to 221/100,000 livebirths in 2011 [1]. Neverthleless, there was a dramatic decrease in June 2015 to 115/100,000 livebirths which was still short of the 2015 Millennium Development Goal (MDG) of 15 per 100,000 livebirths. In 2015, the Philippines ranked 74th among 184 countries for maternal mortality rate (MMR) [2]. The major cause of maternal death in the country has been hemorrhage at 41% [1]. The different causes of maternal deaths worldwide have been attributed to hemorrhage (27%) of which 17% occurred in the postpartum period, sepsis (10.7%), obstructed labor (2.8%), hypertensive disorders (14%), and complications of unsafe abortion (7.9%). Most of these disorders are preventable with early diagnosis and prompt interventions [3]. Placental implantation abnormalities (PIAs) namely, placenta previa, marginal/low lying placenta, placenta accreta vasa previa and velamentous cord insertion account for both intrapartum and postpartum maternal hemorrhages [4]. They are identified by ultrasound, which normally can be done anytime between 18 and 22 weeks [4]. In contrast, the trend for neonatal mortality rate (NMR) of the Philippines or deaths in the newborn before they reach 28 days of life showed a downward trend from 20 per 1000 livebirths in 1990 to 12.6 per 1000 livebirths in 2015. This was comparable to Indonesia's estimated 13.5 neonatal deaths per 1000 livebirths [5]. The top three causes of newborn deaths in the Philippines are prematurity (31%) followed by asphyxia and birth trauma (23%) and congenital anomalies (19%), which are congruent with the worldwide statistics [6]. Nevertheless, PIAs contributed substantially to preterm birth with prematurity rates ranging from 38 to 82% simply because premature termination of pregnancy in many instances may be the definitive management for PIAs [7]. Several studies on maternal health traced the link between neonatal and maternal deaths to the lack of adequate health care during pregnancy [3]. Poor access to obstetric ultrasound in rural areas of developing countries is known to be significantly detrimental to perinatal outcomes [8]. A separate study in 2011 reported not only the under-ultilization of ultrasound imaging in many developing countries but also the lack of trained sonographers as a challenge in delivering quality maternal healthcare [9].

In the Philippines, even the cheapest handheld types are not available in the government birthing facilities. In addition, ultrasound machines can only be found in government Tertiary Hospitals where most Obstetrician (OB)-Sonographers practice. In primary and secondary health facilities, the prenatal management is confined to measuring the vital signs of the pregnant patient, performing physical examination including the Leopold's Maneuver and doing routine blood tests. A study in Botswana, involving 2309 patients, who attended an Ultrasound Service in a district hospital showed fetal demise, spontaneous abortion, low lying placenta and ectopic pregnancy as among the obstetrical pathologies. It found out that offering ultrasound services during the prenatal visits are cost effective and can improve patient care by 30% [10].

Active surveillance of the pregnant patient with abnormal obstetrical images on ultasound can be initiated earlier, reducing the development of conditions to a more catastrophic event. Unnecessary internal examination, which can potentially result to undue vaginal bleeding, can also be avoided by the early identification of abnormal placental implantation. Lastly, adequate preparation such as improving the hemodynamic state of the parturient to withstand heavy blood loss during labor and delivery especially by cesarean section can be appropriately instituted avoiding possible blood transfusions during labor and delivery. A study of Oyelese and colleagues reported 97% (59/61) of infants prenatally diagnosed by ultrasound with vasa previa surviving compared with only 44% (41/94) survivors out of those undiagnosed [11]. Finally, Harris and Marks in 2009 summarized the anecdotal experience of ultrasound in low resource setting. They observed improvement of public health care including maternal care with the deployment of donated ultrasound units. They particularly cited the experience of a Nicaraguan physician who reported a reduction of maternal mortality from 12 deaths per year to 5 per year in his practice. The study recommended doing field trials using ultrasound against a reference validation machine on a scale equal with public health interventions [12].

The objectives of the study were: (1) to ascertain the benefits of early ultrasound imaging of pregnant women in their 20th to 24th weeks age of gestation in detecting PIAs, fetal conditions such as malpresentations and multiple pregnancies; (2) to estimate the agreement between the ultrasound readings of the trainees with their trainers; (3) to validate the readings from the handheld ultrasound (HU) with the reference ultrasound validation machine; (4) to determine the type of birth attendant and place of deliveries of our study population representing both rural and urban sites and (5) to estimate the maternal and neonatal deaths possibly averted from the use of a HU in their prenatal care.

Methods

Study sites and population

Parañaque city, the urban study site and Tagum city, the rural study site, are located in 2 different regions of the Philippines. They were purposively selected as study sites based on their similar MMR of 1 per 1000 livebirths. Parañaque consisting of 17 barangays with a population of

582,000 is a highly urbanized city located in the National Capital Region. Tagum, located in the province of Davao del Norte is an agricultural city rich in mineral deposits, has 23 barangays and a population of 242,000. The study participants were randomly sampled from the list of pregnant women in their 20th to 24th weeks of pregnancies during which time placental localization is more reliably established [5]. Before the 18th weeks age of gestation, 50% of placenta will be low lying and between 18th and 24th weeks age of gestation it is estimated that 2–4% will still remain low lying. Thus, the Society of Obstetrician and Gynecologists of Canada recommends repeating the ultrasound for PIAs by the third trimester to confirm the final localization of the placenta [13]. All the towns locally known as barangays from each study site were included in the sampling frame. The number of samples from each town was proportional to the size of its population. Excluded were pregnant women with known allergy to gel, with concurrent medical or surgical conditions and those who were not able to provide informed consents. Prior to the implementation of the project, the study proposal was reviewed and approved by the National Ethics Committee. The informed consent was written in the local dialect and was administered to all women who were recruited. Women who signed the informed consent were eligible and included in the study.

Study design and sample size

A cross sectional study design was used. The sample size was calculated based on the prevalence of abnormal ultrasound images of 35% in the second trimester of pregnancy reported from an earlier study [14].

Ultrasound technical working group

All cities and municipalities in the country have a community healthcare team (CHT), which is composed of general practitioners, nurses, and midwives. A technical working group (TWG) composed of 10 members of the CHT was identified for each study site to act as coordinators and to undergo training in ultrasound scanning. A total of 20 ultrasound trainees, consisting of 6 doctors, 5 nurses, and 9 midwives from both cities, were selected by their respective City Health Officer and subsequently trained in scanning. The training package was composed of classroom lecture, hands-on training and 2–3 days of actual scanning of the pregnant women recruited by the study. The Training Team administered a pre-test prior to the training proper to establish the baseline knowledge of the selected TWG-trainees on obstetrical ultrasound. All the lectures were delivered by the head of the scanning team who was then the President of the Philippine Society of Ultrasound in Obstetrics and Gynecology (PSUOG). All trainees were taught on how to scan using a mobile handheld General Electric (GE) ultrasound called VScan. The GE VScan has a dual probe that can be used to scan the pelvic and abdominal organs like the liver and the heart. It comes with a docking station and 4 GB micro-SD memory card. The VScan does not have a M-Mode and therefore cannot give an actual count of the fetal heart rate.

The TWG were trained to identify and measure 5 obstetrical ultrasound images namely; viability of the fetus, number of pregnancy, fetal presentation, location of the placenta and amniotic fluid volume (AFV) using maximal vertical pocket. By focusing only on specific obstetrical parameters, we were able to effectively train our community healthcare workers (CHWs) for a short period of time and avoided any possible conflicts with the practice of the credentialed OB–sonographers of the site. After the hands-on training, a written post-test was administered to the TWG-trainees to determine improvement of their knowledge on the principles of ultrasound imaging from baseline.

Ultrasound iBuntis screening intervention

Streamers and banners with the iBuntis Logo were posted in the different health facilities to effectively recruit pregnant volunteers. The demographic and obstetrical data of the pregnant recruits who fulfilled the inclusionary criteria were collected even prior to the free ultrasound sessions which were conducted for three days in urban study site and two days in the rural study site. During the actual ultrasound sessions, the TWG-trainees of each study city performed the initial ultrasound scan using the VScan. Their ultrasound readings were instantly confirmed by the trainers using the same VScan and both their readings further confirmed by the head sonologist of the study using the GE Logic 5 Premium ultrasound as the reference standard. Thus, sources of the disagreements and errors of the trainees were immediately identified, explained and corrected by the trainers. At the end of the study, each trainee on average scanned 30 women.

Patients with abnormal readings were immediately tagged and referred for more intensive prenatal surveillance under an accredited birthing facility or an Emergency Maternal and Neonatal Care unit. The ultrasound results were shared with the participants who were advised to repeat their ultrasound by the 32nd weeks age of gestation. Thereafter, midwives were commissioned to follow up all women for their pregnancy outcomes.

Health outcome measurements

For the purpose of estimating the health outcome, we classified the different abnormal scans into those which can potentially lead to maternal deaths and those which are more likely to cause neonatal deaths. All abnormal ultrasound findings can actually lead to catastrophic events in either mother or neonate or both. Nevertheless, by adopting a specific operational definition of "deaths averted" based on the ultrasound results we can calculate our health outcomes. Thus possible "maternal deaths averted" were estimated as percent possible cases of deaths from PIAs and transverse lie only over the total number of scans, while possible "neonatal deaths averted" were estimated as percent cases of twin, breech presentation and AFV abnormalities over the total number of scans. We likewise assumed that even if abnormal ultrasound images can eventually become normal at birth e.g. breech to cephalic and low-lying to normal placentation, possible catastrophic perinatal outcomes were considered averted by their timely referral to better-equipped hospitals and more targeted prenatal surveillance.

Data collection and management

Using the case report forms (CRF) of the study, data were extracted in the CRF, double encoded into a Google form version of the CRF, and matched for any data entry discrepancies. Any inconsistencies in the Google database were resolved by cross-checking with the CRFs. Access to the Google database was limited to the Principal Investigator and the biostatistician/epidemiologist of the study.

Statistical analysis

We calculated descriptive statistics for all the health outcomes and covariates of the study population. Mean and the standard deviation were used to summarize continuous variables while frequencies and the percentages were used to summarize categorical variables. Association between the study sites (Tagum and Parañaque) and the categorical health outcomes were assessed using either Fisher's Exact test or Pearson's Chi-square test and using Student's t-test for continuous variables. *P*-values ≤ 0.05 were considered statistically significant. STATA v13 (StataCorp, College Station, TX, USA) was used in the analysis.

Results

A total of 462 pregnant women were recruited but only 460 met the inclusionary criteria. Two hundred fifty pregnant women were recruited from the urban Paranaque study site and 210 from the rural Tagum study site. The characteristics of the pregnant women are summarized in Table 1. The women in Paranaque were slightly older than the women in Tagum (mean age in years ± standard deviation (SD): 26.0 ± 6.4 vs. 25.0 ± 6.2, *p*-value = 0.09), and 1 out of 10 women had irregular menstrual cycles for both study sites. Although the duration of training in the urban site took longer than in the rural site, there was no difference in the scores of the pre- and post- test of the trainees or their performances in the actual scanning sessions for both rural and urban sites. A total of 20 CHW trainees with 78 hours of training was produced and 3 training modules were created.

Table 2 shows the possible maternal and neonatal deaths averted in both study sites. One hundred forty-six of the 460 pregnant volunteers (31.7%) had abnormal scans. There was a statistically significant difference in the number of abnormal scans between the urban Parañaque study site and the rural Tagum study site with the former having a higher prevalence of abnormal ultrasound results (37.6% vs. 24.8%, *p*-value <0.01). The distribution of abnormal scans included abnormal AFV (0.6%), twin pregnancy (1.3%), PIAs (3.7%) and fetal malpresentation (26.7%). The most common fetal malpresentation was breech (24.1%) followed by transverse lie (2.6%). The total maternal and neonatal deaths possibly averted at the time of the scanning from both study sites were estimated to be 6.3% and 26.1%, respectively using the predetermined definition. Furthermore, higher percentages of deaths possibly averted were observed in urban Parañaque compared to rural Tagum for both maternal (8.8% vs. 3.4%, *p*-value = 0.02) and neonatal (30% vs. 21.4%, *p*-value = 0.02) deaths. At the time of delivery, 40% of the 111 breech presentations turned to cephalic which decreased the neonatal deaths possibly averted to approximately 14.6% (67/460).

Table 3 summarizes the distributions of the referral to health facility and the place of delivery of the study participants. There was no difference between the two study sites regarding home deliveries of women with abnormal scans (*p*-value = 0.70). However, more women with abnormal findings in the urban study site delivered in hospitals (24.4% vs 14.3%, *p*-value <0.05), and in birthing facilities/lying in (11.6% vs. 8.1%, *p*-value = 0.02), than those residing in the rural study site.

Doctors from the two study sites attended 19.7% of the abnormal birth deliveries followed by midwives (10.0%), and traditional birth attendants (TBA) at 2.0% (Table 4). More pregnancies with abnormal scans were delivered by Physicians in the urban site compared to those in the rural site (24.4% vs. 14.3%, *p*-value = 0.03). Conversely, more pregnancies with normal scans were delivered by midwives in the rural site compared to the urban study site (36.2% vs. 24.8%, *p*-value = 0.03). In addition, neonatal mortality, still birth and congenital anomalies were only observed in the rural study site with prevalence of approximately 10 per 1000 livebirths, 5 per 1000 livebirths and 10 per 1000 livebirths, respectively.

Very good agreement at 95% was observed between the ultrasound readings of the trainee CHWs with those of the credentialed trainers. Furthermore, excellent agreement at 95.7% was also observed between the readings made from the HU and the reference machine. Most of the disagreements were observed on fetal presentation. The trainess-CHWs tend to misdiagnose breech and transverse lie as cephalic (see Table 5 for details).

Table 1 Characteristics of study population from two regions in the Philippines ($N = 460$)

Characteristic	Rural Tagum ($n = 210$)	Urban Parañaque ($n = 250$)	p-value
Age (years), *mean* [SD][a]	25.0 [6.2]	26.0 [6.4]	0.09
Age of 1st menstruation (years), *mean* [SD]	13.1 [1.6]	13.4 [1.7]	0.053
Smoking status, *N* (%)			
Ever	31 (14.8)	36 (14.4)	0.91
Never	179 (85.2)	214 (85.6)	
Contraceptive usage, *N* (%)			
Ever	108 (51.4)	121 (48.4)	0.52
Never	102 (48.6)	129 (51.6)	
Menstrual cycle, *N* (%)[b]			
Irregular	22 (10.5)	27 (10.8)	0.91
Normal	188 (89.5)	223 (89.2)	
Had a pap smear procedure, *N* (%)			
Yes	31 (15.7)	34 (13.6)	0.55
No	166 (84.3)	214 (85.6)	
Missing	13		

[a]*SD* Standard deviation; [b]Irregular menstrual cycle: < 28 days or >35 days

The cost for the intervention in both study sites was 1.7 million pesos (PhP 1.7 M), with a higher cost of the intervention in the rural study site (PhP 981,000.00) compared to the urban study site (PhP 719,000.00). The PhP 262,000.00 difference in cost was due to the air fares spent to conduct the study in Tagum. The capital outlay for the equipment was reasonably priced at PhP 350,000.00 for each study site (see Table 6 for details).

Discussion

Access to prenatal care and services by pregnant women in the Philippines has been restricted mainly due to the following reasons; limitations of diagnostic equipment

Table 2 Maternal deaths and neonatal deaths possibly averted in Parañaque City and Tagum City

Health Outcome	Total ($N = 460$)	Urban Parañaque ($N = 250$)	Rural Tagum ($N = 210$)	p-value
Ultrasound findings (%)				
Normal scans	68.3	62.4	75.2	< 0.01
Abnormal scans	31.7	37.6	24.8	
Maternal deaths possibly averted[a] (%)				
Normal	93.7	91.2	96.6	0.02
Abnormal placentation				
Low lying	2.4	2.4	2.4	
Placenta previa	1.3	2.0	0.5	
Fetal malpresentation				
Transverse	2.6	4.4	0.5	
Neonatal deaths possibly averted[b] (%)				
Normal	74.6	71.2	78.6	0.02
Fetal malpresentation				
Breech	24.1	26.8	20.9	
Oligohydramnios	0.2	0.0	0.5	
Polyhydramnios	0.4	0.8	0.0	
Twins[c]	1.3	2.4	0.0	

[a]maternal deaths averted = maternal deaths due to bleeding from abnormal placental localization and transverse lie; [b]neonatal deaths averted = neonatal deaths due to fetal malpresentation; [c]neonatal deaths averted for twins = actual number of twins × 2

Table 3 Health facility referral and place of delivery based on study site

Outcome parameter	Total (*N* = 460)	Urban Parañaque (*N* = 250)	Rural Tagum (*N* = 210)	*p*-value
Health facility referral (%)				
Hospital	52.4	56.8	47.1	0.11
Birthing facility / Lying in	40.6	36.4	45.7	
Home	7.0	6.8	7.2	
Place of delivery (%)				
Hospital				
Normal cases	32.6	32.4	32.9	0.046
Abnormal cases	19.8	24.4	14.3	
Birthing facility / Lying in				
Normal cases	30.7	24.8	37.6	0.02
Abnormal cases	10.0	11.6	8.1	
Home				
Normal cases	5.0	5.2	4.8	0.70
Abnormal cases	2.0	1.6	2.4	

and treatment modalities in the health facilities, the nature of its geography being an archipelago with bodies of water separating hospitals from their clients, cost of health care and the lack of maternal health advocacy. The project was named iBuntis, a local and short term for "Information Pregnancy". We observed that almost all abnormal ultrasound findings seen between the 20th and 24th weeks age of gestation have not given rise to any clinical signs and symptoms that necessitated emergency referrals to a specialist or hospital. But with the ultrasound scanning done earlier, abnormal findings were shared with the City Health Officers of both study sites. This allowed the tagging of all the pregnant participants at risk for complications during labor and delivery to allow closer surveillance. These referrals could have helped pregnant women since there were no maternal deaths reported from both study sites.

The results of our study showed that screening of high-risk pregnancies could provide more targeted follow-up and management of pregnancies. It is worth mentioning that only 42.6% (40/94) of patients with abnormal scans in the urban study site and none in the rural study site went for the repeat scan. We hypothesize the reason for failing to do so was the lack of funds to pay for the repeat ultrasound. In spite of the issuance of an administrative order that prohibited home birth delivery prior to the conduct of the iBuntis study, 6.2% (9/146) of the abnormal cases still delivered at home. The observed 6.2%, however, is lower than the reported 9.1% of births attended at home by TBA in 2015 [15]. Nevertheless, more effective information campaigns on the benefits of hospital and birthing facility delivery could be requested from the Department of Health and the local governments. Furthermore, 93.8% (137/146) of the

Table 4 Types of birth attendants according to study site

Outcome parameter	Total (*N* = 460)	Urban Parañaque (*N* = 250)	Rural Tagum (*N* = 210)	*p*-value
Obstetrician (%)				
Normal cases	33.3	32.4	34.3	0.03
Abnormal cases	19.7	24.4	14.3	
Total	53.0	56.8	48.6	
Midwife (%)				
Normal cases	30.0	24.8	36.2	0.03
Abnormal cases	10.0	11.6	8.1	
Total	40.0	36.4	44.3	
Traditional birth attendant (%)				
Normal cases	5.0	5.2	4.8	0.70
Abnormal cases	2.0	1.6	2.4	
Total	7.0	6.8	7.2	

Table 5 Agreement between the handheld ultrasound and the reference bigger ultrasound machine for selected Obstetrical ultrasound parameters ($N = 460$)[a]

Ultrasound parameter	In agreement [N, (%)]	Not in agreement [N, (%)]
Fetal presentation	440 (95.7%)	20 (4.3%)[b]
Amniotic fluid	458 (99.6%)	2 (0.4%)
Location	459 (99.8%)	1 (0.2%)
Fetal number	460 (100.0%)	0 (0.0%)

[a]Handheld ultrasound: GE VScan and Reference standard ultrasound: GE Logic 5 Premium
[b]Not in agreement breakdown: Cephalic-Breech (9), Cephalic-Transverse (4), Breech-Transverse (3), Transverse-Breech (2), and Breech-Cephalic (2)

abnormal scans delivered at either the referral hospitals or birthing facilities. We could attribute the effective high referral outcome to women going with additional information in the form of an ultrasound reading about their conditions.

Our study successfully showed that all CHWs from doctors, nurses to midwives are highly trainable and competent in using the HU. Capacitating CHWs to perform screening ultrasound for 5 obstetrical parameters is highly tenable. Brunette et al. reported a similar finding among midwives in Uganda [16]. Midwives were successfully trained on the use of a low-cost, portable and easy-to-use ultrasound. As a consequence of their training, they were able to effectively identify high risk conditions for referrals to bigger hospitals and birthing facilities. With the advancing technology for smaller and mobile ultrasound machines and their lower cost, our local governments may eventually be able to procure handheld ultrasounds as part of their armamentarium for good prenatal care. Nevertheless, more studies in the cost-effectiveness of ultrasounds in rural and urban settings are still needed. Interestingly, we learned that ultrasound screening could influence the decision to use postpartum family planning methods. About 30–35% of women who were scanned asked for the sex of their unborn child and articulated their intention to practice postpartum contraception, or even surgical sterilization, if the child they are carrying carries the sex that they or their husbands wish for. In our study, we also learned that HU should not be used to scan for congenital defects. With a focused ultrasound screening using a 3.5-in. monitor, congenital anomalies could be easily missed. A more extensive training in obstetrical imaging is required for one to develop the ability to detect congenital anomalies using the bigger ultrasound. Based on the Birth Defects Surveillance of the Philippines of 2011, congenital anomalies rank third in the list of common causes of death in infancy in the country [17]. In our study, all congenital anomalies were observed in the rural site, Tagum. A more comprehensive environmental exposure assessment study among pregnant women should be done in similar rural study sites.

Table 6 Cost of intervention for the two study sites

Outcome parameters	Total	Urban Parañaque	Rural Tagum
Cost in PhP			
Equipment	700,000.00	350,000.00	350,000.00
Training	570,000.00	285,000.00	285,000.00
Travel	292,000.00	15,000.00	277,000.00
Consultants	138,000.00	69,000.00	69,000.00
Total	1,700,000.00	719,000.00	981,000.00

Our study showed that the handheld ultrasound at the "point of care" might successfully screen for abnormal obstetrical conditions, which can potentially lead to maternal and neonatal deaths or complications. Using surrogate indicators, 6.3% of maternal deaths and 14.6% of neonatal deaths were possibly averted by the early ultrasound screening. We also observed that socio-cultural beliefs could be stronger determinants than knowledge and logical reasoning for making decision on childbirth and labor. This was manifested by one of our patients who was diagnosed to have a fetus in breech presentation but refused to deliver in the hospital despite warnings that she and her child were at risk for complications and birth injuries respectively. We recommend more studies on the psyche, beliefs and socio-cultural factors affecting women to have a safe labor and delivery.

One limitation of the study is the limited number of study sites due to restricted funding. However, our study design enabled us to explore the contrast between pregnant women living in an urban setting vs. a rural setting. A more expanded ultrasound intervention study is warranted to verify the results of our project. We recommend a scale up study to other regions especially to geographically isolated areas of the country through their Local Government Officials. We also recommend doing the screening in a larger number of pregnant women against a control group without the procedure to estimate its cost effectiveness in averting possible maternal and neonatal deaths.

Conclusion

Very few pregnant women in the rural areas of low to low-middle income countries actually have any information about the location of their placentas and the conditions of their fetuses in the prenatal period. Absence of information lowers the chance of pregnant women avoiding catastrophic events during their labor and delivery. General practitioners, nurses and midwives were highly trainable and reliable in performing ultrasound scanning for five obstetrical parameters namely, fetal number and viability, fetal presentations, amniotic fluid volume and placental localization. Identification of these conditions can possibly avert maternal deaths and neonatal deaths. Lastly, the Local Government Units and the CHWs are key players in improving pregnancy outcomes in the country.

Abbreviations

AFV: Amniotic fluid volume; CHT: Community Health Team; CHW: Community Health Worker; GE: General Electric; HU: Handheld Ultrasound; LGU: Local Government Unit; MMR: Maternal Mortality Rate/Ratio; OB: Obstetrician; TBA: Traditional Birth Attendant; TWG: Technical Working Group

Acknowledgements

Aside from the grant support given by Grand Challenges Canada, the authors would like to acknowledge the help provided by the following: GE Philippines Inc., the Department of Pharmacology and Toxicology University of the Philippines Manila, the Department and Institute of Clinical Epidemiology University of the Philippines Manila, Margarita Moran Floirendo, Municipal Health Officers, Technical Working Groups, and Mayors of Parañaque City and Tagum City, the iBuntis Research Team and Volunteers, and all the pregnant women participants.

Funding

This study was supported by a grant from Grand Challenges Canada (Cycle 6, Grant # 0547-01-10). The funding body, Grand Challenges Canada, had no role in the design of this study and did not have any role during its execution, analyses, interpretation of the data, or decision to submit results for publication.

Authors' contributions

GVD: study concept, training of technical working groups, data collection, data analysis, drafting of manuscript, manuscript revision, and approval of final version. RTR: study concept, training of technical working groups, data collection, approval of final version. AEH: study concept, training of technical working groups, and approval of final version. LMVC: study concept, data collection, and approval of final version. MJTJ: study concept, and approval of final version. MCC: study concept, training of technical working groups, data collection, and approval of final version. ATN: study concept, training of technical working groups, data collection, and approval of final version. ESB: study concept, data collection, data analysis, drafting of manuscript, manuscript revision, and approval of final version. All the authors approved the submission of the final paper.

Competing interests

The authors declare that they have no competing interests.

Author details

[1]Department of Pharmacology and Toxicology, College of Medicine, University of the Philippines-Manila, Manila, Philippines. [2]Department of Clinical Epidemiology, College of Medicine, University of the Philippines-Manila, Manila, Philippines. [3]Institute of Clinical Epidemiology, National Institutes of Health, University of the Philippines- Manila, Manila, Philippines. [4]Department of Obstetrics and Gynecology, Makati Medical Center, Makati, Philippines. [5]Department of Obstetrics and Gynecology, College of Medicine, University of the Philippines- Manila, Manila, Philippines. [6]Department of Obstetrics and Gynecology, Manila Doctors Hospital, Manila, Philippines. [7]Department of Obstetrics and Gynecology, College of Medicine, Manila Central University FDT Medical Foundation, Caloocan, Philippines.

References

1. Maternal and newborn health country profiles: Philippines. UNICEF. https://www.unicef.org/philippines/MNH_Philippines_Country_Profile.pdf.
2. Philippines Maternal Mortality Rate. 2015. https://www.indexmundi.com/philippines/maternal_mortality_rate.html.
3. Filippi V, Chou Ronsmans C, et.al, Level and causes of maternal mortality and morbidity.In: Black RE,Laxminarayan R, Temmerman M. et al.,editors. Reproductive, maternal, newborn and child health: diseases control priorities, Third Edition (Volume 2). Washington (DC): The International Bank for Reconstruction and Development/The World Bank; 2016 Apr 5. Chapter 3. Available from https://www.ncbi,nih.gov/books/NBK361917/. doi:https://doi.org/10.1596/978-1-4648-0348-2_ch3.
4. Vintzileos AM, Ananth CV, Smulian JC. Using ultrasound in the clinical management of placental implantation abnormalities. Am J Obstet Gynecol. 2015;213(4 Suppl):S70–7. https://doi.org/10.1016/ajog.2015.05.059.
5. World Data Atlas. Philippines neonatal mortality rate (deaths per/1000 livebirths). Retrieved January 15, 2018. https://knoema.com/atlas/Philippines/Neonatal-mortality-rate?compareTo=ID.
6. Mortality rate, neonatal (per 1,000 live births). The World Bank. https://data.worldbank.org/indicator/SH.DYN.NMRT.
7. Vahanian SA. Vintzelios. Placental implantation abnormaties: a modern approach. Curr Opin Obstet Gynecol. 2016;28(6):477–84. https://doi.org/10.1097/GCO.0000000000000319.
8. Stanton K,Mwanri L."Global maternal and child health outcomes: the role of obstetric Ultrasosund in low resource settings." world J Prev Med2013, 1(3): 22-29.
9. Wiafe YA, Odoi AT, Dassah ET. The role of obstetric ultrasound in reducing maternal and perinatal mortality, Ultrasound Imaging - Medical Applications, Minin IV and Minin OV (Ed.), ISBN: 978-953-307-279-1, INTECH, https://doi.org/10.5772/22847. https://www.intechopen.com/books/ultrasound-imaging-medical-applications/the-role-of-obstetric-ultrasound-in-reducing-maternal-and-perinatal-mortality.
10. Bussman H, Koen E, Arhin- Tenkorang D, Munyadzwe G, Troeger J. Feasibility of an ultrasound service on district health care level in Botswana. Tropical Med Int Health. 2001;6(12):1023–31.
11. Oyelese Y. Placenta previa: the evolving role of ultrasound. Ultrasound Obstet Gynecol. 2009;34:123–6. https://doi.org/10.1002/uog.7312.
12. Harris RD, Marks WM. Compact ultrasound for improving maternal and perinatal care in low-resource. J Ultrasound Med. 2009;28(8):1067–76.
13. SOGC clinical practice guideline: diagnosis and Management of Placenta Previa no. 189 (2007). Principal Author; lawrence Oppenheimer.Maternal Fetal medicine Committee. http://sogc.org/wp-content/uploads/2013/01/189E-CPG-March2007.pdf
14. Reddy U, Filly R, Copel J. Prenatal imaging: ultrasound and Magntic resonance imaging. Obstet Gynecol. 2008;112(1):145–57. PMCID: PMC2788813
15. Philippine Statistics Authority. Philippine Live Births: 2015 retrieved Dec 27,2017. https://psa.gov.ph/content/philippine-live-births-2015.
16. Brunette W., Hicks M., Hope A., Ruddy G., Anderson R., Kolko B. Reducing maternal mortality: an ultrasound system for village midwives. http://ieeexplore.ieee.org/xpl/login.jsp?tp=&arnumber=6103613&url=http%3A%2F%2Fieee
17. Padilla CD, Paz C-d, Cavan B, Abarquez C, Sur A, Sales R, Posecion W, Orbillo L, Basilio J. Establishment of the Philippines birth defect surveillance. Acta Medica Philippina. 2011;40(4):12–9.

7

Quality medicines in maternal health: results of oxytocin, misoprostol, magnesium sulfate and calcium gluconate quality audits

Chimezie Anyakora[1*], Yetunde Oni[2], Uchenna Ezedinachi[1], Adebola Adekoya[1], Ibrahim Ali[2], Charles Nwachukwu[2], Charles Esimone[3], Victor Abiola[2] and Jude Nwokike[1]

Abstract

Background: The high level of maternal mortality and morbidity as a result of complications due to childbirth is unacceptable. The impact of quality medicines in the management of these complications cannot be overemphasized. Most of those medicines are sensitive to environmental conditions and must be handled properly. In this study, the quality of oxytocin injection, misoprostol tablets, magnesium sulfate, and calcium gluconate injections was assessed across the six geopolitical zones of Nigeria.

Method: Simple, stratified random sampling of health facilities in each of the political zones of Nigeria. Analysis for identification and content of active pharmaceutical ingredient was performed using high-performance liquid chromatography procedures of 159 samples of oxytocin injection and 166 samples of misoprostol tablets. Titrimetric methods were used to analyze 164 samples of magnesium sulfate and 148 samples of calcium gluconate injection. Other tests included sterility, pH measurement, and fill volume.

Results: Samples of these commodities were procured mainly from wholesale and retail pharmacies, where these were readily available, while the federal medical centers reported low availability. Approximately, 74.2% of oxytocin injection samples failed the assay test, with the northeast and southeast zones registering the highest failure rates. Misoprostol tablets recorded a percentage failure of 33.7%. Magnesium sulfate and Calcium gluconate injection samples recorded a failure rate of 6.8% and 2.4%, respectively.

Conclusion: The prevalence of particularly of oxytocin and misoprostol commodities was of substandard quality. Strengthening the supply chain of these important medicines is paramount to ensuring their effectiveness in reducing maternal deaths in Nigeria.

Background

Complications due to pregnancy are among the leading causes of maternal deaths worldwide. According to a World Health Organization (WHO) 2015 report, approximately 830 women die every day from preventable causes related to pregnancy and childbirth and 99% of these deaths occur in low-resource countries [1]. The global distribution of maternal deaths is influenced by two regions, sub-Saharan Africa and southern Asia, which account for the majority of all maternal deaths [2]. In 2015, two countries, Nigeria and India, accounted for more than one-third of all global maternal deaths, with approximately 58,000 maternal deaths (19%) in Nigeria and 45,000 maternal deaths (15%) in India [3]. Ten countries accounted for nearly 59% of global maternal deaths: in addition to Nigeria and India, they are the Democratic Republic of Congo (22,000), Ethiopia (11,000), Pakistan (9700), Tanzania (8200), Kenya (8000), Indonesia (6400), Uganda (5700), and Bangladesh (5500).

A high percentage of women in these regions deliver at home or outside a health facility without access to

* Correspondence: CZA@usp.org
[1]Promoting the Quality of Medicines Program, USP, Rockville, MD, USA
Full list of author information is available at the end of the article

obstetric care or a skilled birth attendant. This makes them more vulnerable to complications related to childbirth [4]. Therefore, there is increased interest in finding alternative ways to make low-cost treatments available to improve women's health in these low-resource countries.

Say et al. reported that, between 2003 and 2009, direct causes were responsible for nearly 72.5% of maternal deaths while indirect causes were responsible for 27.5% of maternal deaths [5]. Postpartum hemorrhage (PPH) is a leading cause of maternal morbidity and mortality [6–8] and accounted for 27.1% of maternal mortality. PPH may be defined as a vaginal loss of blood ≥500 mL immediately after labor or within 24 h after birth [6, 9]. It is usually caused by excessive bleeding due to lack of efficient uterine contraction (uterine atony), vaginal or cervical tears, or tears of the genital system [10–12]. Anemia during pregnancy has been associated with PPH [13, 14]. WHO recognizes injectable oxytocin as the safest and most effective medicine central to the prevention and treatment of PPH [15, 16]. It is currently on the WHO Essential Medicines List [17] and the United Nations Commission on Life-Saving Commodities list of 13 critical commodities [18]. Oxytocin is widely available in low income countries and is fairly inexpensive. Yet challenges in health sector infrastructure and health service delivery can create barriers to oxytocin use [19]. Most countries require that oxytocin injection be administered by trained health care workers, so women delivering at home or with a traditional birth attendant may not have access to oxytocin [16].

In 2013, the Promoting the Quality of Medicines (PQM) program—funded by the U.S. Agency for International Development (USAID) and implemented by United States Pharmacopeia (USP)—conducted a study in Ghana in collaboration with the Ghanaian Food and Drug Authority. The research team found that 55.6% of the 169 oxytocin samples analyzed were found to contain less active pharmaceutical ingredient than label claim. In addition, 39 of 40 samples (97.5%) that were tested also failed the test for sterility [20]. In 2014, an unpublished study carried out in ten regional zones in Ghana showed similar results. In 2016, Torloni et al. conducted a systematic review on the quality of oxytocin in low- and middle-income countries (LMICs), synthesizing studies that contained results of quality tests of 559 samples of oxytocin [21]. The most common reason for failure was an insufficient amount of active pharmaceutical ingredient (API). The 2015 WHO survey of the quality of medicines identified by the United Nations Commission showed a 64.0% failure of oxytocin samples when tested against pharmacopeial specifications, including appearance, identification, assay, related substances, pH measurement, and extractable volume [22].

Besides the challenges with the quality of oxytocin, other factors that hinder the use of oxytocin in low-resource regions include the need for refrigeration, intravenous and intramuscular injection, and lack of trained providers for administration. Oxytocin can be viewed as a tracer medicine for gauging the performance of regulatory systems in LMICs for several reasons, and marketing approval from the local authority provides insight into premarketing and inspection capacity. Oxytocin is time and temperature sensitive; exposure to high temperatures degrades the product. If countries have reliable post-marketing surveillance (PMS) systems, good distribution and storage practices, they can ensure the integrity of the product throughout the supply chain.

Prevention and treatment of PPH in low-resource settings by conventional uterotonics has been challenging, as the desired impact is not being achieved [23–25]. Prostaglandins have been considered an alternative. Misoprostol is a heat-stable prostaglandin E1 analogue used in the prevention and treatment of peptic ulcer disease caused by prostaglandin-synthetase inhibitors. It has been shown to be a potent uterotonic [25] with the ability to increase uterine tone and decrease postpartum bleeding [26]. Misoprostol has been studied as an alternative to oxytocin due to its low cost, stability at room temperature, wide availability, and ease of administration. It can be administered sublingually, orally, vaginally, and rectally [27–29].

The second most common cause of maternal mortality, preeclampsia/eclampsia (PE/E) is a hypertensive, multisystem disorder of pregnancy with no known underlying cause and is usually associated with raised blood pressure and proteinuria [30–32]. In 1992, a global estimate of 50,000 maternal deaths were attributed to eclampsia [33]. In Nigeria, eclampsia is a major cause of obstetric complications, [34, 35] reported to have contributed to 46.3% and 43% of maternal deaths in Kano State [36] and Jigawa State [37], respectively.

Although delivery remains the ultimate treatment for preeclampsia, [38, 39] magnesium sulfate is the drug of choice for preventing eclamptic seizures and also has the additional benefit of reducing the incidence of placental abruption [40, 41]. Occasionally, the administration of magnesium sulfate results in an accidental overdose leading to respiratory paralysis, central nervous system depression and cardiac arrest. Intravenous calcium gluconate, an antidote that quickly reverses the effects of magnesium toxicity, may be required when moderate to severe toxicity occurs [42–44].

With a population greater than 170 million people, Nigeria is a very attractive market for pharmaceuticals and other regulated products. Over 60% of medicines are imported into the country, due to the gap created by inadequate in-country production of essential medicines. With a maternal mortality ratio of 814 per 100,000 live births, it is obvious that Nigeria has a weak health care delivery system, particularly in the area of maternal health. This is exacerbated by the availability of poor-quality medicines, due to either inadequate storage and distribution or poor manufacturing practices. Hence, constant monitoring of the quality of medicines in circulation is a public health necessity. As is the case with most LMICs, quality remains an issue, and the impact of poor-quality medicines cannot be overemphasized. In the case of the uterotonics and drugs for preeclampsia, the implication for poor-quality treatment can prove dire. In this study, quality levels of four maternal commodities in the six geopolitical zones of Nigeria were assessed.

Methods

Sampling

To determine sample size, the following criteria were taken into account: population size; confidence level with an assumption of a normal 95% distribution of sample values; and degree of variability in the quality of oxytocin, magnesium sulfate, calcium gluconate injections, and misoprostol tablets distributed across the study sites.

The following factors were carefully considered in drafting the sampling plan:

- Availability of oxytocin, magnesium sulfate, calcium gluconate injections, and misoprostol at the federal medical centers (FMC), state hospitals (SH), primary health care centers (PHCC), and midwife clinic (MWC) levels
- Budgetary and time constraints
- Geographical access
- The laboratory's standard operating procedures for testing to ensure adequate samples for triplicate testing and handling of out-of-specification occurrences

Table 1 describes distribution of the samples across the different levels of sampling sites. These included FMCs, SHs, PHCCs, MWCs, wholesale pharmacies, retail pharmacies, and patent and proprietary medicine vendors (PPMVs). A total of 234 samples per commodity were determined as an adequate sample size that would represent the true situation in this study. Even though the PPMVs are not permitted to stock these prescription-only commodities, sampling was conducted due to previous records of illegal stocking of ethical pharmaceutical products.

Sampling was carried out in six regions across the country during the period May 23–28, 2016: Abia State for the southeast, Edo State for the south-south, Ogun

Table 1 Sample Distribution

Level of Sampling	No. of Outlets	No. of Samples from Each Outlet	Quantity of Commodity per Sample
Level 1: Patent Medicine Stores	5 patent stores	1 sample of different brands or lots from EACH outlet	Sample A: 10 ampoules each of oxytocin, calcium gluconate, and magnesium sulfate + 20 tablets of misoprostol
Level 2: Wholesale and Retail Pharmacy Stores	4 pharmacies	2 samples of different brands or lots from EACH outlet	Sample A: 30 ampoules each of oxytocin, calcium gluconate and magnesium sulfate + 60 tablets of misoprostol
			Sample B: 30 ampoules each of oxytocin, calcium gluconate and magnesium sulfate + 60 tablets of misoprostol
Level 3: Midwife Clinics	5 MWCs	2 samples of different brands or lots from EACH outlet	Sample A: 10 ampoules each of oxytocin, calcium gluconate and magnesium sulfate + 20 tablets of misoprostol
			Sample B: 10 ampoules each of oxytocin, calcium gluconate and magnesium sulfate + 20 tablets of misoprostol
Level 4: Primary Health Care Centers	5 PHCCs	2 samples of different brands or lots from EACH outlet	Sample A: 10 ampoules each of oxytocin, calcium gluconate and magnesium sulfate + 30 tablets of misoprostol
			Sample B: 10 ampoules each of oxytocin, calcium gluconate and magnesium sulfate + 30 tablets of misoprostol
Level 5: State Hospital Stores	1 SH	4 samples of different brands or lots	Sample A: 15 ampoules each of oxytocin, calcium gluconate and magnesium sulfate + 30 tablets of misoprostol
			Sample B: 15 ampoules each of oxytocin, calcium gluconate and magnesium sulfate + 30 tablets of misoprostol
			Sample C: 15 ampoules each of oxytocin, calcium gluconate and magnesium sulfate + 30 tablets of misoprostol
			Sample D: 15 ampoules each of oxytocin, calcium gluconate and magnesium sulfate + 30 tablets of misoprostol
Level 6: FMC Warehouse	1 FMC	2 samples of different brands or lots	Sample A: 15 ampoules each of oxytocin, calcium gluconate and magnesium sulfate + 30 tablets of misoprostol
			Sample B: 15 ampoules each of oxytocin, calcium gluconate and magnesium sulfate + 30 tablets of misoprostol

Table 2 Gradient Elution for Oxytocin

Time (min)	Mobile phase A (% *v/v*)	Mobile phase B (% v/v)	Comments
0–5	100	0	Isocratic
5–20	70	30	Linear gradient
20–50	30	70	Linear gradient
50–51	60	40	Return to initial composition
51–65	100	0	Re-equilibration

State for the southwest, Kwara State for the north-central, Kaduna State for the northwest, and Bauchi State for the northeast.

At the point of sampling, samples were maintained at the stated manufacturers' storage conditions while Oxytocin samples were stored in a cold box to ensure the 2 °C–8 °C storage temperature rule was preserved. The temperature of the cold box was constantly monitored and documented until arrival of the products in the laboratory.

Identification and quantification

Packages of the sampled products were first inspected for correct labelling and packaging according to the requirements of the regulatory authority. These requirements include name of drug product, list of active ingredient, batch number, National Agency for Food and Drug Administration and Control (NAFDAC) number, expiry date, storage conditions, indication for use, name and address of manufacturer, and visibility of particulate matter in injectable.

Content analysis

Analysis of the API was conducted using the respective compendia methods (USP 39) for oxytocin and USP Pharmacopeial Forum Vol. 26 (5) [Sept–Oct 2000] for misoprostol tablets. Titrimetric method was used for magnesium sulfate and calcium gluconate, as recommended in the current official monographs (BP 2016 and USP 39). Other tests that were carried out to ascertain the quality of these samples included sterility, identification, pH measurement, and fill volume.

High-performance liquid chromatography (HPLC) analyses were conducted on Dionex Ultimate 3000 system and Hitachi Lachrom with Chromeleon and EZChrom software, respectively. Dionex Ultimate 3000 was employed for the analysis of misoprostol, while Hitach Lachrom was employed for oxytocin analysis. The HPLC systems consisted of a quaternary analytical pump, autosampler, and ultraviolet (UV) detector. For misoprostol, the column used was an Ascentis C8 (150 mm × 4.6 mm i.d.; 3 μm particle size); UV detection was performed at 200 nm, while the injection volume was maintained at 100 μL. An online isocratic mobile phase containing a filtered and degassed mixture of methanol, water, and acetonitrile (40:35:25) was employed at a flow rate of 1.5 mL/min and run time of 15 min. The peak responses of the standard and sample solution chromatographs were recorded at a retention time of about 5.50 min.

In the analysis of oxytocin, the column used was C18 (120 mm × 4.6 mm i.d. with a 5 μm particle size). UV detection was performed at 220 nm, and the injection volume was maintained at 100 μL. The system was equilibrated with ratio 7:3 gradient mixtures of mobile phase A (0.1 M monobasic sodium phosphate) and mobile phase B (acetonitrile and water in ratio 1:1) (Table 2). A flow rate of 1.5 mL/min was employed, with a run time of approximately 10 min for oxytocin.

Results

Samples collected consisted of four commodities from six levels of health facilities (Table 3). The expected number of samples as derived from the sample size calculation could not be achieved because the

Table 3 Total Number of Products Sampled from the Health Facilities

Facility	Oxytocin	Misoprostol	Magnesium Sulfate	Calcium Gluconate	Total
Pharmacy	73	79	65	68	285
MWC	46	39	37	28	150
PHCC	37	31	32	31	131
Patent Medicine Store	26	32	22	14	94
SH Store	16	13	16	9	54
FMC	12	8	11	11	42
Total	210	202	183	161	756

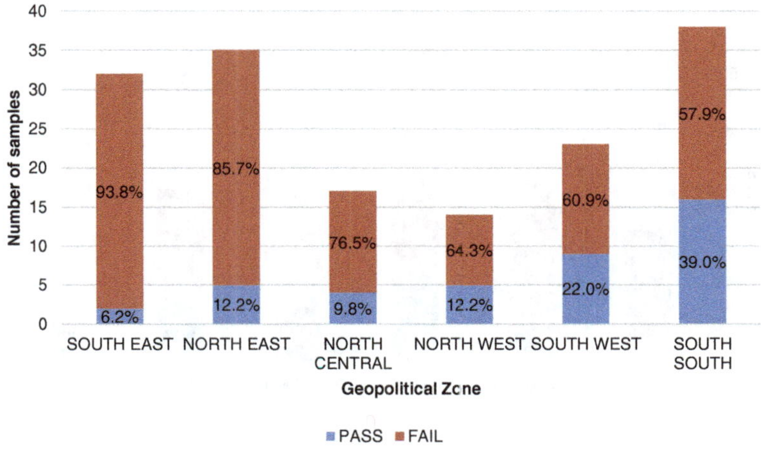

Fig. 1 Percentage Failure of Oxytocin Samples by Geopolitical Zone

availability of these products in most of the public health facilities was limited.

In addition, due to damaged samples and incomplete packaging information, the number of analyzed products for each commodity varies with the number of sampled products. It is worthy to note that owing to the relative difference in the number of samples obtained from the different regions, reported failure rates must be interpreted independently. Analysis of the sample data was performed using the R Language and Environment for Statistical Computing.

Oxytocin

A total of 159 samples of oxytocin were analyzed and subjected to registration verification. It was observed that all the samples were registered with the national medicines regulatory authority. Labelling information regarding dosage form, brand name, active ingredient, and batch number were provided. Expiry dates of the samples were recorded and found to be within a year at the time of sampling. Although all samples passed visual inspection and complied with the specification from monographs for other parameters tested, the percentage composition of the active ingredient varied between 0.0% and 163.7%. HPLC assay results showed that 74.2% (118/159) did not meet the specification for assay (between 90.0% and 110.0%) as indicated in monograph USP 39. Figure 1 gives a summary of these results categorized by regions of collection.

According to the package labels, the majority of samples were imported, with 60.4% manufactured in China, 12.6% in India, 15.1% in Germany, and none in Nigeria. Figure 2 shows the percentage of samples from different countries and their failure rates.

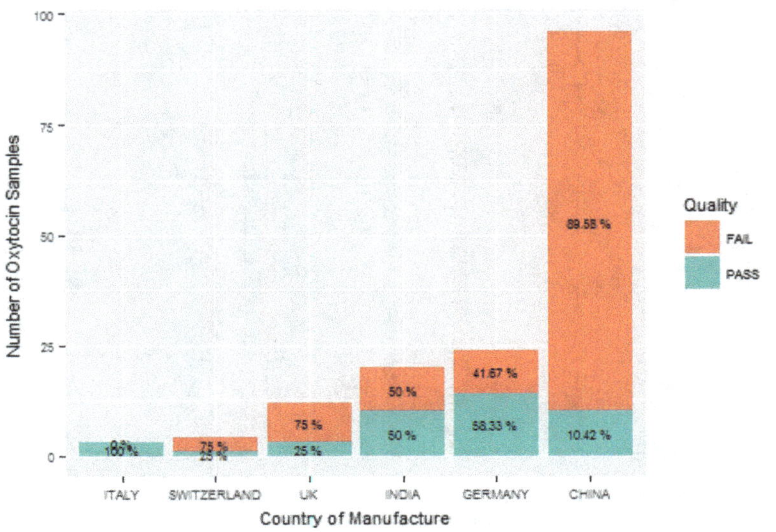

Fig. 2 Quality of Oxytocin by Country of Manufacture

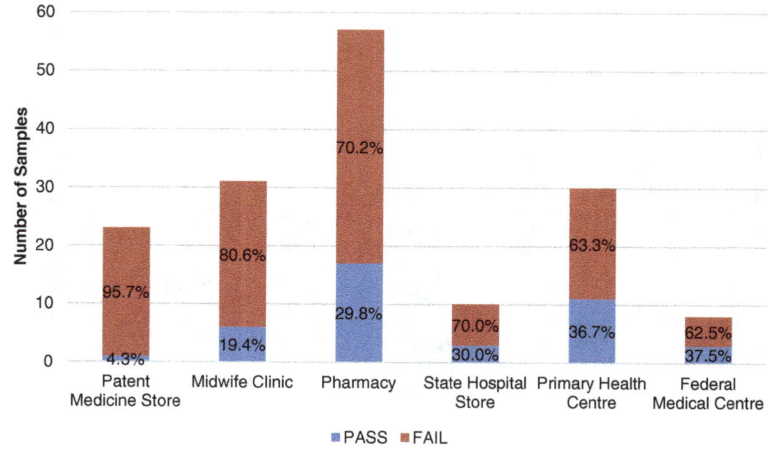

Fig. 3 Percentage Failure of Oxytocin per Level of Health Facility

In this study, samples from the patent medicine store were shown to have the highest percentage of failed oxytocin, with a 95.7% (22/23) fail, followed closely by the midwife clinic at 80.6% (25/31), as shown in Fig. 3.

Due to the effect of higher temperatures on oxytocin injection, storage conditions at the site of sampling were recorded. As shown in the boxplot in Fig. 4, storage temperature ranges for oxytocin samples were observed to be higher in the northern regions, with over 50% of outlets in each collection site of the region recording highs of 30 °C–33 °C and lows of 8 °C–11 °C. Higher storage temperatures ranges were observed in samples from private health facilities compared to those from the public sector in all regions of the geopolitical zones. Although high temperatures were also observed for samples that passed the assay, this was only a small subsection of the samples. Recommended storage temperature range of 2 °C–8 °C was observed in a number of facilities in the southern regions, where a greater number of samples passed the assay test.

Misoprostol

A total of 166 samples of misoprostol were subjected to registration verification. It was observed that all samples were registered with the national medicines regulatory authority. Labelling information regarding dosage form, brand name, active ingredient, and batch number were provided. Expiry dates of the samples were recorded and found to be within a year at the

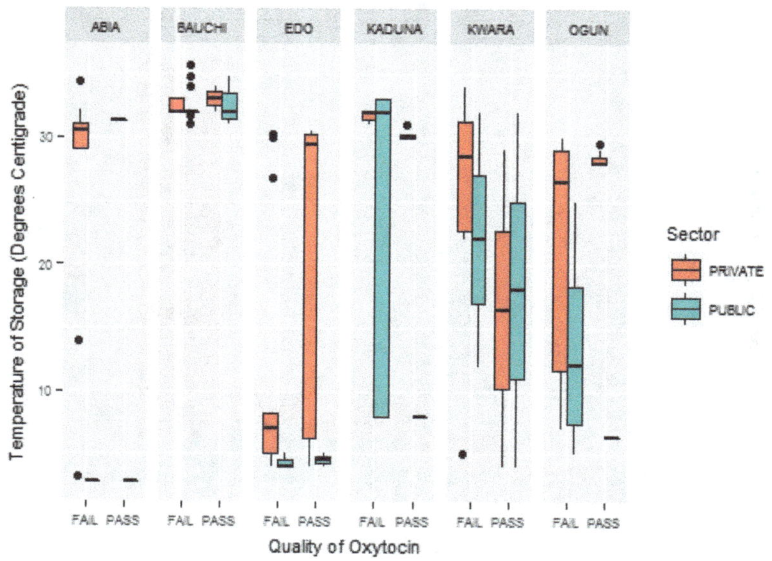

Fig. 4 Storage Conditions of Oxytocin and Quality Effect from Each Geopolitical Zone

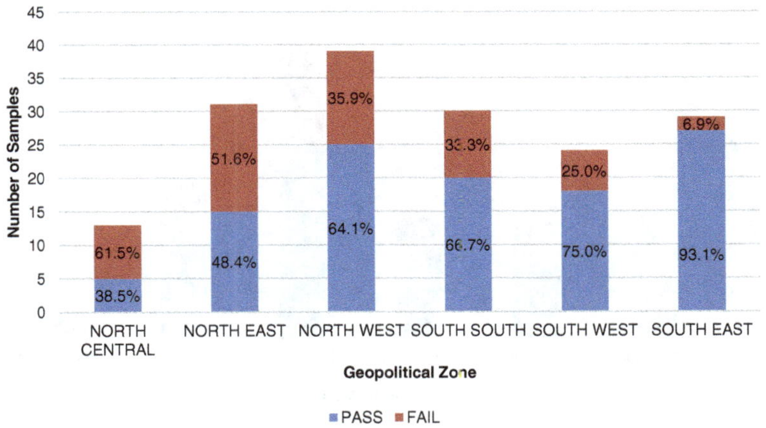

Fig. 5 Percentage Failure of Misoprostol by Geopolitical Zone

time of sampling. Although all samples passed visual inspection, the percentage composition of the active ingredient varied grossly. HPLC assay results showed that 33.7% (56/166) did not meet the monograph specification for assay content (between 90.0% and 110.0%). Figure 5 gives a summary of these results categorized by regions of collection.

According to the package labels, the majority of the samples were imported, with 62.7% manufactured in India, 25.3% in the United Kingdom, 7.8% in Korea, and 4.2% in Nigeria. Figure 6 shows the percentage of samples from different countries and their failure rates.

In this study, samples from the state hospital store were shown to have the highest percentage of failed misoprostol tablets, with a 50.0% (5/10) fail, followed closely by PHCCs with a fail of 42.9% (12/28). The midwife clinics and patent medicine stores recorded a percentage failure of 37.0% (10/27) and 21.2% (7/33), respectively, while the retail and wholesale pharmacy observed a 34.9% (22/63) fail. No failure was recorded from the samples obtained from the FMCs, as shown in Fig. 7.

Storage conditions have been shown to play a major role in the quality of misoprostol tablets, with absorption of moisture being the foremost concern. Minimum storage temperature of the products was found in the south-south and southeast regions, at 20.5 °C and 26.0 °C as illustrated in Fig. 8. The boxplots show that storage temperatures of samples procured from the northern region of Kaduna and Kwara were above 30 °C. Although 60% of the samples were sampled from the private sector, there was no distinction between the storage temperatures of the samples from the public and the private sectors.

The quality of misoprostol tablets varied by geopolitical zone, with the northern part recording the highest prevalence of poor-quality misoprostol. However, the southern zones did not perform considerably better, with

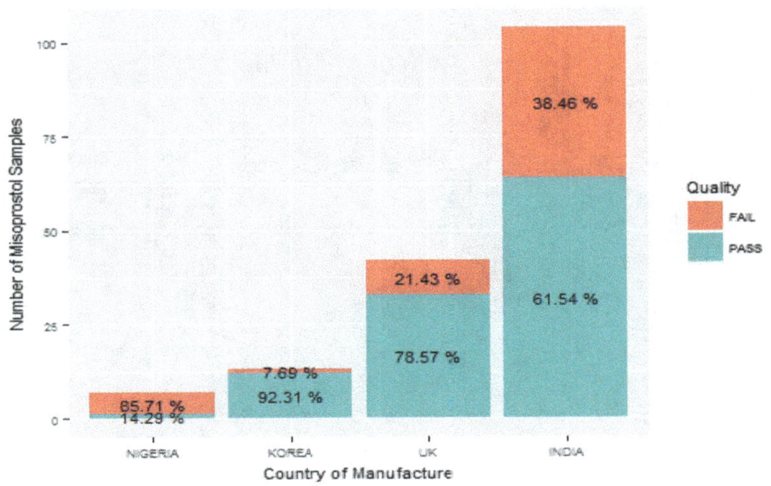

Fig. 6 Percentage Failure of Misoprostol by Country of Manufacture

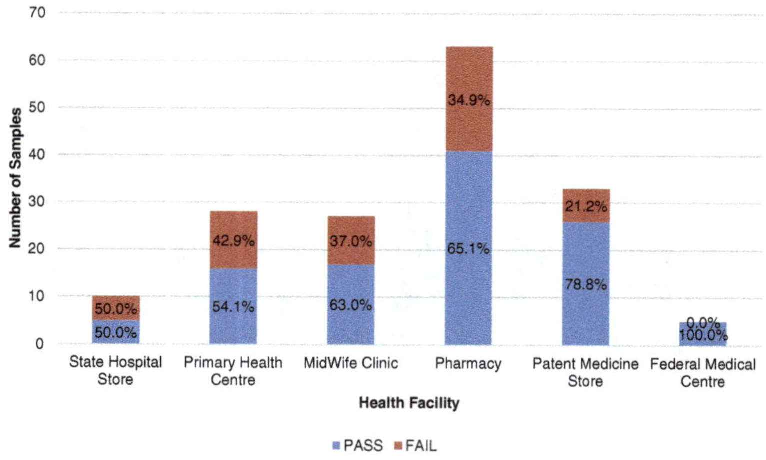

Fig. 7 Percentage Failure of Misoprostol Tablets per Level of Health Facility

percentage failures of 33.3% and 25.0% for the south-south and southwest zones, respectively.

Magnesium sulfate

A total of 163 samples were subjected to registration, verification and analyzed for the presence of API and sterility. A total of 160 magnesium sulfate samples were shown to have passed the test, while four samples failed to meet the monograph specification range of 93.0% and 107.0% of the labelled amount of magnesium sulfate. Figure 9 gives the distribution of these samples across different geopolitical zones.

Calcium gluconate

A total of 148 samples were analyzed for the presence of API and sterility, and 138 samples of calcium gluconate were shown to have passed the test, while 10 samples failed to meet the monograph specification range of 95.0% and 105.0% of the labelled amount of calcium gluconate. Figs. 10 and 11 give the distribution of these samples across different levels of facilities and in different geopolitical zones, respectively.

Discussion

Injectable oxytocin and misoprostol tablets recorded percentage failures of 74.2% and 33.7%, respectively. In contrast, magnesium sulfate and calcium gluconate injections were both found to be of rather good quality, with 2.4% and 6.8% failure rates, respectively.

The high failure rate of first-line PPH treatment portends a serious health implication and may be a contributing factor in the high maternal mortality ratio in Nigeria.

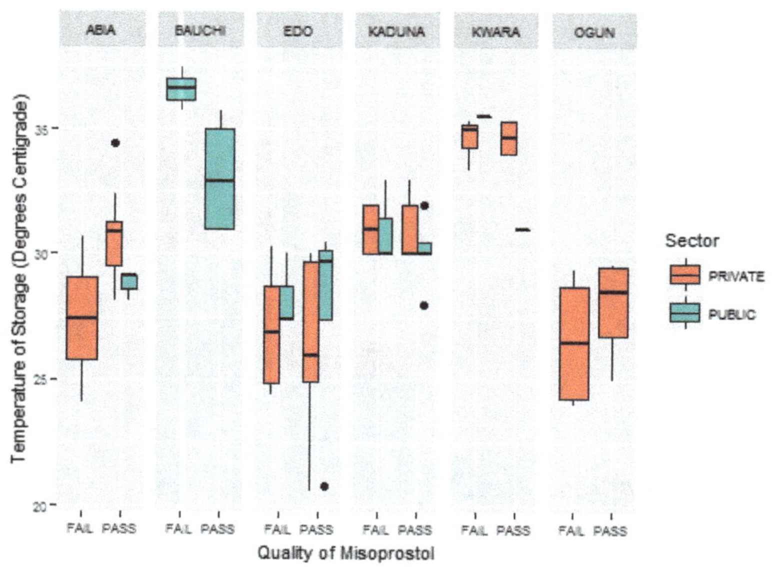

Fig. 8 Storage Conditions of Misoprostol Tablets and Quality Effect from Each State

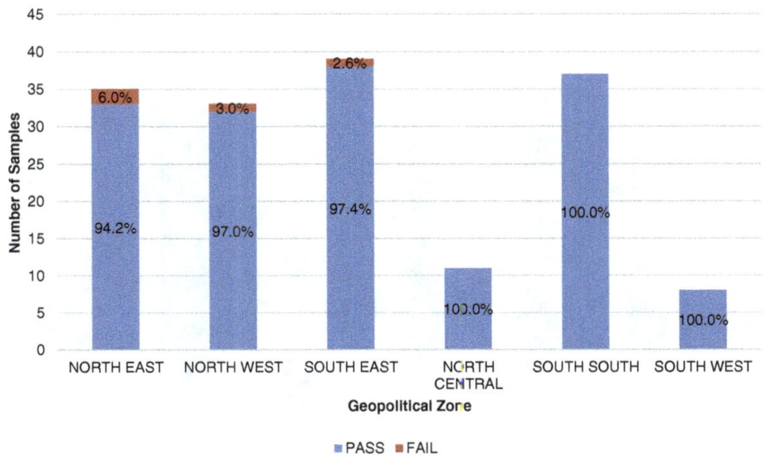

Fig. 9 Percentage Failure of Magnesium Sulfate by Geopolitical Zone

The southeastern and northeastern part of the country recorded the highest failure rate of 25%, while lower failure rates were observed in the south-south and southwest regions. WHO recommends that oxytocin be refrigerated or stored at a temperature of 2 °C–8 °C but low-resourced countries may lack facilities required for proper storage of these products, so storage conditions were equally assessed in the health facilities where sampling was carried out. This result is logical as can be seen from Fig. 4 where the average storage temperature of Oxytocin in the southeastern and northeastern part of Nigeria were above 30 °C unlike the situation in the other regions of the country. Likely causes of this troubling failure rate could be degradation as a result of improper storage as well as poor manufacturing practices.

Misoprostol was observed to have high failure rates in the northeast and south-south regions of the country. Storage conditions of misoprostol tablets though not as critical as the conditions of Oxytocin, is affected by temperature and humidity and is recommended to be stored at a temperature range of 25 °C–30 °C. This recommended temperature was observed in about 50% of the sites, while the others recorded storage temperatures above 30 °C. Furthermore, one of the sampled products was observed to be falsified, as no active ingredient was found.

The northern region of the country reported most of the failure rates of magnesium sulfate, while calcium gluconate injections sampled in the northwest and southeast regions showed relatively poorer quality products. In comparing failure rates across geographic zones and across levels in the supply chain, it is instructive to know that sample sizes were not the same in the various geographic zones and levels;

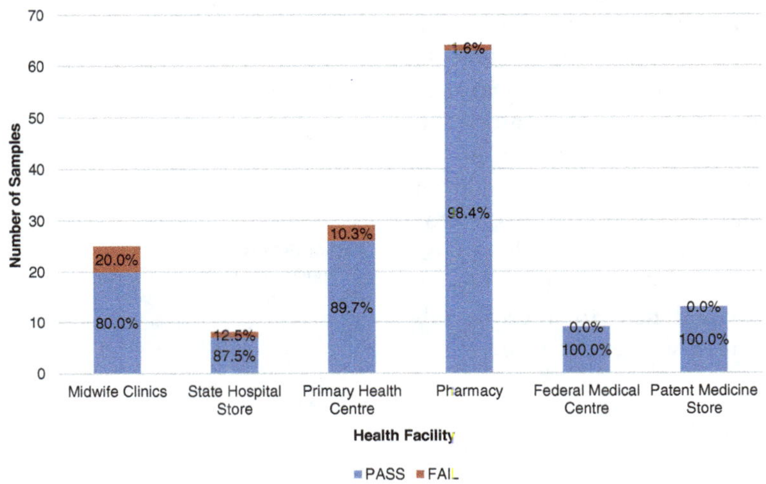

Fig. 10 Percentage Failure of Calcium Gluconate by Facility

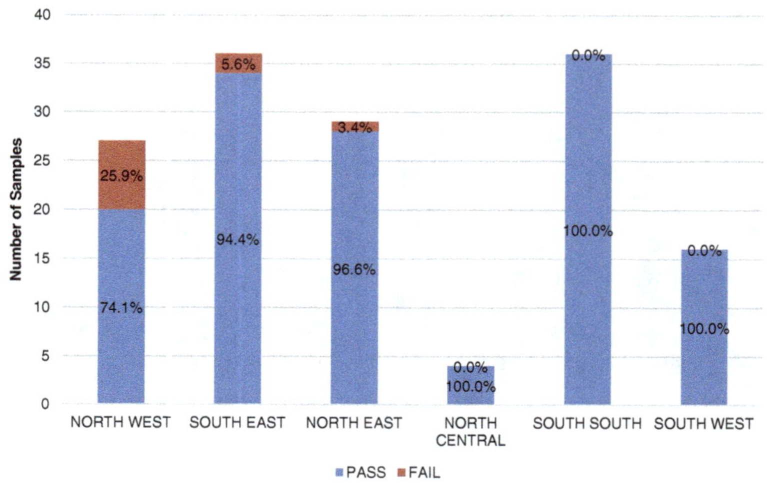

Fig. 11 Percentage Failure of Calcium Gluconate by Geopolitical Zone

therefore, differences in failure rates should be interpreted with caution. As a result, absolute failure rates are more interpretive than relative failure rates.

Limitations

A baseline study of the quality of the studied commodities was not established prior to the study. The prevalence of poor-quality medicines may also have been attributed to the initial quality, but this issue was not addressed by our study. In addition, while post-partum hemorrhage is a major cause of maternal deaths, there are no reliable data correlating the prevalence of maternal deaths in Nigeria with the quality of the medicines used in the treatment of post-partum hemorrhage.

Conclusion

The level of substandard oxytocin injections and misoprostol tablets was significantly high. The storage conditions could be a possible source of this level of failure as both oxytocin injections and misoprostol tablets degrade rapidly if poorly stored. Stronger regulatory action by the Medicines Regulatory Authority (MRA), engagement and education of all key players in the pharmaceutical supply chain could ensure they have a more full understanding of the storage conditions of these commodities. Also, more frequent post-marketing surveillance of these maternal health commodities could help to improve substandard medication given to women in need.

Abbreviations

API: Active pharmaceutical ingredient; FMC: Federal medical center; HPLC: High-performance liquid chromatography; LMIC: Low- and middle-income country; MCH: Maternal and child health; MWC: Midwife clinic; NAFDAC: National Agency for Food and Drug Administration and Control; PE/E: Preeclampsia/eclampsia; PHCC: Primary health care center; PMS: Post-marketing surveillance; PPH: Postpartum haemorrhage; SH: State hospital; UV: Ultraviolet; WHO: World Health Organization

Acknowledgements

The authors are grateful to the team of NAFDAC staff who participated in sampling and testing during this study.

Funding

This study was funded by the U.S. Agency for International Development (USAID) Mission in Nigeria through the PQM program of USP.

Authors' contributions

CA, JN, IA, CN. AA CE and YO designed the study. CA, IA, AA, UE, CN and VA executed the study, including coordinating the sampling and testing. UE, AA and CA wrote the first draft of the manuscript. All authors corrected the draft and approved the final version of the manuscript.

Authors' information

C. Anyakora is the Chief of Party in Nigeria for the USP PQM program. A. Adekoya and U. Ezedinachi are USP PQM staff in Lagos, Nigeria. Y. Oni is the acting Director General of NAFDAC. I. Ali, C. Nwachukwu, and V. Abiola are staff of NAFDAC. C. Esimone is a staff of the Faculty of Pharmacy, Nnamdi Azikiwe University. J. Nwokike is the Director of the USP PQM program.

Competing interests

There is no competing interest. C. Anyakora, U. Ezedinachi, A. Adekoya, and J. Nwokike are USP employees working on the Promoting the Quality of Medicines (PQM) program. Y. Oni, I. Ali, C. Nwachukwu, and V. Abiola are NAFDAC employees.

Author details

[1]Promoting the Quality of Medicines Program, USP, Rockville, MD, USA. [2]National Agency for Food and Drug Administration and Control, Abuja, Nigeria. [3]Faculty of Pharmacy, Nnamdi Azikiwe University, Awka, Nigeria.

References

1. WHO. Maternal mortality. Fact sheet No. 348 http://www.who.int/mediacentre/factsheets/fs348/en/. Updated November 2015.
2. WHO (World Health Organization). b. Trends in Maternal Mortality: 1990 to 2013, Estimates by WHO, UNICEF, UNFPA, the World Bank and the United Nations population division. Geneva: WHO; 2014.

3. Filippi V, Chou D, Ronsmans C, Graham W, Say L. Levels and Causes of Maternal Mortality and Morbidity. In: Black ER, Laxminarayan R, Temmerman M, Walker N, editors. Reproductive, Maternal, Newborn, and Child Health: Disease Control Priorities Third Edition, vol. 2. Washington DC: The International Bank for Reconstruction and Development/The World Bank; 2016. Chapter 3.
4. Hamid R. Misoprostol: an essential medicine for managing postpartum hemorrhage in low-resource settings? Int J Gynecol Obstet. 2011;114(3):209–10.
5. Say L, Chou D, Gemmill A, Tuncalpo O, Moller A-B, et al. Global causes of maternal death: a WHO systematic analysis. Lancet Glob Health. 2014;2(6):e323–33.
6. Kumar N. Postpartum Hemorrhage; a Major Killer of Woman: Review of Current Scenario. Obstet Gynecol Int J. 2016;4(4):00116.
7. Olowokere AE, Adekeye OA, et al. The prevalence, management and outcome of primary postpartum haemorrhage in selected health care facilities in Nigeria. International Journal of Nursing and Midwifery. 2013;5(3):28–34.
8. Ononge S, Mirembe F, Wandabwa J, Campbell OMR. Incidence and risk factors for postpartum hemorrhage in Uganda. Reprod Health. 2016;13:38.
9. Active Management of the Third Stage of Labour: Prevention and Treatment of Postpartum Hemorrhage. SOGC Clinical Practice Guideline, 2009. http://sogc.org/wp-content/uploads/2013/01/gui235CPG0910.pdf
10. Walraven G, Blum J, Dampha Y, Sowe M, Morison L, Winikoff B. Misoprostol in the management of the third stage of labour in the home delivery setting in rural Gambia; a randomised controlled trial. International Journal of Obstetrics and Gynaecology. 2005;112:1277–83.
11. Chandhiok N, Dhillon BS, Datey S, Mathur A, Saxena AC. Oral misoprostol for prevention of postpartum hemorrhage by paramedical workers in India. Int J Gynaecol Obstet. 2006;92:170–5.
12. Mousa HA, Blum J, Abou El Senoun G, Shakur H, Alfirevic Z. Treatment for primary postpartum haemorrhage. Cochrane Database of Systematic Reviews 2014, Issue 2.
13. Frass KA. Postpartum haemorrhage is related to the haemoglobin levels at labor: observational study. Alexandria Journal of Medicine. 2015;51(4):333–7.
14. Kavle JA, Stoltzfus RJ, Witter F, Tielsch JM, Khalfan SS, Caulfield LE. Association between Anaemia during pregnancy and blood loss at and after delivery among women with vaginal births in Pemba Island, Zanzibat, Tanzania. J Health Popul Nutr. 2008;26(2):232–40.
15. WHO. WHO recommendations for the prevention and treatment of postpartum haemorrhage. http://apps.who.int/iris/bitstream/10665/75411/1/9789241548502_eng.pdf
16. Jhpiego. 2014. Business case: investing in production of high-quality oxytocin for low-resource settings. Publication prepared by C. Schocken through the Reproductive Health Supplies Coalition. Available at http://reprolineplus.org/oxytocin-case. Accessed 3 Aug 2016.
17. WHO. WHO Model List of Essential Medicines, 16th List (Updated). Geneva: WHO; 2010. http://www.who.int/medicines/publications/essentialmedicines/en/index.html
18. United Nations. United Nations Commission on life-saving Commodities for Women and Children; Commissioner's report 2012. New York: United Nations; 2012.
19. Accelovate. Brief: how can we increase global utilization of oxytocin for treatment of postpartum hemorrhage? Baltimore: Jhpiego; 2015. Accessed at: www.jhpiego.org/accelovate
20. Karikari BE. Post-market quality surveillance project maternal health care products on the Ghanaian market. Ghana Food and Drugs Authority: Accra; 2013.
21. Torloni MR, Gomes FC, Kartoglu UH, Metin GA, Widmer M. Quality of oxytocin available in low- and middle-income countries: a systemic review of the literature. Br J Obstet Gynaecol. 2016;123(13):2076–86.
22. WHO. Survey of the quality of medicines identified by the United Nations Commission on Life-Saving Commodities for Women and Children, 2015. https://extranet.who.int/prequal/sites/default/files/documents/UNCoLSC_2015.pdf.
23. Hofmeyr GJ, Ferreira S, Nikodem VC, et al. Misoprostol for treating postpartum haemorrhage: a randomized controlled trial. BMC Pregnancy and Childbirth. 2004;4:16.
24. McCormick ML, Sanghvi HC, Kinzie B, McIntosh N. Preventing postpartum haemorrhage in low-resource settings. Int J Gynaecol Obstet. 2002;77:267–75.
25. Alfirevic A, Blum J, Walraven G, Weeks A, Winikoff B. Prevention of postpartum hemorrhage with misoprostol. Int J Gynecol Obstet. 2007; 99(Suppl 2):198–201.
26. Oladapo, Olufemi T. Misoprostol for preventing and treating postpartum hemorrhage in the community: A closer look at the evidence. International Journal of Gynecology and Obstetrics. 2012;119(2):105–11.
27. Caliskan E, Dilbaz B, Meydanli MM, Ozturk N, Narin MA, Haberal A. Oral Misoprostol for the third stage of labor: a randomized controlled trial. Obstet Gynecol. 2003;101(5 pt 1):921–8.
28. Norman JE, Thong KJ, Baird DT. Uterine contractility and induction of abortion in early pregnancy by misoprostol and mifepristone. Lancet. 1991;338:1233–6.
29. Hofmeyr GJ, Ferreira S, Nikodem VC, et al. Misoprostol for treating postpartum haemorrhage: a randomized controlled trial [ISRCTN72263357]. BMC Pregnancy and Childbirth. 2004;4:16.
30. Moodley J, Daya P. Eclampsia: a continuing problem in developing countries. Int J Gynecol Obstet. 1994;44(1):9–14.
31. Uzan J, Carbonnel M, Piconne O, Asmar R, Ayoubi J-M. Pre-eclampsia: pathophysiology, diagnosis, and management. Vasc Health Risk Manag. 2011;7:467–74.
32. American College of Obstetricians and Gynecologists. ACOG practice bulletin: Diagnosis and management of preeclampsia and eclampsia. Number 33, January 2002. Obstet Gynecol. 2002;99(1):159–67.
33. Duley L. Maternal mortality associated with hypertensive disorders of pregnancy in Africa, Asia, Latin America and the Caribbean. BJOG. 1992; 99(7):547–53. https://doi.org/10.1111/j.1471-0528.1992.tb13818.
34. Kullima A, Kawuwa MB, Audu B, Usman H, Geidam AD. A 5-year review of maternal mortality associated with eclampsia in a tertiary institution in northern Nigeria. Ann Afr Med. 2009;8(2):81–4. https://doi.org/10.4103/1596-3519.56233.
35. Oladapo OT, Lamina MA, Fakoya TA. Maternal deaths in sagamu in the new millennium: a facility-based retrospective analysis. BMC Pregnancy Childbirth. 2006;6:6.
36. Society of Gynaecology and Obstetrics of Nigeria: Status of emergency obstetric service in six states of Nigeria – A needs assessment report, 2004.
37. Tukur J, Rai'u, Gill KS. Pattern of eclampsia in a tertiary health facility situated in a semi-rural town in northern Nigeria. Annals of African Medicine. 2008; 6(4):164–7.
38. Moser M. Working Group Report on High Blood Pressure in Pregnancy. J Clin Hypertens. 2001;3:75–88.
39. ACOG Committee On obstetric practice. ACOG practice bulletin. Diagnosis and management of preeclampsia and eclampsia. No. 33, January 2002. American College of Obstetricians and Gynecologists. Obstet Gynecol. 2002;99:159–67.
40. Duley L, Gülmezoglu AM, Henderson-Smart DJ. Magnesium sulphate and other anticonvulsants for women with pre-eclampsia. Cochrane Database Syst Rev. 2003;2:CD000025.
41. Magpie Trial Collaboration Group. Do women with preeclampsia, and their babies, benefit from magnesium sulphate? The magpie trial: a randomised placebo controlled trial. Lancet. 2002;359:1877–90.
42. Australian Medicines Handbook. Magnesium sulphate: Drugs in pre-eclampsia and eclampsia: AMH. 2014.
43. Agus ZS, Lau K. Disorders of magnesium metabolism. In: Arieff AI, RA DF, editors. Fluid, electrolyte, and acid-base disorders. 2nd ed. New York: Churchill Livingstone; 1995. p. 475–92.
44. Burridge N, Collard N, Symons K and Society of Hospital Pharmacists of Australia (issuing body). Australian injectable drugs handbook (Sixth edition). Collingwood, Vic: The Society of Hospital Pharmacists of Australia; 2014.

Evaluation of a novel vital sign device to reduce maternal mortality and morbidity in low-resource settings: a mixed method feasibility study for the CRADLE-3 trial

Nicola Vousden[1*], Elodie Lawley[1], Hannah L. Nathan[1], Paul T. Seed[1], Adrian Brown[2], Tafadzwa Muchengwa[4], Umesh Charantimath[3], Mrutyunjaya Bellad[3], Muchabayiwa Francis Gidiri[5], Shivaprasad Goudar[3], Lucy C. Chappell[1], Jane Sandall[1], Andrew H. Shennan[1] and on behalf of the CRADLE Trial Collaborative Group

Abstract

Background: The CRADLE-3 trial is a stepped-wedge randomised controlled trial aiming to reduce maternal mortality and morbidity by implementing a novel vital sign device (CRADLE Vital Sign Alert) and training package into routine maternity care in 10 low-income sites. The MRC Guidance on complex interventions proposes that interventions and implementation strategies be shaped by early phase piloting and development work. We present the findings of a three-month mixed-methodology feasibility study for this trial, describe how this was informed by the MRC guidance and the study design was refined.

Methods: The fidelity, dose, feasibility and acceptability of implementation and training materials were assessed in three representative non-trial sites (Zimbabwe, Ethiopia, India) using multiple-choice questionnaires, evaluation of clinical management (action log), healthcare provider (HCP) semi-structured interviews and focus groups 4–10 weeks after implementation. Simultaneously, the 10 sites included in the main trial (eight countries) collected primary outcome data to inform the power calculation and randomisation allocation and assess the feasibility of data collection.

Results: The package was implemented with high fidelity (85% of HCP trained, $n = 204$). The questionnaires indicated a good understanding of device use with 75% of participants scoring > 75% ($n = 97$; 90% of those distributed). Action logs were inconsistently completed but indicated that the majority of HCP responded appropriately to abnormal results. From 18 HCP interviews and two focus groups it was widely reported that the intervention improved capacity to make clinical decisions, escalate care and make appropriate referrals. Nine of the ten main trial sites achieved ethical approval for pilot data collection. Intensive care was an inconsistent marker of morbidity and stroke an infrequent outcome and therefore they were removed from the main trial composite outcome. Tools and methods of data collection were optimized and event rates used to inform randomisation.

Conclusions: This feasibility study demonstrates that the components of the intervention were acceptable, methods of implementing were successful and the main trial design would be feasible. Qualitative work identified key moderators that informed the main trial process evaluation. Changes to the training package, implementation strategy, study design and processes were identified to refine the implementation in the main trial.

(Continued on next page)

* Correspondence: Nicola.vousden@kcl.ac.uk
[1]Department of Women and Children's Health, School of Life Course Sciences, Faculty of Life Sciences and Medicine, King's College London, London SE1 7EH, UK
Full list of author information is available at the end of the article

(Continued from previous page)

Keywords: Complex intervention, Maternal mortality, Low resource, Feasibility, Pilot, Implementation

Background

Maternal mortality remains a challenge in the post-Millennium Development Goal (MDG) era, especially in low resource settings where in 2013, 800 women died every day from complications of pregnancy and childbirth [1]. The most common causes of maternal mortality worldwide are hypertensive disorders, obstetric haemorrhage, sepsis and abortion complications. There are simple interventions that are readily available to treat these conditions. However, in low-resource settings, delays in presenting to care, reaching care and receiving this care all contribute to high maternal mortality. Measurement of vital signs is the first step in recognising women at risk of deterioration and therefore in initiating life-saving treatments [2]. Despite this, access to accurate equipment to measure vital signs and adequate healthcare provider (HCP) training on escalation pathways are frequently lacking in low and middle income countries (LMIC) [3].

The CRADLE-3 trial aims to determine whether implementation of a novel vital sign alert (VSA) device into routine maternity care at both community and facility levels, will reduce a composite outcome of maternal mortality and morbidity in LMIC. This is a stepped wedge randomised controlled trial (RCT) based in seven low-income and one middle-income country over 20 months. The CRADLE VSA is a semi automated device that measures blood pressure, pulse and calculates the mothers risk of shock. It has been extensively validated for accuracy [4, 5] and usability [6] and the need defined in this context through field work and stakeholder engagement.

The trial development was informed by the Medical Research Council (MRC) guidance for complex interventions [7]. Although the stages of development and evaluation can take many different forms, it is recommended that key uncertainties in the design are systematically studied in a development phase. Procedures should be tested for their acceptability and the likely rates of recruitment estimated to inform sample size calculations. The guidance also states that a mixture of qualitative and quantitative methods is likely to be needed in order to understand barriers to participation and estimated responses. Guidance on how best to undertake this was provided by Moore et al. in 2015 [8].

Whilst the MRC guidance is heavily cited there are few published papers that consider its practical application during this stage especially taking into context the challenges of working in multiple LMIC. Prior to the CRADLE 3 trial start a mixed-methodology feasibility study was undertaken to finalise the intervention and implementation processes which were guided by the Expert Recommendations for Implementing Change (ERIC) project [9]. Potential causal mechanisms and contextual factors that may influence the success of the trial were also identified. A logic model was created to describe these components and to identify the key research questions that inform the process evaluation of the main trial [10]. Through presenting results of this feasibility study, we aim to provide a worked example of the application of the MRC guidance in finalising the subsequent trial protocol and process evaluation.

Method

The study took place over 3 months from November 2015 to January 2016 with a further 3 months to analyse and adapt the intervention and protocol prior to the trial start in April 2016. It consisted of three key objectives:

1. Exploration of the acceptability and feasibility of the CRADLE programme components and the development of its implementation strategies by a mixed-method evaluation in three non-trial sites representative of the 10 main trial clusters.
2. Collection of primary outcome data in the 10 main trial clusters in order to evaluate the methods of data collection, and assess factors related to the randomisation programme (number of deliveries per month) and the sample size calculation.
3. Utilise results to optimize final CRADLE 3 protocol including training materials and implementation strategy for main trial.

Setting

Implementation was undertaken in three areas representative of the main trial clusters. These were a convenience sample of facilities meeting the study's inclusion criteria but geographically distant to avoid contamination of the main trial. All facilities approached agreed to participate. These were sites based around Ramdurg in Karnataka, India, Bishoftu in Ethiopia, and Masvingo in Zimbabwe. In accordance with the 10 main trial clusters (list in Additional file 1) these included one or more secondary or tertiary facilities that provided comprehensive emergency obstetric care and the surrounding primary care facilities that referred to these higher facilities and were urban or semi-urban.

Participants

The CRADLE VSA was incorporated into routine maternity care. All HCPs working in these services were eligible for training and all women identified as pregnant or within the 6 weeks post-partum period, presenting for antenatal, intrapartum or postpartum care within the three areas were eligible for inclusion.

Intervention

The intervention, described in accordance with the TiDieR guidance [11], included two key components. The Microlife CRADLE VSA is a novel device that accurately measures blood pressure and pulse [4, 5, 12] and calculates the pregnant mother's risk of hypovolaemic or septic shock [13, 14]. It has been specifically developed to meet the World Health Organisation's criteria for use in a low resource setting. A traffic light Early Warning System display alerts users to abnormalities in the vital signs results. The lights are triggered by standard thresholds of hypertension as well as by shock index (heart rate divided by systolic blood pressure) [13], as shown in Table 1. The CRADLE VSA was incorporated into routine maternity care.

Primary, secondary and tertiary facilities were allocated devices according to their delivery rate, staffing numbers and number of beds per ward. Pre-existing BP devices were removed from clinical areas, unless existing equipment has functionality designed for that area e.g. repeated automated measures in a high dependency area. This was supported with a CRADLE training package consisting of short animated film, interactive sessions, booklet and posters. There were two sets of training materials available, one for facility HCP and one for community HCP with very limited resources or no formal training.

Table 1 Thresholds that trigger the CRADLE VSA Early Warning System

Hypertension Thresholds		
Light and Arrow Results	Category	Blood Pressure (mmHg)
RED LIGHT & UP ARROW	Severe hypertension	≥ 160 and / or ≥ 110
YELLOW LIGHT & UP ARROW	Hypertension	≥ 140 & ≤ 159 and / or ≥ 90 & ≤ 109
GREEN LIGHT	Normal	< 140 and < 90
Shock Index (SI) Thresholds		
Light and Arrow Results	Category	Shock Index (HR / sBP)
RED LIGHT & DOWN ARROW	Severe shock	≥ 1.7
YELLOW LIGHT & DOWN ARROW	Shock	≥ 0.9 and < 1.7
GREEN LIGHT	Normal	< 0.9

The CRADLE package content covered:

- How to use the CRADLE VSA.
- Maintenance of the CRADLE VSA.
- Basic overview of clinical assessment and management of pre-eclampsia/eclampsia and shock in relation to the traffic light alerts.

The local implementation team and research team delivered one-off interactive group training sessions lasting 2–4 h to local stakeholders and representative HCP from each of the clinical areas in the cluster. This included a presentation on the background of the CRADLE VSA and the importance of measuring vital signs in pregnancy. This was followed by a demonstration of the features and use of the CRADLE VSA and small group practice using the CRADLE VSA. Training finished with interactive clinical scenarios exploring the use of the CRADLE VSA with available guidance and resources.

Attendees were given training materials and CRADLE VSA devices to disseminate to their clinical areas. The implementation team attended each clinical area over the subsequent days (depending on cluster size) to support dissemination and hold interactive sessions.

The core components of the intervention (provision of the CRADLE VSA devices, animated films, posters and content of the training presentation) were standardized across all sites. The way the core components were delivered was adapted to meet the needs of the site. This intervention can be described as complex [7] because it comprises multiple interacting components that require considerable shift in the behavior of recipients. It is also being implemented at multiple levels of low-resource health services and will affect multiple outcome measures [7]. In the main trial, the intervention will be compared to routine maternity care with clinical assessment and management according to local guidelines. Vital signs measurement is normally undertaken with a variety of blood pressure devices where these are available, which are rarely validated in pregnancy.

Study design

For this feasibility study, the 10 clusters involved in the main trial collected the primary outcome as defined at that time: a composite of maternal mortality or major morbidity (one of maternal death, Intensive Care Unit admission (or predefined equivalent), eclampsia, stroke, or hysterectomy, with no double counting). Data were collected from existing healthcare facility registers, maternity records, maternal mortality reports and healthcare providers at the discretion of the local research team. Anonymised data were recorded onto a paper form and transferred by the research team onto a purpose-built online database (MedSciNet).

The components of the mixed methodology assessment of the acceptability and feasibility of the CRADLE programme components, undertaken in the three non-trial sites are shown in Table 2.

In order to explore potential mediators of action a purposive sample of HCP were requested to complete action logs of clinical practice to evaluate their referral practice. In these action logs, HCP were requested to record any "yellow" or "red" Early Warning System with the action they took, for example 'administered anti-hypertensives and referred to hospital today'. This was compared to baseline information of available resources to interpret how HCP had understood and interpreted the training. Questionnaires assessing knowledge of when and how to use the CRADLE VSA and how to interpret the results were filled after training by a random sample of participants.

We undertook semi-structured interviews and focus groups (guides available on request) 4–10 weeks after implementation. This time was selected to allow sufficient experience of the VSA in clinical practice whilst allowing time to make improvements to the intervention within the funding timeline. The aim of these was to further knowledge on the acceptability of the device features gained from a previous observational study of the CRADLE VSA (CRADLE 2) [15] by exploring the feasibility of implementing the CRADLE package and how incorporating it into routine care might change behaviour. Participants were selected through purposive sampling to ensure representation of different HCP cadres in hospital and community care. Participants were approached face-to-face and gave written informed consent to participate in the qualitative study. The interviews were recorded and transcribed verbatim for further analysis and field notes were recorded. Snowball sampling was utilised until data saturation was achieved in each site. Two data coders that were independent to the interviewers undertook analysis using QSR NVivo 11 software (QRS, Vic, Australia). We used the framework method with a coding framework that draws upon the study objectives, logic model and interview guide [16, 17]. New concepts initiated by participants that could not be categorized within the initial scheme were coded using an inductive approach and added to the framework. The COnsolidated criteria for REporting Qualitative research (COREQ) Checklist was used to report the methodology and findings [18].

Results

Development of trial tools

We developed the training materials and data collection tools based on the experiences of the previous CRADLE projects [4, 5, 12–14]. It was necessary to create a training package that could be disseminated quickly in multiple contexts and easily understood by every cadre of HCP with different resources available. Therefore, we selected animated film as the main component so that voice overs could be translated at minimal additional cost and it could be disseminated widely onto smart phones by Bluetooth. Feedback from end-users, health service managers and implementation experts was incorporated.

We created a logic model to depict the components of the intervention, how they may interact to produce change and what the anticipated outcome of that change may be (Fig. 1) [10, 19]. This was developed based on the evidence described in the introduction with input of the research team and key stakeholders. These included representative healthcare professionals and service managers from our low-income trial sites and implementation experts. The moderating factors and anticipated changes to practice in the logic model were utilized to inform the process evaluation outcome measures.

Feasibility of implementation

The intervention was implemented in three regional hospitals, one from each site, together with 61 associated primary healthcare facilities. The proportion of staff trained and the duration of training is shown in Table 3. In India and Ethiopia, we translated the training materials and in India the graphics of the poster and booklets were altered to be more culturally appropriate. In all countries the guidance for management of pre-eclampsia, haemorrhage and shock, which was based on WHO guidelines [20, 21],

Table 2 Outcomes, method of measurement and time of measurement in the CRADLE-3 feasibility study

Outcome		Method of Measurement	Time of measurement
Feasibility	Fidelity	Duration of training	At training
	Dose	Proportion of staff trained	At training
		Number of facilities included	At training
	Adaptations to fit context	Observation of training	At training
	Understanding of training materials	Questionnaires ($n = 30$ each site)	Post training
		Action Log of Clinical Practice ($n = 30$ each site)	For 1 month post training
Acceptability		Stakeholder Interviews ($n = 5$ each site)	3 months post implementation
		Stakeholder Focus Group ($n = 1$ each site)	3 months post implementation

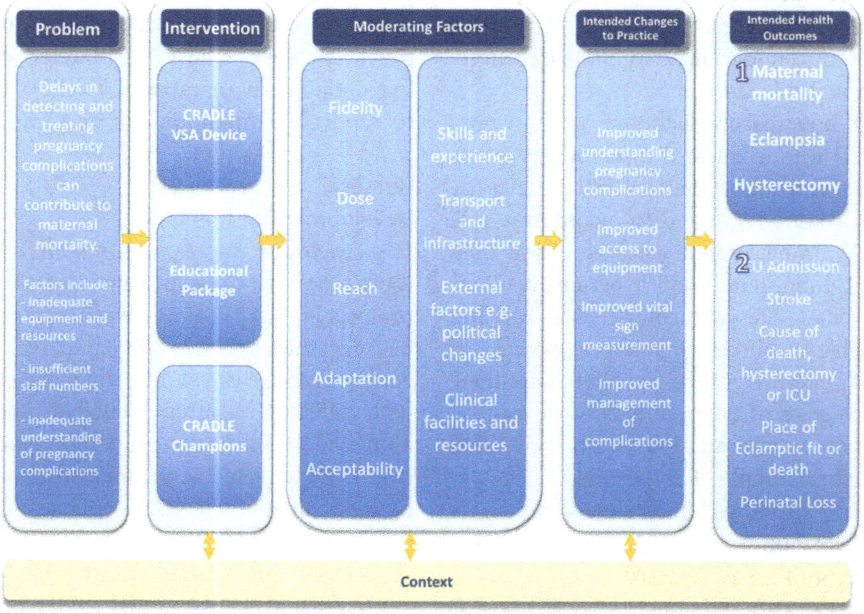

Fig. 1 Logic model for the CRADLE-3 intervention

was adapted to incorporate locally available resources and infrastructure.

In total, 108 questionnaires were distributed and 97 fully completed by HCP and analysed, 16% by HCP working in primary level facilities and 84% in secondary level facilities. This represents 48% of those trained. Of these, five were doctors, 78 were nurses and midwives and 15 were allied HCP. The majority of respondents had more than 5 years of service (1–5 years $n = 28$, 29%; 6–10 years $n = 35$, 36%; > 10 years $n = 34$, 35%). Results indicated a good understanding use of the VSA and interpretation of results with 73 participants (75%) scoring more than 75% correct answers. HCP working in secondary care scored higher in questions on how to act in response to abnormal vital signs than HCP working in primary care (74% ($n = 60$) scoring over 75% correct compared to 56% ($n = 9$) of clinic participants.

Action logs were distributed to 90 HCP and completed by 68 (76%). The level of detail completed was diverse with many participants failing to complete details on medication given or the time frame taken for action. This was reported to be due to the additional burden of work required to complete these logs and this is explored further in the discussion. Analysis of these records was therefore challenging and results should be interpreted with caution. It was possible to determine that in total, 62 red lights were recorded, indicating severely abnormal vital signs. The majority ($n = 50$, 81%) had optimal care appropriate for the available resources. Of the 12 that did not, five were referred to hospital but within a longer timeframe and seven were reported to look well so no further action was taken.

The action logs demonstrated varying practice in response to a yellow light with a downward pointing arrow. This result indicates a relative low blood pressure compared to the heart rate. In Ramadurg, India, the majority of these patients were referred to higher level care, compared to fewer in Bishoftu, Ethiopia. This variance highlighted ambiguity in the training materials. This was explored widely with stakeholders and changes made to the training materials accordingly. A yellow down light may be caused by multiple clinical causes of varying importance (such as maternal anaemia which can be common in pregnancy) and therefore greater emphasis was made on assessment of the patient's clinical condition in the final training materials.

Table 3 Fidelity and dose of implementation

Study Site	Number of primary health care facilities involved	Proportion of HCP trained	Duration of training	Devices Distributed
Masvingo, Zimbabwe	21	90% ($n = 92$)	8 days	62
Bishoftu, Ethiopia	3	85% ($n = 37$)	3 days	29
Ramadurg, India	37	95% ($n = 75$)	2 days	53

Acceptability of the intervention and implementation strategies

A total of 18 interviews and two focus group were undertaken across the three sites in January and February 2016.

Participants were approached face to face and provided written informed consent. The participants had limited prior relationship with the researchers from training and outreach support visits. Individual interviews were undertaken with nine nurses, five midwives, one maternity manager, two health assistants and one doctor. The median age of participants was 25–34 years ($n = 12$) (18–24, $n = 1$; 34–44, $n = 3$; 45–54, n-2), the most common number of years of service was 1–5 ($n = 8$) (6–10 years, $n = 5$; 11–15 years, $n = 2$; > 15, $n = 3$). Findings are presented under themes below. Interviews and focus groups were undertaken in private, quiet locations near the participant's place of work with no non-participant observers to ensure confidentiality and allow for an open discussion. Sessions lasted between 15 and 75 min and were undertaken, translated and transcribed by experienced local research coordinators (clinical background) following training from the trial coordinator and senior social scientist (JS).

Use of CRADLE VSA in clinical decision making

It was widely reported that the CRADLE VSA package improved capacity to make decisions about which women require treatment and referral. This was true for HCP in the community who initiated referral as well as those working in facilities who initiated treatment or escalated care to senior staff. The suggested reasons for this were varied. HCP who were previously using auscultatory BP devices reported lack of confidence in accurately auscultating the Korotkoff sounds and therefore reported regularly rounding the BP to the nearest ten or delaying taking action. This was alleviated by the digital display of systolic and diastolic blood pressure and pulse on the CRADLE VSA.

> *"There, if we get high BP, we used to think and get the BP checked by others, as we had less confidence in that machine. We used to ask others saying that it has shown high BP in our machine and we want to check by you also. Here with this device (CRADLE VSA) we can take decision immediately." Staff Nurse, Hospital, India*

HCP also reported that the Early Warning System alerted them to abnormalities in the results which may otherwise not be recognised. This was reported to be mainly because in pressured environments with fatigued staff abnormal results may be missed whereas a red light is an instantly recognisable alarm. This, in combination with the training materials was felt to provide valuable guidance in the action required to manage abnormalities. The majority of HCP reported that this has improved the time taken to recognise pregnancy complications and initiate treatment or referral. These views are illustrated in the quote below:

> *"Yes, more interventions are done and done in a more prompt manner because of the indicators which one can easily refer to and take action promptly. Interventions are done early or immediately because of the indicators that alert the clinicians. They are forced to act quickly even if they refer, but they will have taken some action" Staff Nurse Masvingo, Zimbabwe*

Whilst the majority of HCP felt that the results are accurate and the lights beneficial, there were two HCP who reported that they did not always act on the lights because they were confused. They felt that the yellow light was reported too frequently when patients appeared well. The quote below demonstrates this:

> *"But what we are observing is that for majority of women it is showing yellow with down arrow. But the patient is stable, normal, she is not sick and she is well. In such situations we feel "why it so? The woman is normal, but still why it is showing yellow down"?" Staff nurse, PHC, India.*

Other HCP acknowledged that this was a common result but demonstrated understanding of potential causes and how to manage this result. This finding triangulates the results of the Action Log and is explored further in the discussion.

Aid of the CRADLE VSA in escalating care and referral

Nursing HCP reported that when they were previously using auscultatory devices they reported doubt or being challenged when referring cases to medical staff. The improved confidence in the vital signs measurement and the understanding conveyed by the training package was beneficial in escalating care to senior staff. This was also true in convincing women and their families of the need for further monitoring or referral.

> *"It is helpful in providing immediate care to the patient. As everything is given there (booklets and poster) like the patient has to be referred within 4 hours or within 1 week...etc., we call the attenders and convince them, to refer the patient at the earliest." Staff Nurse, Gokak, India*

The majority of HCP reported an increase in the number of vital sign abnormalities detected; however, the reported impact on the rate of referrals varied between countries. All participants from India reported an increase in the number of referrals. The number of hypertensive patients referred was increased as mild hypertension was considered more seriously. The number of patients with low blood pressure detected and referred was also noted to increase. In Zimbabwe and Ethiopia responses were mixed with some reporting a reduction in referrals due to improved understanding of vital signs and confidence in initiating treatment peripherally. A quote to illustrate this is:

> *"because of the indicators the referrals have decreased, now we know when to refer and we now don't refer all patients for the sake of referring."*
> *Nurse, Clinic, Zimbabwe*

Use of results to finalise implementation strategies

The MRC Guidance and supporting documents highlight that the pilot data should be used to shape the intervention and implementation strategies. Following the completion of this feasibility study, the experiences of implementation and input from a stakeholder meeting across all sites in February 2016 were used to agree a number of changes prior to the main trial. The choice of implementation strategy was guided by the Expert Recommendations for Implementing Change project [9] with the aim of improving understanding of the training materials and overcoming identified barriers to use. Table 4 presents the key issues experienced through the feasibility study alongside quotes to support this and the implementation strategies or changes we have selected.

A key implementation strategy that we selected as a result of the feasibility findings was the identification and training of CRADLE champions. These are clinical staff and local leaders who receive more in-depth training about device and are equipped with the tools to support the use of the VSA in their area. Whilst we wanted the trial to remain pragmatic and replicable, this strategy was chosen to support ongoing local training and build local capacity for maintenance. The importance of the support of the implementation team on the effectiveness of the intervention was also noted during the study and added to the logic model as a core component of the intervention. In order to maintain the pragmatic trial design, it was decided not to quantify this support but for the research team to observe it during the routine monthly site monitoring and be aware of its potential impact.

Main trial primary outcomes

As the main trial has a stepped wedge design with an intervention incorporated into routine care, cluster level consent instead of individual was appropriate. This was agreed as preferable by all sites during the development work. All ten trial sites gained ethical and local approval for participation in the main trial. Nine of them achieved this before or during the feasibility phase and were therefore able to commence data collection, with six sites completing a full 3 months of data collection. During this formative phase a total of 844 outcome

Table 4 Barriers to measuring the vital signs and using the VSA and actions made prior to the main trial

Issue from Feasibility study	Supporting quotes from Interviews and Focus Group	Changes required after feasibility study
Understanding of yellow light with down arrow	*"When the pregnant woman comes to us she is well and it shows yellow down (laughs); in that case how to interpret?" Staff Nurse, India*	- Training materials updated to explain the reason for each colour light. - Guidance updated to place greater emphasis on how to assess the woman to decide *if* further action or referral is required.
Problems with charging the VSA	*"... some workers say that the battery life is good but I have to charge it for daily. If I have to go for BP check-up today I have to charge it first." Staff Nurse, India*	- Interactive training session developed which incorporates guidance on charging and accountability for charging. - Including explanation that more than 100 readings can be taken even when the battery low sign is showing and overcharging will damage the battery.
Provision of Charger	*"the package should include the charger rather than USB cable only so that we can charge it easily" Staff Nurse, Zimbabwe*	Chargers provided in addition to the cable that comes as standard in the package.
High staff turnover / incapacity to train all staff at once	*"Initially, we faced difficulty. There were nurses using it during the night shift and they were not trained." Staff Nurse, Bishoftu*	Designated CRADLE Champions in each facility identified to provide ongoing local training and support for CRADLE VSA
Unsupportive seniors	*"Recently during an ANC clinic he inquired which device we are using; we said "we are using the CRADLE device given by the research unit" then he said "oh... it shows yellow down to all pregnant women, so better do not use it"." SN, India*	- Designated CRADLE Champions identified to provide ongoing local training and support for CRADLE VSA - Engage Local Opinion leaders prior to implementation
Need for equipment	*"...no BP machines at all, the one we had was no longer working." Staff Nurse, Zimbabwe*	Ensure adequate supply of VSA available

events (any one of eclampsia, maternal death, hysterectomy, ICU admission or stroke) occurred in 681 women from nine of the ten sites. On average, the number of women experiencing events each month varied from five in Gokak, India to 63 in Zomba and South-Eastern Malawi (median 19.6, standard deviation 19.6). The most common outcome was eclampsia ($n = 386$, 46%) followed by ICU admission ($n = 271$, 32%), hysterectomy and maternal death ($n = 96$, 11%; $n = 91$, 11% respectively) and stroke ($n = 2$, 0.2%). The tools for data collection were found to be appropriate. Methods of data collection were discussed and optimised based on the existing resources available in each site. Outcomes were triangulated across multiple sources (including referral registers, ward registers, patient records, local mortality and morbidity records, active case finding) to ensure data completeness and all outcomes checked to avoid double counting.

These outcomes had been intended as unequivocal markers of severe maternal mortality and morbidity. However, during the process of data collection it became apparent that ICU admission was dependent on availability of services which varied greatly between clusters and therefore this was not a reliable proxy marker of maternal morbidity. The number of strokes reported across all sites was just two, both from one site. It was therefore prospectively decided that for the main trial the composite primary outcome would include only eclampsia, maternal death and emergency hysterectomy. Given that the size of clusters varies greatly, it was agreed that the number of deliveries would be counted as a surrogate denominator so that results for the main trial could be presented as an event rate per 10,000 deliveries. These prospective amendments were added to the trial registry (ISRCTN41244132).

Randomisation and power calculation

An estimated event rate from the data was used to inform the randomisation sequence and power calculation of the main trial. With so few centres to be randomised there was a risk of unbalance – for example that by chance the centres with the highest event rates might be allocated to the intervention at the end of the study, giving a false impression of a low event rate in centres which received the intervention early, and hence a biased estimate of the treatment effect. Although the planned analysis would correct for this, to further minimize the problem, a restricted form of randomisation was used, so that the rank correlation between the initial event rate, and the order of randomisation was zero. For logistic reasons, the two centres outside Africa: Cap Hatien (Haiti) and Gokak (India) were treated as one centre for randomisation (but not for analysis).

First the overall rate of the primary outcome was determined in the nine clusters and each cluster given a corresponding rank r between 1 and 9. Then a provisional list l of the order of intervention was determined for each cluster using computer-generated random numbers based on an arbitrary random number seed. Spearman's rank correlation rho between r and l was determined. If the rank correlation was not equal to 0, the list was discarded, and the process repeated until an acceptable order was determined. The first acceptable randomly-generated list was retained. This resulted in a near-zero Pearson's product-moment correlation of – 0.019 between the event rate and the order of randomisation.

Based on these data, our sample size estimation was carried out by the trial statistician, using Stata version 13.1 and the methods of Hemming and Girling [22]. For the purpose of the power calculation, an assumption that there are at least 4000 deliveries per cluster per month was made (or 8000 per cluster period of 2 months) and at least nine clusters, each observed for 20 months (ten time periods of 2 months each). Our feasibility data indicated a baseline event rate of 1% and we have anticipated a 25% reduction in this to 0.75% post intervention. We would require a total of 2450 outcome events with a coefficient of variation of 0.4 and an Intra Cluster Correlation of 0.0085, to have power of 95%.

Discussion

This paper aims to describe the mixed methodology feasibility study exploring the acceptability and feasibility of introducing the CRADLE package into routine maternity care in LMIC along with the feasibility of the main trial data collection processes. The key findings are that the intervention can be delivered with high fidelity and dose and incorporated into routine maternity care successfully in different contexts without major adaptation. In addition, we have confirmed that the methods of collecting the main outcome data are feasible and can be maintained for consistency and this data has successfully been used to improve the study design, randomisation and power calculation.

The MRC framework stresses the importance of quality development work to avoid problems with acceptability, compliance, recruitment and retention. Yet methodological research suggests that pilot studies are often poorly performed and few are published [23]. Most published examples of complex interventions demonstrate valuable learning from pilots; for example, the exploratory RCT of an intervention to reduce alcohol related harm demonstrated that whilst the trial was methodologically feasible, poor enthusiasm resulted in low fidelity thus the conclusion that the intervention would need to be enforced in future work [24]. However, published description of its use in the field of maternity and in LMIC is scarce.

One key learning from our feasibility study was the practicalities of a pragmatic process evaluation in a low-resource setting. The MRC supporting guidance provides explanation for each of the key dimensions of implementation that could be measured and guides researchers to select the most important questions to investigate. Whilst this is a strength of the framework as it ensures comprehensive evaluation of implementation, it provides little guidance on how to select suitable outcome measures for each dimension. This is especially challenging when working in a resource-poor environment with additional burden of high workload and heterogeneous routine data collection. In this feasibility study, measuring multiple components compared to baseline was not possible within the short time frame. The proportion of people trained centrally and time taken for training were selected as simple surrogates of fidelity and dose. However, in the qualitative work the majority of HCP reported the VSA was easy to use and it was possible to commence use just on reading the training materials so the extent that these measures may impact the effectiveness of the program is unknown. In the main trial the number of core components delivered in training and how they were adapted to context were added to the measure of fidelity.

The MRC Guidance advises using the logic model to identify causal assumptions and guide selection of research questions. In the CRADLE Logic model the assumed changes to practice include improving access to equipment therefore in the trial we will capture the proportion of HCP that have access to a working BP machine before and after implementation. A further assumed change is improving vital sign measurement and management of complications. In this feasibility study, the action log of referral practice was poorly received and completed due to the extra burden of work it demanded. For the main trial, we chose to explore change in practice during the qualitative work rather than during structured observation due to the large variety of normal practice in different countries. The qualitative work also highlighted that number of women referred to higher level care was a potential key moderator. Therefore, after stakeholder discussion across our sites we agreed to measure the proportion of women presenting for maternity care that had their blood pressure measured and the proportion that were referred to higher level care. Due to the intensity of this data collection it was agreed this would be measured for a period of 4 weeks before implementation and 4 weeks, 3 months after the device was introduced to allow time for familiarization of the VSA in routine maternity care. We found the process of identifying potential factors that may impact on the success of the trial and tailoring outcome measures accordingly was achievable for a team of predominantly newcomers to the field of implementation. It was also beneficial in assuring that assumptions are shared between stakeholders.

Strengths and limitations of the study

We describe the feasibility testing of the CRADLE intervention prior to a fully powered trial. This was guided by the MRC guidance and was undertaken over a 6-month period; results are therefore applicable to others working in restricted funding periods. Feasibility and pilot research is often skipped or inadequate to fully inform the main trial and rarely published to inform others researching similar areas. In a situation where a complete development phase is not possible due to the stepped wedge design we demonstrated that our event rate in the main trial sites is sufficient to have adequate power. We undertook formal qualitative analysis to explore the acceptability of the program components and feasibility of implementation. We did not collect cost-effectiveness data in the feasibility study but will collect this data for an economic evaluation in the full trial. We did not assess knowledge of vital signs measurement prior to training and therefore results should be interpreted with caution.

Conclusions

This feasibility study demonstrates that the components of the intervention were acceptable and the methods of implementing successful. Qualitative work identified key moderators that have informed the main trial process evaluation. Changes to the training package, implementation strategy, study design and processes were identified to optimize the main trial implementation. Carrying out these changes in practice, (for example to the data collection forms, database and graphics of the training materials were challenging) within the six-month allocated time frame of this feasibility study. If larger changes had been required, for example to the components of the intervention which would require re-testing, this would not have been possible. Funders recommending that a development phase is incorporated into a standard 3-year funding period might therefore take into consideration the time taken to undertake the work, analyse results and incorporate changes into the study to ensuring meaningful improvements can be made.

Concurrently assessing the feasibility of the trial outcomes in the 10 main trial sites and the implementation processes in geographically distant sites was necessary to avoid contamination of the trial area. Whilst undertaking this in multiple sites required additional work, it allowed for greater understanding of how the intervention could be adapted in each context and how the main trial will run. The MRC Guidance and supporting documents provided a valuable tool to guide the overall design of this study and the development of the process evaluation for the main trial. This study presents a real world worked example that has utilised this guidance to refine the intervention, main trial outcomes and process measures.

Abbreviations

COREQ: COnsolidated criteria for reporting qualitative research; ERIC: Expert recommendations for implementing change; HCP: Health care provider; LMIC: Low and middle income countrie; MDG: Millennium development goal; MRC: Medical research council; RCT: Randomised controlled trial; SI: Shock index; VSA: Vital sign alert; WHO: World Health Organisation

Acknowledgements

John Hopkins Public Health and implementation department, JHPIEGO, contributed $10,000 towards the development of the training videos and provided academic input and review during their development. We would like to acknowledge all authors of the CRADLE Trial Collaborative Group for their contribution to this work: Kate E Duhig, King's College London, UK Natasha L Hezelgrave, King's College London, UK; Umesh Charantimath, KLE University's J N Medical College, India; Chandrappa C Karadiguddi, KLE University's J N Medical College, India;Sphoorthi S Mastiholi, KLE University's J N Medical College, India; Geetanjali M Mungarwadi, KLE University's J N Medical College, India; Feiruz Surur, St Paul's Millennium Medical School,Ethiopia; Lomi Yadeta, Maternity Worldwide, Ethiopia; Yonas Guchale, Maternity Worldwide, Ethiopia; Violet Mambo, University of Zimbabwe, Zimbabwe; Sebastian Chinkoyo, Ndola Teaching Hospital, Zambia; Thokozile Musonda, Ndola Teaching Hospital, Zambia; Christine Jere, Ndola Teaching Hospital, Zambia; Bellington Vwalika, University of Zambia, Zambia; Mercy Kopeka, University Teaching Hospital, Zambia; Martina Chima, University Teaching Hospital, Zambia; Josephine Miti, University Teaching Hospital, Zambia; Rebecca Best, Welbodi Partnership, Sierra Leone; Matthew Clarke, Welbodi Partnership, Sierra Leone; Jesse Kamara, Welbodi Partnership, Sierra Leone; Jeneba Conteh, Princess Christian Maternity Hospital, Sierra Leone; Patricia Sandi, Princess Christian Maternity Hospital, Sierra Leone; Margaret Sesay, Princess Christian Maternity Hospital, Sierra Leone; Fatmata Momodou, Princess Christian Maternity Hospital, Sierra Leone; Julius Wandabwa, Busitema University, Uganda; James Ditai, Sanyu Africa Research Institute, Uganda; Nathan Mackayi Odeke, Sanyu Africa Research Institute, Uganda; Annettee Nakimuli, Makerere University College of Health Sciences, Uganda; Josaphat Byamugisha, Makerere University College of Health Sciences, Uganda; Dorothy Namakula, Mulago National Referral Hospital, Uganda; Noela Kalyowa, Mulago National Referral Hospital, Uganda; Doreen Birungi, Mulago National Referral Hospital, Uganda; Emily Nakirijja, Mulago National Referral Hospital, Uganda; Carwyn Hill, Hope Health Action, Haiti; Grace Greene, Hope Health Action, Haiti; Adeline Vixama, Hope Health Action, Haiti; Paul Toussaint, Hospital Convention Baptiste d'Haiti, Haiti; Grace Makonyola, Maternity Worldwide, Malawi; Doreen Bukani, Maternity Worldwide, Malawi; Monice Kachinjika, Maternity Worldwide, Malawi; Jane Makwakwa, Maternity Worldwide, Malawi.

Jane Sandall and Paul Seed were supported by the National Institute for Health Research (NIHR) Collaboration for Leadership in Applied Health Research and Care South London at King's College Hospital NHS Foundation Trust. Lucy Chappell is supported by the National Institute for Health Research Professorship, (RP-2014-05-019). The views expressed are those of the author(s) and not necessarily those of the NHS, the NIHR or the Department of Health.

Funding

This study is funded by Medical Research Council (UK), Department for International Development (UK) and Department of Biotechnology (India) through the Department for International Development (UK) Global Research Programme: Addressing the health needs of women and children in the most disadvantaged populations globally. Neither funding body had any role in the design of the study or collection, analysis, and interpretation of data or in writing the manuscripts.

Authors' contributions

AS is primary investigator for the CRADLE-3 trial and has academic oversight in all actions. SG and FG are co-PIs for India and low –resource settings respectively. JS is senior social scientist who has supported NV and EL to design and undertake the process evaluation and qualitative components of this study. PS as trial statistician has undertaken all statistical work. AB, TM, BM and UC have overseen data collection in their sites. NV as trial coordinator has overseen all data collection, created training package and data collection tools with assistance from EL. LC and HN are co-investigators supporting trial management. All authors have contributed to the writing of this paper.

Ethics approval and consent to participate

Ethical approval has been granted by the Biomedical Sciences, Dentistry, Medicine and Natural & Mathematical Sciences Research Ethics Subcommittee at King's College London (LRS-14/15–1484). Local ethical approval from each cluster has been granted by:

- Ethiopian Public Health Institute, Ethiopia: EPHI6.4/185
- K.L.E Society's Jawaharlal Nehru Medical College, Belgaum, India: MDC/IECHSR/2015–16/A-59
- Medical Research Council of Zimbabwe; Zimbabwe: MRCZ/A/1999

Institutional level consent was sought prior to implementation of the CRADLE intervention. Informed written consent was sought from HCP participating in interviews, focus group discussions and the action logs of clinical practice.

Competing interests

The CRADLE VSA has been developed by Microlife with academic input from King's College London and funding from Bill and Melinda Gates. The device is provided at manufacturing cost for this trial and is available to purchase at low cost to all LMIC. King's College London receive no funds from the sale of devices to LMIC.

Author details

[1]Department of Women and Children's Health, School of Life Course Sciences, Faculty of Life Sciences and Medicine, King's College London, London SE1 7EH, UK. [2]Maternity Worldwide Community Base, 113 Queens Road, Brighton BN1 3XG, UK. [3]Women's and Children's Health Research Unit, KLE Academy of Higher Education and Research Jawaharlal Nehru Medical College, Belgaum, Karnataka 590010, India. [4]Morgenster Mission Hospital, Masvingo, Zimbabwe. [5]Department of Obstetrics and Gynaecology, College of Health Sciences, University of Zimbabwe, Harare, Zimbabwe.

References

1. World Health Organisation. Trends in maternal mortality: 1990 to 2013. Estimates by WHO, UNICEF, UNFPA, the World Bank and the United Nations population division. 2015 http://apps.who.int/iris/bitstream/10665/194254/1/9789241565141_eng.pdf?ua=1. [Accessed 20th November 2017].
2. World Health Organisation. The world health report 2005: make every mother and child count, vol. 2005. Geneva: World Health Organization.
3. Baker EC, van der Westhuizen A, Duhig KE, Shennan A. Can a low-resource-use blood pressure device impact on global maternal mortality? Hypertension in pregnancy : official journal of the International Society for the Study of Hypertension in Pregnancy. 2011;30(3):359–63.
4. Nathan HL, de Greeff A, Hezelgrave NL, Chappell LC, Shennan AH. An accurate semiautomated oscillometric blood pressure device for use in pregnancy (including pre-eclampsia) in a low-income and middle-income country population: the microlife 3AS1-2. Blood Press Monit. 2015;20(1):52–5.
5. Nathan HL, de Greeff A, Hezelgrave NL, Chappell LC, Shennan AH. Accuracy validation of the microlife 3AS1-2 blood pressure device in a pregnant population with low blood pressure. Blood Press Monit. 2015;20(5):299–302.
6. Nathan HL, Boene H, Munguambe K, Sevene E, Akeju D, Adetoro OO, et al. The CRADLE vital signs alert: qualitative evaluation of a novel device designed for use in pregnancy by healthcare workers in low-resource settings. Reprod Health. 2018;15(1):5.
7. Craig P, Dieppe P, Macintyre S, Michie S, Nazareth I, Petticrew M. Developing and evaluating complex interventions: the new Medical Research Council guidance. BMJ. 2008;337:a1655.
8. Moore GF, Audrey S, Barker M, Bond L, Bonell C, Hardeman W, et al. Process evaluation of complex interventions: Medical Research Council guidance. BMJ. 2015;350:h1258.

9. Powell BJ, Waltz TJ, Chinman MJ, Damschroder LJ, Smith JL, Matthieu MM, et al. A refined compilation of implementation strategies: results from the expert recommendations for implementing change (ERIC) project. Implement Sci. 2015;10(1):21.
10. W.K. Kellogg Foundation. Logic Model Development Guide: Using logic models to bring together planning, evaluation and action. 2004 https://www.wkkf.org/resource-directory/resource/2006/02/wk-kellogg-foundation-logic-model-development-guide. [Accessed 20th November 2017].
11. Hoffmann TC, Glasziou PP, Boutron I, Milne R, Perera R, Moher D, et al. Better reporting of interventions: template for intervention description and replication (TIDieR) checklist and guide. BMJ. 2014;348:g1687.
12. de Greeff A, Nathan H, Stafford N, Liu B, Shennan AH. Development of an accurate oscillometric blood pressure device for low resource settings. England: Blood Press Monit. 13; 2008. p. 342–8.
13. Nathan HL, El Ayadi A, Hezelgrave NL, Seed P, Butrick E, Miller S, et al. Shock index: an effective predictor of outcome in postpartum haemorrhage? BJOG. 2015;122(2):268–75.
14. El Ayadi AM, Nathan HL, Seed PT, Butrick EA, Hezelgrave NL, Shennan AH, et al. Vital sign prediction of adverse maternal outcomes in women with hypovolemic shock: the role of shock index. PLoS One. 2016;11(2):e0148729.
15. Nathan HL, Boene H, Munguambe K, Sevene E, Akeju D, Adetoro OO, Charanthimath U, Bellad MB, de Greeff A, Anthony J, Hall DR, Steyn W, Vidler M, von Dadelszen P, Chappell LC, Sandall J, Shennan AH, and the CLIP Working Group. The CRADLE vital signs alert: qualitative evaluation of a novel device designed for use in pregnancy by healthcare workers in low-resource settings. BMC Reproductive Health. 2018;15(1):5.
16. Ritchie JLJ. Qualitative research practice: a guide for social science students and researchers. London: Sage; 2003.
17. Gale NK, Heath G, Cameron E, Rashid S, Redwood S. Using the framework method for the analysis of qualitative data in multi-disciplinary health research. BMC Med Res Methodol. 2013;13:117.
18. Tong A, Sainsbury P, Craig J. Consolidated criteria for reporting qualitative research (COREQ): a 32-item checklist for interviews and focus groups. Int J Qual Health Care. 2007;19(6):349–57.
19. Kirby D. BDI logic models: a useful tool for designing, strengthening and evaluating programs to reduce adolescent sexual risk taking, pregnancy, HIV and other STDs. 2004 http://recapp.etr.org/recapp/documents/BDILOGICMODEL20030924.pdf. [Accessed 14th June 2017].
20. World Health Organisation. WHO recommendations for prevention and treatment of pre-eclampsia and eclampsia. 2011 http://apps.who.int/iris/bitstream/10665/44703/1/9789241548335_eng.pdf. [Accessed 3rd April 2017].
21. World Health Organisation. WHO recommendations for the prevention and treatment of postpartum haemorrhage. 2012 http://apps.who.int/iris/bitstream/10665/75411/1/9789241548502_eng.pdf. [Accessed 30th October 2017].
22. Hemming K, Girling A. A menu-driven facility for power and detectable-difference calculations in stepped-wedge cluster-randomized trials. Stata J. 2014;14(2):363–80.
23. Eldridge SM, Ashby D, Feder GS, Rudnicka AR, Ukoumunne OC. Lessons for cluster randomized trials in the twenty-first century: a systematic review of trials in primary care. Clinical Trials. 2004;1(1):80–90.
24. Moore SC, Murphy S, Moore SN, Brennan I, Byrne E, Shepherd J, et al. An exploratory randomised controlled trial of a premises-level intervention to reduce alcohol-related harm including violence in the United Kingdom. BMC Public Health. 2012;12:412.

The relationship between maternal anxiety and cortisol during pregnancy and birth weight of chinese neonates

Fenling Fan[1†], Yuliang Zou[2*†], Yushun Zhang[1], Xiancang Ma[3], Junbo Zhang[1], Cai Liu[2], Jie Li[2], Meili Pei[2], Yu Jiang[2] and Anthony M. Dart[4*]

Abstract

Background: To determine the relationship between maternal anxiety and cortisol values and birth weight at various stages of pregnancy.

Methods: Two hundred sixteen pregnant Chinese women were assessed for anxiety and depression and had measurement of morning fasting serum cortisol. Women were assessed either in the first (71), second (72) or third (73) trimester. Birth weights of all children were recorded.

Results: There were significant negative correlations between anxiety level and birth weight of − 0.507 ($p < 0.01$) and − 0.275 ($p < 0.05$) in trimesters 1and 2. In trimester 3 the negative relation between anxiety and birth weight of −.209 failed to reach significance ($p = 0.070$). There was no relation between depression and birth weight in any trimester ($p > 0.5$ for all). Maternal cortisol was significantly inversely related to birth weight in trimester 1 ($r = -0.322$) and with borderline significance in trimester 2 ($r = -0.229$). Anxiety score and maternal cortisol were significantly correlated in each trimester ($r = 0.551, 0.650, 0.537$). When both anxiety score and maternal cortisol were simultaneously included in multiple regression analyses only anxiety score remained significant.

Conclusion: Whilst both maternal anxiety score and maternal cortisol are inversely related to birth weight the associations with anxiety score were more robust perhaps indicating the importance of mechanisms other than, or in addition to, maternal cortisol in mediating the effects of anxiety. The findings indicate the importance of measures to reduce maternal anxiety, particularly of a severe degree, at all stages of pregnancy.

Keywords: Pregnancy, Anxiety, Cortisol, Trimester, Birth weight

Background

It is well recognised that low birth weight, generally defined as < 2.5 kg (Kg), is associated with deleterious effects in adult life, including increased susceptibility to cardiovascular disease [1–4]. In addition it has been shown that even in the 'normal' birth weight range inverse relationships exist between birth weight and a range of health outcomes such as blood [5] pressure. Thus aside from any immediate consequences of variation in birth weight, understanding the causes of this variation are of importance to health in later life.

A number of factors are known to affect birth weight [6]. These include maternal cigarette smoking, maternal nutrition, foetal abnormalities, maternal diabetes and others. Psychological disturbances are common during pregnancy and can include features of both anxiety and depression. Estimates of their prevalence have varied widely probably depending in part on the nature of the instruments as well maternal background. Studies from the UK reported anxiety in 22% and depressive symptoms in 19% of women during

* Correspondence: zouyuliangfl@126.com; a.dart@alfred.org.au
†Fenling Fan and Yuliang Zou contributed equally to this work.
[2]Department of Gynaecology and Obstetrics, the First Affiliated Hospital of Medical College, Xi'an Jiaotong University, Xi'an 710061, China
[4]Department of Cardiovascular Medicine, The Alfred, Baker Heart and Diabetes Institute, Melbourne, Vic 3004, Australia
Full list of author information is available at the end of the article

pregnancy [7]. Other studies have reported rates of up to 60% for anxiety and 30% for depressive symptoms [8, 9]. A number of studies have examined the relationship between maternal psychological wellbeing and birth outcomes. A majority [10–14], but not all [15, 16] have reported that increased state anxiety in mothers, assessed using a variety of instruments, is associated with prematurity and/or low birth weight. Some studies have found relationships between birth outcomes and stressful life events but not state anxiety [17, 18]. The relationship between maternal state anxiety and distribution of birth weights in term infants has been less well studied with less consistent results [12]. Association between maternal depression and birth outcomes have also been reported [19].

We recently demonstrated an inverse relation between maternal circulating cortisol levels and birth weight [20]. Anxiety is a complex state with multiple physiological associations including changes in levels of stress hormones, activity of the autonomic system and effects on the cardiovascular system including uterine artery resistance [21]. A previous study using foetal biometry reported an inverse association between urinary cortisol and estimated birth weight [12]. Interestingly in this study anxiety state was not significant in multivariate analysis. We have here examined the associations between both anxiety and maternal cortisol and measured birth weight to investigate the extent to which the associations of birth weight with anxiety might be mediated by concomitant changes in maternal cortisol.

Methods

Full details of the cohort have been given previously [20, 22]. In brief, levels of anxiety were assessed by questionnaire in 231 pregnant Chinese women attending a major university hospital for antenatal care. 15 women were lost to follow-up, leaving 216 included in the final data analysis. All gave birth in hospital and birth weight were obtained from hospital records. All women were in their first (only) pregnancy. Women were assessed at a single time point during the first (71), second (72) or third trimester (73). In addition, fasting blood was drawn from the women between 9 am and 11 am for measurement of serum cortisol. Pregnancy duration at time of cortisol measurements (weeks) were 8.4 ± 1.6, 20.9 ± 4.4 and 33.8 ± 3.1. The study was approved by the Ethics Committee, the 1st Affiliated Hospital of Xi'an Jiaotong University. Written informed consent was obtained.

Assessment of anxiety & depression

Anxiety was assessed with The Hamilton Anxiety Scale (HAMA). A psychologist or trained physician asks 14 semi-structured questions, 7 related to psychological anxiety symptoms and 7 related to somatic anxiety symptoms, and then provides a score according to a 5-point scale for each item (0 - Not at all; 1 – Mild; 2 – Moderate; 3 – Severe; 4 - Very Severe). The total scores are used for assessment (Mild Anxiety: 18–25; Moderate Anxiety: 26–30; Severe Anxiety: > 30).

The HAMD is the most widely used outcome scale for depression studies. The 24-item HAMD questionnaire is the most common version used in mainland China scoring 5 points for each item as described for HAMA. The total scores are then used to quantify depression (Mild Depression: 10–19; Moderate Depression: 20–29; Severe Depression: > 30). The two scales were translated and rigorously tested with different populations in mainland China. Their reliability and validity were assessed and approved by the responsible authority (Shanghai Mental Health Center).

Measurement of serum cortisol

Venous blood samples were taken between 9 and 11 am, in the fasting state. The samples were immediately put on ice and the obtained serum was frozen at – 80° centigrade (C). Samples were subsequently thawed for determination of cortisol levels by radioimmunoassay (Jiuding Biotechnology, Tianjin, China) at the hospital chemical pathology department and in accordance with the manufacturer's instructions. Coefficient of variation within each batch was < 5%.

Statistical analysis

Statistical analysis was undertaken with SPSS v19. Group data is presented as mean ± sd. Associations between variables were assessed using Spearman correlation coefficient for correlations involving levels of anxiety and Pearson correlation coefficient for other associations. Multiple regression analysis was performed using stepped entry and removal. Analysis was conducted separately for each trimester to evaluate whether effects of anxiety or cortisol were trimester dependent.

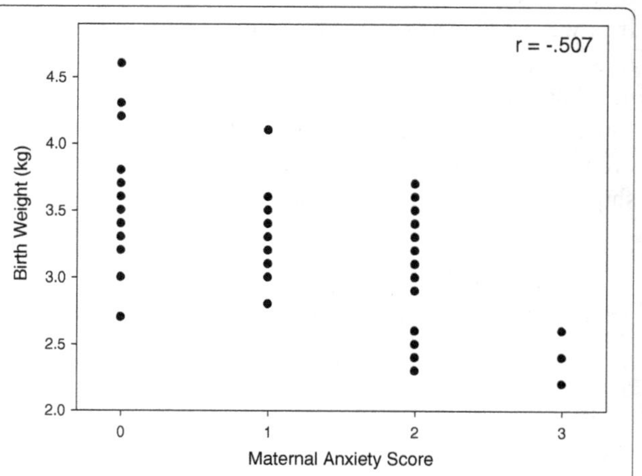

Fig. 1 The figure shows the relationship between maternal anxiety score and birth weight for mothers recruited in the first trimester. r Spearman rank coefficient

Table 1 The Table shows Pearson correlation coefficients (r) between birth weight and maternal serum cortisol separately for each trimester. Respective p values are shown in brackets

	Maternal Cortisol (nmol/l)		
	Trimester 1	Trimester 2	Trimester 3
Birth Weight (Kg)	−0.322 ($p = 0.006$)	−0.229 (0.053)	− 0.192 (0.103)

Results

Mothers were aged 26.4 ± 3.2 years, had pre-pregnancy weight of 53.4 ± 4.0 Kg and height of 160 ± 3.6 cm (cm). All mothers were in their first (only) pregnancy and were from metropolitan areas. All were of Han Chinese ethnicity and gave birth in the first affiliated hospital of Xi'an Jiaotong University. None of the mothers drank alcohol or smoked cigarettes during the pregnancy (and only 4 reported smoking prior to pregnancy), none were diabetic or hypertensive. All pregnancies proceeded to term. Birth weights of the children were 3.25 ± 0.47, 3.36 ± 0.33 and 3.43 ± 0.38 Kg, for those whose mothers were recruited in the first, second and third trimester respectively. There were no significant correlations between pre-pregnancy maternal weight and childrens birth weight (− 0.078) nor between maternal height and childrens birth weight (− 0.082).

Mild, moderate and severely elevated anxiety scores were present in 30.9, 29.5 and 5.6% of mothers recruited in trimester 1, 22.2, 8.3 and 2.7% of mothers recruited in trimester 2 and 32.8, 6.8% and 0% of mothers recruited in trimester 3. Respective rates for anxiety of any degree were 66.0%, 33.2 and 39.6%. Depression of any degree was found in 47, 54.1 and 47.9% for trimesters 1, 2 and 3 respectively. Moderate or severe depression was present in 12.6%, 11.1 and 8.2% of trimester 1, 2 and 3 respectively. Whilst 33.4, 23.6 and 23.2% were found to have both anxiety and depression (of any degree). There were significant negative correlations between anxiety level and birth weight of − 0.507 ($p < 0.01$) and − 0.275 ($p < 0.05$) in trimesters 1 (Fig. 1) and 2. In trimester 3 the negative relation between anxiety and birth weight of −.209 failed to reach significance ($p = 0.070$). However, there were no significant correlations between levels of depression and birth weight in any trimester($p > 0.5$ for all).

Maternal cortisol values were 341 ± 85, 371 ± 66 and 411 ± 7 nmoles/litre (nmol/l) in trimesters 1, 2 and 3 respectively. In order to examine whether the effects of anxiety could be mediated by changes in maternal cortisol we firstly examined the dependence of birth weight on cortisol. As seen in Table 1 there were significant correlations between birth weight and cortisol in the first trimester and borderline significant correlations in the second but not in the third trimester. We then examined whether changes in cortisol were related to levels of anxiety (Table 2, Fig. 2) which was significant for all trimesters.

We then undertook multiple analysis separately for each trimester with birth weight as the dependant variable and including anxiety level, depression level, maternal cortisol, maternal height and maternal weight as independent variable. In these analyses maternal anxiety was the only significant term with all other variables having $p > 0.5$ (Table 3).

Discussion

This study confirms an inverse relation between maternal anxiety and birth weight. As previously reported there was also an inverse relation between maternal cortisol and birth weight [20]. The effects of anxiety and maternal cortisol were more evident in early compared with late pregnancy. This is the first study in which the effects of maternal anxiety and circulating cortisol on measured birth weight were evaluated in the same mothers. As expected there was a strong correlation between anxiety level and circulating cortisol.

The significant association between maternal anxiety and maternal cortisol combined with the association between maternal cortisol and birth weight is compatible with the notion that the effects of anxiety on birth weight are mediated through maternal cortisol in the first and possibly also in the second trimester. However, when both parameters were included in multiple regression analyses only the effects of maternal anxiety remained significant. Whilst this may be an indication that factors other than maternal cortisol mediate (or contribute to) the link between maternal anxiety and birth weight, it might also be an indication that the assessment by questionnaire of anxiety at one time point during pregnancy is a better reflection of the prevailing psychological status of the mother than a single cortisol assessment is of the prevailing level of cortisol. In contrast to the current findings Diego et al. found that urinary cortisol but not anxiety state was predictive of estimated (fetal biometry) birth weight when both were entered into multivariate analysis. Interestingly this

Table 2 The Table shows Spearman rank correlation coefficients (r) between maternal cortisol and anxiety score, separately for each trimester. Respective p values are shown in brackets

	Maternal Cortisol (nmol/l)		
	Trimester 1	Trimester 2	Trimester 3
Maternal Anxiety Score	0.551 ($p < 0.001$)	0.650 ($p < 0.001$)	0.537 ($p < 0.001$)

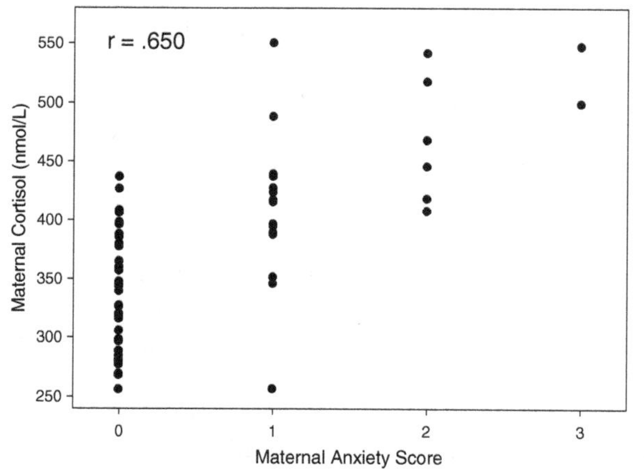

Fig. 2 The figure shows the relationship between maternal anxiety score and maternal cortisol for mothers recruited in the second trimester. r Spearman rank correlation

study was conducted in the second trimester when anxiety is less prevalent [21, 23]. Depression was also common in this cohort but there was no relation between depression and birth weight.

Whilst maternal corticosteroids are subject to the effects of placental 11β hydroxysteroid dehydrogenase type 2 it is known that there is sufficient trans placental transfer of cortisol to affect foetal growth and physiology. Thus hydrocortisone infusion during pregnancy in sheep affects not only foetal growth but also foetal cardiac parameters and blood pressure [24]. Human studies have also reported effects of maternal cortisol on infant neuro and cognitive development [25–28]. Previous studies have indicated that although the placenta itself may be a source of ACTH like peptides maternal ACTH does not appear to access the foetal circulation [29–32].

Other concomitants of heightened anxiety, such as alterations in the maternal autonomic nervous system, might also contribute to the effects of anxiety. Catecholamines in the maternal circulation seem unlikely to access the foetal circulation given the evidence that placental clearance of catecholamines is extensive with significant activity of catechol-O-methyl transferase and monoamine oxidase activity present in placental tissue [33–35]. In addition the placenta is known to contain the noradrenaline uptake transporter [36]. However, there may be effects on placental vascular function leading to impaired foetal growth. Changes in maternal haemodynamic parameters associated with stress may also be relevant. Anxiety in the non-pregnant state has also been associated with a range of other effects including on immune function, circulating cytokines and other hormones which may affect placental function [37–41].

Birth weight is known to be affected by a number of factors in addition to anxiety and it is possible that the effects of anxiety are also mediated by one or more of these [6]. For example, anxiety may be expected to influence maternal nutrition which is a well-recognised factor influencing birth weight. Whilst cigarette smoking is a potent influence on birth weight and will likely be affected by anxiety maternal cigarette smoking will not be a factor in the current study as none of the pregnant women smoked cigarettes during the pregnancy (and indeed very few were cigarette smokers prior to pregnancy). The mothers could have been exposed to second hand cigarette smoke given the high prevalence of cigarette smoking among Chinese males [42] but this was not quantified in the current study. Effects on maternal caffeine and alcohol intake are also not likely to be responsible given the very low consumption of coffee amongst Chinese women and the avoidance of alcohol during pregnancy.

The current study cannot determine whether the anxiety scores determined during pregnancy were representative of the non-pregnant state or were predominantly related to pregnancy as anxiety scores were not available in the mothers at other times. Estimates of the prevalence of anxiety and depression during pregnancy in other cohorts have varied. In a study from the UK anxiety was found in approximately 22% and depression in 19% of women during pregnancy [7]. Studies from Finland and South America have reported anxiety rates of between 16 and 60% [8, 9] whilst overall rates of psychosocial stress 40–84% have been reported amongst pregnant Chinese women [43]. In addition to ethnic or cultural factors these differences most likely also relate to differences in the instruments used to detect and quantify anxiety and depression. However, all

Table 3 The table shows results from multiple regression analyses with birth weight as the dependent variable and including maternal anxiety, maternal depression, maternal cortisol, maternal height, maternal weight as independent variables

Anxiety					
	Overall r	Unstandardised Coefficient		Standardised Coefficient	p
		B	SEM		
Trimester 1	.591	−.300	.049	−.591	< 0.001
Trimester 2	.355	−.154	.049	−.365	0.002
Trimester 3	.373	−.228	.067	−.373	< 0.001

Analysis used stepped entry (PIN 0.05) and removal (POUT 0.1). Anxiety was the only significant independent variable in each of the trimesters. Respective significance values (p) for cortisol were .895, .804 and .887 in trimesters 1, 2 and 3 respectively

studies find anxiety to be common during pregnancy and more prevalent than for women in the non-pregnant state.

Variation in levels of anxiety during pregnancy has also been reported with higher prevalence's in the 1st and 3rd trimesters [23, 44]. In agreement with the findings reported here levels are higher in the 1st than the 3rd trimester in primigravidae.

Conclusion

The findings from this, and other, studies suggest that measures to lessen anxiety during pregnancy may have an effect on birth weight and thus on the health of off-spring in later life. The effects of heightened anxiety appear not to be fully explained by changes in maternal cortisol.

Abbreviations

C: Centigrade; cm: centimetres; Kg: Kilogram; nmol/L: nanomoles/litre; sd: Standard deviation

Acknowledgements

We greatly thank all the participants and their families for their participation in this study.

Funding

Xi'an Science and Technology Project, China (GG04137).
National Nature Science Foundation of China (NSFC 81170294).
Clinic Research Award of First Affiliated Hospital of Xi'an Jiaotong University, China (XJTU1AHCR2014-019).
The funding body was not involved in the design of the study and collection, analysis and interpretation of data and in writing the manuscript.

Authors' contributions

FF: contributed to study design, analysis and interpretation of data. YZ: contributed to study design, acquisition and interpretation of data. YZ: contributed to data analysis and drafting of manuscript. XM: contributed to study design, assessment and analysis of psychological tests. JZ: contributed to data acquisition. CL: contributed to data acquisition. JL: contributed to data collection and analyses. MP: conceived study and contributed to laboratory analyses. YJ: contributed to study design and coordination and helped to draft the manuscript. AD: has made contribution to data analyses, drafting of the manuscript and has given final approval of the version to be published. All authors have read and approved the final version of the manuscript.

Competing interests

The authors declare that they have no competing interests.

Author details

[1]Department of Cardiovascular Medicine, the First Affiliated Hospital of Medical College, Xi'an Jiaotong University, Xi'an 710061, China. [2]Department of Gynaecology and Obstetrics, the First Affiliated Hospital of Medical College, Xi'an Jiaotong University, Xi'an 710061, China. [3]Department of Psychology and Psychiatry, the First Affiliated Hospital of Medical College, Xi'an Jiaotong University, Xi'an 710061, China. [4]Department of Cardiovascular Medicine, The Alfred, Baker Heart and Diabetes Institute, Melbourne, Vic 3004, Australia.

References

1. Barker DJ, Winter PD, Osmond C, Margetts B, Simmonds SJ. Weight in infancy and death from ischaemic heart disease. Lancet. 1989;2(8663):577–80.
2. de Jong F, Monuteaux MC, van Elburg RM, Gillman MW, Belfort MB. Systematic review and meta-analysis of preterm birth and later systolic blood pressure. Hypertension. 2012;59(2):226–34.
3. Lackland DT, Egan BM, Ferguson PL. Low birth weight as a risk factor for hypertension. J Clin Hypertens (Greenwich). 2003;5(2):133–6.
4. Pereira JA, Rondo PH, Lemos JO. Pacheco de Souza JM, Dias RS: the influence of birthweight on arterial blood pressure of children. Clin Nutri. 2010;29(3):337–40.
5. Law CM, Shiell AW. Is blood pressure inversely related to birth weight? The strength of evidence from a systematic review of the literature. J Hypertension. 1996;14(8):935–41.
6. Kramer MS. Determinants of low birth weight: methodological assessment and meta-analysis. Bull World Health Org. 1987;65(5):663–737.
7. Heron J, O'Connor TG, Evans J, Golding J, Glover V, Team AS. The course of anxiety and depression through pregnancy and the postpartum in a community sample. J Affective Disord. 2004;80(1):65–73.
8. Faisal-Cury A, Rossi Menezes P. Prevalence of anxiety and depression during pregnancy in a private setting sample. Archives of Women's Mental Health. 2007;10(1):25–32.
9. Kurki T, Hiilesmaa V, Raitasalo R, Mattila H, Ylikorkala O. Depression and anxiety in early pregnancy and risk for preeclampsia. Obstet Gynecol. 2000; 95(4):487–90.
10. Beydoun H, Saftlas AF. Physical and mental health outcomes of prenatal maternal stress in human and animal studies: a review of recent evidence. Paediatr Perinat Epidemiol. 2008;22(5):438–66.
11. Copper RL, Goldenberg RL, Das A, Elder N, Swain M, Norman G, Ramsey R, Cotroneo P, Collins BA, Johnson F, et al. The preterm prediction study: maternal stress is associated with spontaneous preterm birth at less than thirty-five weeks' gestation. National Institute of Child Health and Human Development maternal-fetal medicine units network. Am J Obstet Gynecol. 1996;175(5):1286–92.
12. Diego MA, Jones NA, Field T, Hernandez-Reif M, Schanberg S, Kuhn C, Gonzalez-Garcia A. Maternal psychological distress, prenatal cortisol, and fetal weight. Psychosom Med. 2006;68(5):747–53.
13. Ding XX, Wu YL, Xu SJ, Zhu RP, Jia XM, Zhang SF, Huang K, Zhu P, Hao JH, Tao FB. Maternal anxiety during pregnancy and adverse birth outcomes: a systematic review and meta-analysis of prospective cohort studies. J Affective Disord. 2014;159:103–10.
14. Rondo PH, Ferreira RF, Nogueira F, Ribeiro MC, Lobert H, Artes R. Maternal psychological stress and distress as predictors of low birth weight, prematurity and intrauterine growth retardation. Eur J Clin Nutr. 2003;57(2):266–72.
15. Andersson L, Sundstrom-Poromaa I, Wulff M, Astrom M, Bixo M. Neonatal outcome following maternal antenatal depression and anxiety: a population-based study. Am J Epidemiol. 2004;159(9):872–81.
16. Sjostrom K, Valentin L, Thelin T, Marsal K. Maternal anxiety in late pregnancy and fetal hemodynamics. Eur J Obstet Gynecol Reprod Biol. 1997;74(2):149–55.
17. Dancause KN, Laplante DP, Oremus C, Fraser S, Brunet A, King S. Disaster-related prenatal maternal stress influences birth outcomes: project ice storm. Early Human Dev. 2011;87(12):813–20.
18. Newton RW, Hunt LP. Psychosocial stress in pregnancy and its relation to low birth weight. Br Med J (Clin Res Ed). 1984;288(6425):1191–4.
19. Grote NK, Bridge JA, Gavin AR, Melville JL, Iyengar S, Katon WJ. A meta-analysis of depression during pregnancy and the risk of preterm birth, low birth weight, and intrauterine growth restriction. Arch Gen Psychiatry. 2010; 67(10):1012–24.
20. Fan F, Zou Y, Zhang Y, Zhang J, Ma X, Liu Y, Geng J, Li J, Liu K, Dart AM. Effects of maternal cortisol during pregnancy on Children's blood pressure responses. Neuroendocrinology. 2016;103(3–4):282–90.
21. Teixeira JM, Fisk NM, Glover V. Association between maternal anxiety in pregnancy and increased uterine artery resistance index: cohort based study. BMJ. 1999;318(7177):153–7.

22. Fan F, Zou Y, Tian H, Zhang Y, Zhang J, Ma X, Meng Y, Yue Y, Liu K, Dart AM. Effects of maternal anxiety and depression during pregnancy in Chinese women on children's heart rate and blood pressure response to stress. J Hum Hypertens. 2016;30(3):171–6.
23. Lee AM, Lam SK. Sze Mun Lau SM, Chong CS, Chui HW, Fong DY: prevalence, course, and risk factors for antenatal anxiety and depression. Obstet Gynecol. 2007;110(5):1102–12.
24. Jensen EC, Gallaher BW, Breier BH, Harding JE. The effect of a chronic maternal cortisol infusion on the late-gestation fetal sheep. J Endocrinol. 2002;174(1):27–36.
25. Talge NM, Neal C, Glover V, Early Stress TR. Prevention science network F, neonatal experience on C, adolescent mental H: antenatal maternal stress and long-term effects on child neurodevelopment: how and why? J Child Psychol Psychiat Allied Dis. 2007;48(3–4):245–61.
26. de Weerth C, van Hees Y, Buitelaar JK. Prenatal maternal cortisol levels and infant behavior during the first 5 months. Early Hum Dev. 2003;74(2):139–51.
27. Davis EP, Sandman CA. The timing of prenatal exposure to maternal cortisol and psychosocial stress is associated with human infant cognitive development. Child Dev. 2010;81(1):131–48.
28. Bergman K, Sarkar P, Glover V, O'Connor TG. Maternal prenatal cortisol and infant cognitive development: moderation by infant-mother attachment. Biol Psychiatry. 2010;67(11):1026–32.
29. Allen JP, Cook DM, Kendall JW, McGilvra R. Maternal-fetal ACTH relationship in man. J Clin Endocrinol Metab. 1973;37(2):230–4.
30. Frim DM, Emanuel RL, Robinson BG, Smas CM, Adler GK, Majzoub JA. Characterization and gestational regulation of corticotropin-releasing hormone messenger RNA in human placenta. J Clin Invest. 1988;82(1):287–92.
31. Migeon CJ, Prystowsky H, Grumbach MM, Byron MC. Placental passage of 17-hydroxycorticosteroids: comparison of the levels in maternal and fetal plasma and effect of ACTH and hydrocortisone administration. J Clin Invest. 1956;35(5):488–93.
32. Miyakawa I, Ikeda I, Maeyama M. Transport of ACTH across human placenta. J Clin Endocrinol Metab. 1974;39(3):440–2.
33. Barnea ER, MacLusky NJ, DeCherney AH, Naftolin F. Catechol-o-methyl transferase activity in the human term placenta. Am J Perinatol. 1988;5(2):121–7.
34. Bzoskie L, Blount L, Kashiwai K, Tseng YT, Hay WW Jr, Padbury JF. Placental norepinephrine clearance: in vivo measurement and physiological role. Am J Phys. 1995;269(1 Pt 1):E145–9.
35. Saarikoski S. Fate of noradrenaline in the human foetoplacental unit. Acta Physiol Scand Suppl. 1974;421:1–82.
36. Ramamoorthy S, Prasad PD, Kulanthaivel P, Leibach FH, Blakely RD, Ganapathy V. Expression of a cocaine-sensitive norepinephrine transporter in the human placental syncytiotrophoblast. Biochemistry. 1993;32(5):1346–53.
37. Arranz L, Guayerbas N, De la Fuente M. Impairment of several immune functions in anxious women. J Psychosom Res. 2007;62(1):1–8.
38. Kiecolt-Glaser JK, McGuire L, Robles TF, Glaser R. Psychoneuroimmunology: psychological influences on immune function and health. J Consult Clin Psychol. 2002;70(3):537–47.
39. Maes M, Song C, Lin A, De Jongh R, Van Gastel A, Kenis G, Bosmans E, De Meester I, Benoy I, Neels H, et al. The effects of psychological stress on humans: increased production of pro-inflammatory cytokines and a Th1-like response in stress-induced anxiety. Cytokine. 1998;10(4):313–8.
40. Pitsavos C, Panagiotakos DB, Papageorgiou C, Tsetsekou E, Soldatos C, Stefanadis C. Anxiety in relation to inflammation and coagulation markers, among healthy adults: the ATTICA study. Atherosclerosis. 2006;185(2):320–6.
41. Zakowski SG, McAllister CG, Deal M, Baum A. Stress, reactivity, and immune function in healthy men. Health Psychol. 1992;11(4):223–32.
42. Li Q, Hsia J, Yang G. Prevalence of smoking in China in 2010. N Engl J Med. 2011;364(25):2469–70.
43. Gou W-L, Wu LF: Delivery Science [in Chinese]. 1st Editorial Beijing, China: republic Health Press 2003:625–628.
44. Teixeira C, Figueiredo B, Conde A, Pacheco A, Costa R. Anxiety and depression during pregnancy in women and men. J Affective Dis. 2009; 119(1–3):142–8.

10

Inequalities in maternal health care utilization in Benin

Sanni Yaya[1*], Olalekan A. Uthman[2], Agbessi Amouzou[3], Michael Ekholuenetale[4] and Ghose Bishwajit[1]

Abstract

Background: Ensuring equitable access to maternal health care including antenatal, delivery, postnatal services and fertility control methods, is one of the most critical challenges for public health sector. There are significant disparities in maternal health care indicators across many geographical locations, maternal, economic, socio-demographic factors in many countries in sub-Sahara Africa. In this study, we comparatively explored the utilization level of maternal health care, and examined disparities in the determinants of major maternal health outcomes.

Methods: This paper used data from two rounds of Benin Demographic and Health Survey (BDHS) to examine the utilization and disparities in factors of maternal health care indicators using logistic regression models. Participants were 17,794 and 16,599 women aged between15–49 years in 2006 and 2012 respectively. Women's characteristics were reported in percentage, mean and standard deviation.

Results: Mean (±SD) age of the participants was 29.0 (±9.0) in both surveys. The percentage of at least 4 ANC visits was approximately 61% without any change between the two rounds of surveys, facility based delivery was 93.5% in 2012, with 4.9% increase from 2006; postnatal care was currently 18.4% and contraceptive use was estimated below one-fifth. The results of multivariable logistic regression models showed disparities in maternal health care service utilization, including antenatal care, facility-based delivery, postnatal care and contraceptive use across selected maternal factors. The current BHDS showed age, region, religion were significantly associated with maternal health care services. Educated women, those from households of high wealth index and women currently working were more likely to utilize maternal health care services, compared to women with no formal education, from poorest households or not currently employed. Women who watch television (TV) were 1.31 (OR = 1.31; 95% CI = 1.13–1.52), 1.69 (OR = 1.69; 95% CI = 1.20–2.37) and 1.38 (OR = 1.38; 95% CI = 1.16–1.65) times as likely to utilize maternal health care services after adjusting for other covariates.

Conclusion: The findings would guide stakeholders to address inequalities in maternal health care services. More so, health care programmes and policies should be strengthened to enhance accessibility as well as improve the utilization of maternal care services, especially for the disadvantaged, uneducated and those who live in hard-to-reach rural areas in Benin. The Benin government needs to create strategies that cover both the supply and demand side factors at attain the universal health coverage.

Keywords: Antenatal care, Postnatal care, Contraceptive use, Institutional delivery, Inequalities, Benin, Demographic and health survey, Cross-sectional study

* Correspondence: sanni.yaya@uOttawa.ca
[1]School of International Development and Global Studies, University of Ottawa, Ottawa, Canada
Full list of author information is available at the end of the article

Background

The steps towards achieving the third United Nations (UN) Sustainable Development Goals (SDGs), to reduce maternal morbidity and mortality and achieve universal health coverage to include access to essential health care services by 2030 have been a great issue in developing countries, even with the existence of health care interventions. Though there are numerous health care implementation projects to promote safe motherhood worldwide, maternal morbidity and mortality remain a notable hitch in health care programme and policy making particularly in low-income countries. In spite of the vast efforts by the global community to lessen the burden of mortality as a result of pregnancy and delivery, the rate of death due to pregnancy related complications is worrisome [1]. Developing countries have been reported to account for about 99% of the global maternal mortality, while sub-Saharan Africa (SSA) countries record approximately 62% and having Maternal Mortality Ratio (MMR) of 510 maternal deaths per 100,000 live births [2, 3]. The challenge of unfair distribution of health care services is gaining global attention in the area of public health, with evidence of the disadvantaged sections of the society, having worst health conditions [1]. Like other sub-Saharan countries, Benin is having an unfair share in maternal health care. A country with Total Fertility Rate (TFR) of 5.3, is ranked the 34th in the world with maternal death [4].

Inadequate of access to antenatal, intrapartum and postnatal health care services are among the prominent reasons for high maternal and child morbidities and mortalities in SSA and the world at large [5, 6]. Maternal health care services continue to be important indicators for monitoring the improvement of maternal health outcomes, as well as maternal mortality. In addition, antenatal care, institutional health delivery with skilled birth attendant, and postnatal care strengthen prompt management and treatment of pregnancy related complications to reduce maternal mortality. Besides the benefits of institutional based delivery in the prevention of maternal death, more women give birth utilizing alternative places such as home and Traditional Birth Attendants (TBA) who are not knowledgeable in modern obstetric care [7]. One of the major pillars of the Safe Motherhood Initiative is antenatal care, which helps to provide interventions that are essential for positive pregnancy outcomes [8]. World Health Organization (WHO) remark that receiving antenatal care not less than four times increases the odds of receiving valuable health care promotion and preventive maternal health care interventions during antenatal visits [9, 10]. Furthermore, family planning is also a vital indicator of the Safe Motherhood Initiative to reduce pregnancy related complications and death in developing countries [10].

Essential emergency obstetric health care services are required to access key equitable resources across regions, socio-economic strata and geographical locations [11]. Maternal health care services encompass a wide range of clinical procedures and care provided to women during pregnancy. As a matter of necessity, all pregnant women should have access to quality antenatal care regardless of their economic, cultural, geographical and social background. Interestingly, antenatal care performs a crucial role in ensuring a healthy baby and mother during pregnancy and after delivery. This care is given to pregnant women to optimize quality health outcomes, such as normal birth weight, reduction in maternal and child death and low postpartum anemia [12]. More so, countries that have achieved success in improving maternal health care services and reducing maternal morbidity mortality overall, are still faced with the challenges of large inequities among various sections of the populations. The groups of women that are disadvantaged tend to have more morbidity and mortality, and inadequate access to safe motherhood services, acceptable and affordable health care services to enhance safe pregnancy and delivery [13]. Efforts have been made to reduce health inequities across all facets of the populations, on subnational, national and global levels, and ensure equal opportunities to all members of communities to achieve good health [14]. However, most health care systems are inequitable, benefiting the wealthy than the underprivileged [15].

There are significant disparities in maternal health care indicators across many geographical locations, maternal, economic, socio-demographic factors in many developing countries [16]. Whereas equity has been indicated as a prominent target within the health sectors, huge disparities exist in coverage of maternal and child health care services between the well-off and disadvantaged in low income countries. The inequalities and inequities across various strata of the society have become key determinants of maternal and child health [17, 18]. Obtaining equal access to maternal health care including antenatal, delivery and postnatal services, is one of the most critical concerns in public health programmes and policies shared in virtually everywhere in the world, and demands that women with the same maternal needs should receive the same access to health care services [19].

In this study, inequities in the determinants of major maternal health outcomes including antenatal care, institutional delivery with skilled birth attendance and utilization of modern contraception were examined using Benin Demographic and Health Survey (BDHS) dataset. We presented comparative analyses of the outcome variables in two separate BDHS to assess disparities in the utilization of these services.

Methods

Data extraction

Data for this study were derived from two rounds of Demographic and Health Survey in Benin that provided information on antenatal care, institutional delivery and contraceptive use. The datasets have one record for every eligible woman as defined by the household schedule. The questionnaire contains all the data collected from the individual woman for whom information on antenatal care, delivery and contraceptive usage and some variables from the household were elicited. The 2006 and 2012 Benin Demographic and Health Survey (BDHS) data contains 17,794 and 16,599 cases (units of analysis), which in this file is the woman. BDHS performed cross-sectional analyses using nationally representative data, to collect information on demographic, health, and nutrition indicators. The survey is majorly funded by the United States Agency for International Development (USAID). The two rounds of BDHS utilized a multi-stage, stratified sampling design, with households as the sampling unit. Within each sample household, all eligible women were interviewed [20].

Outcome variables

In this study, we used four outcome measures of maternal health care utilization extracted from the BDHS. Firstly, we derived the; "number of antenatal care (ANC) visits during pregnancy", this was grouped as 4 or more ANC visits vs below 4 ANC visits. ANC visits is a measure of skilled pregnancy care received by women during most recent pregnancy. Secondly, we extracted the "place of delivery (home vs health facility)". This was measured as a binary outcome for 1, if a woman delivered in a health facility (where skilled delivery attention is available) and 0, if otherwise. In addition, postnatal care was measured by "respondents health's checked after discharge/delivery at home" Lastly, women's "contraceptive use"; was obtained as binary indicator taking 1 if the "woman ever used a contraceptive method" and 0, if otherwise.

Explanatory variables

The utilization of ANC visits, facility-based delivery and contraceptive use are known to depend on a set of determinants, such as demographic, economic, other proximate and social factors. Empirical literature on the factors pertinent to maternal health care services basically helped to select the variables of study. These variables age of individual woman (15–19, 20–24, 25–29, 30–34, 35–39, 40–44 and 45–49 year), geographical region (Alibori, Atacora, Atlantique, Borgou, Collines, Couffo, Donga, Littoral, Mono, Queme, Plateau and Zou), type of residence (rural vs urban). Educational attainment was categorized as those having no formal education, primary, secondary and higher education. Religious beliefs included; Christianity, Islam, traditional and other religion, while access to health information was measured using frequency of reading newspaper or magazine, listening to radio and watching TV. The wealth scores is obtained by principal components analysis, based on a list of household assets as specified by DHS, which include, number of household members, wall and roof materials, floor types, access to potable water and sanitation, type of cooking fuel, ownership of television, radio, motorcycle, refrigerator amongst others. Based on the weighted wealth scores, households were grouped into five wealth quintiles; poorest, poorer, middle, richer and richest. Furthermore, parity was measured by the number of children ever born by each individual woman; categorized as 1–4 and > 4 children.

Ethical considerations

We did the analyses using publicly available data from demographic health surveys. Ethical procedures were the responsibility of the institutions that commissioned, funded, or managed the surveys. All DHS surveys are approved by ICF international as well as an Institutional Review Board (IRB) in respective country to ensure that the protocols are in compliance with the U.S. Department of Health and Human Services regulations for the protection of human subjects.

Statistical analysis

Summary statistics including percentage and means (±standard deviation) were used to examine the distribution of socio-demographic, economic distal and proximate maternal characteristics. To adjust for data representation, we used complex survey module (svyset) for all analyses to account for clustering, stratification and sample weight. In addition, the percentages of outcome variables were presented in bar chart. The factors associated with ANC visits, facility-based delivery, postnatal care and contraceptive use were examined using logistic regression models. The bivariate analysis conducted to examine the factors that were added in the multivariable regression models involved a simple regression with each explanatory variable. Therefore, factors, which were statistically significant in the crude regression models, were added in the multivariable regression models to adjust for possible confounders. An α level of 0.05 was considered statistically significant. All analyses were conducted using STATA 14.0.

Results

Sample characteristics

In this study, the characteristics of respondents were explored for 2006 and 2012 respectively. The mean ages of respondents were similar (29.0 ± 9.1/9.0) between the years of survey. The basic socio-demographic characteristics of the respondents were presented in Table 1.

Table 1 Characteristics of respondents. Benin DHS 2006–12

Variable	2006		2012	
	n (17,794)	%	*n* (16,599)	%
Age (Mean ± SD)	29.0 ± 9.1		29.0 ± 9.0	
15–19	3036	17.1	2922	17.6
20–24	3117	17.5	2820	17.0
25–29	3640	20.5	3147	19.0
30–34	2801	15.7	2720	16.4
35–39	2151	12.1	2185	13.2
40–44	1626	9.1	1667	10.0
45–49	1423	8.0	1138	6.9
Region				
Alibori	1197	6.7	1000	6.0
Atacora	1506	8.5	1476	8.9
Atlantique	1988	11.2	1866	11.2
Borgou	1535	8.6	1323	8.0
Collines	1234	6.9	1256	7.6
Couffo	1530	8.6	1225	7.4
Donga	893	5.0	950	5.7
Littoral	1831	10.3	1949	11.7
Mono	1196	6.7	1043	6.3
Quémé	2142	12.0	1811	10.9
Plateau	862	4.8	1046	6.3
Zou	1880	10.6	1654	10.0
Type of place of residence				
Urban	7471	42.0	7070	42.6
Rural	10,323	58.0	9529	57.4
Educational attainment				
No formal education	11,577	65.1	10,383	62.6
Primary	3460	19.4	2766	16.7
Secondary	2595	14.6	3219	19.4
Higher	162	0.9	231	1.4
Religion				
Christianity	9484	53.4	9226	55.6
Islam	3878	21.8	3919	23.6
Traditional	3178	17.9	2284	13.8
Others	1210	6.8	1170	7.0
Read newspaper/magazine				
Yes	1701	9.6	2140	12.9
No	15,957	90.4	14,459	87.1
Listen to radio				
Yes	14,499	81.7	10,525	63.4
No	3257	18.3	6074	36.6
Watch TV				
Yes	6398	36.1	7556	45.5
No	11,320	63.9	9043	54.5

Table 1 Characteristics of respondents. Benin DHS 2006–12 *(Continued)*

Variable	2006		2012	
	n (17,794)	%	*n* (16,599)	%
Wealth index				
Poorest	3357	18.9	3139	18.9
Poorer	3347	18.8	3274	19.7
Middle	3448	19.4	3433	20.7
Richer	3753	21.1	3511	21.2
Richest	3889	21.9	3242	19.5
Parity				
1–4	8379	60.7	8377	66.9
> 4	5435	39.3	4145	33.1
Women decision making power				
Low	4140	35.1	2534	35.4
Moderate	7664	64.9	2741	38.2
High			1892	26.4
Currently working				
Yes	14,114	79.6	10,643	64.1
No	3628	20.4	5956	35.9
Sex of household head				
Male	14,353	80.7	13,326	80.1
Female	3441	19.3	3273	19.7

Prevalence of maternal health care utilization.

In this study, four outcomes were measured namely; antenatal care of at least 4 visits, facility-based delivery, postnatal care and utilization of contraceptive methods. The percentage of 4 or more antenatal visits was 61.4% in 2006, and 61.1% in 2012, which showed that there was no increase in the level of antenatal care visits over time. Facility-based delivery was reported as 88.6% in 2006 which had 4.9% increase by 2012. Postnatal care 15.2% in 2006, but increased to 18.4% in 2012. Further, the percentage of contraceptive use was 17.2% in 2006, however reduced to 14% in 2016 (see Fig. 1 for details).

The results showed that women aged 35–49 years had increase in the odds of facility-based delivery, compared to women aged 15–19 years. Further, women aged 45–49 years had 45% significant reduction in the odds of contraceptive use, compared to women aged 15–19 years after adjusting for other covariates (OR = 0.55; 95% CI = 0.33–0.93). Also, geographical region was significantly associated with ANC visits, facility-based, postnatal care and contraceptive use. Rural women had 17% reduction in the odds of contraceptive use, compared to the urban women after adjusting for other covariates (OR = 0.83; 95% CI = 0.70–0.98). Educated women were more likely to utilize ANC visits, facility-based and postnatal care,

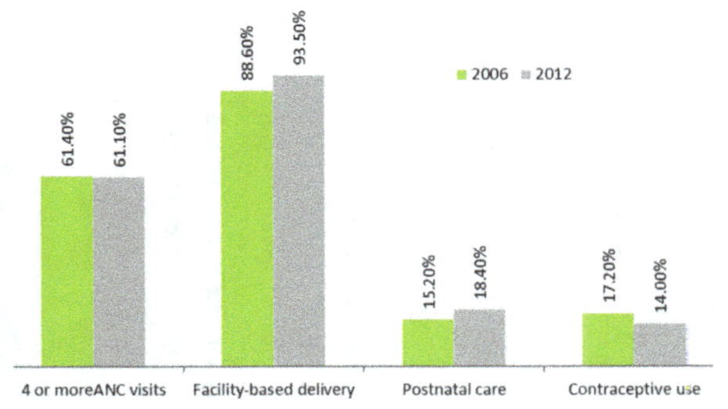

Fig. 1 Prevalence of antenatal care, contraceptive use and facility-based delivery among women of reproductive age in Benin

compared to women with no formal education after adjusting for other covariates.

Women with higher wealth index had significant increase in the odds of adequate ANC visits, facility-based delivery and contraceptive use. Number of children ever born was significantly associated with maternal health care services; women who had above 4 children had significant reduction in adequate ANC visits and facility-based delivery respectively, compared to women who had 1–4 children (ANC- OR = 0.71; 95% CI = 0.61–0.82; facility-based delivery- OR = 0.59; 95% CI = 0.48–0.72). Notwithstanding, women who had above 4 children were 1.48 times as likely to have contraceptive use, compared to women who had 1–4 children (OR = 1.48; 95% CI = 1.27–1.71). Women with moderate decision-making power were 1.26 times as likely to have contraceptive use, compared to women with low decision-making power. Also, women from female headed households were 1.58 times more likely to utilize facility-based delivery, compared to women from male headed households (OR = 1.58; 95% CI = 1.18–2.11). See Table 2 for details.

For 2012, women aged 45–49 years had higher odds of facility-based, compared to women aged 15–19 years after adjusting for other covariates. Respondents aged 35–44 years also had increase in the odds of contraceptive use, compared to those aged 15–19 years. The region and religion of respondents was significantly associated with adequate ANC visits, facility-based delivery, postnatal care and contraceptive use. The respondents with high decision-making power were 1.47 times as likely to have facility-based delivery, compared to women with low decision-making power after adjusting for other covariates (OR = 1.47; 95% CI = 1.03–2.10). Further, women who were currently working or employed had higher odds of ANC visits, facility-based delivery and contraceptive use. Women from female headed households were 2.04 times as likely to have facility-based delivery, compared to other counterpart after adjusting for other covariates (OR = 2.04; 95% CI = 1.14–3.67).

Discussion

Main findings

This study has become the foremost to explore and examine prominent indicators of maternal health care service utilization in Benin, and thus utilized two rounds of nationally representative data set from 2006 and 2012 surveys. The main outcome measures under study were ANC visits, institutional delivery, postnatal care and contraceptive use among women of reproductive age. The prevalence of ANC at least 4 or more visits, facility-based delivery, postnatal care and contraceptive use among women of reproductive age were relatively the same in both rounds of survey. The estimates are consistent with literature from other sub-Saharan Africa countries where maternal health care indicators need more improvement [21–23]. Furthermore, socio-demographic, economic and proximate determinants were the main predictors of maternal healthcare services. Age, geographical region, place of residence, level of education, religious beliefs, use of media, wealth index and parity were significant predictors for the disparity in access to skilled pregnancy care and fertility control [22–25].

In addition, this study found disparities in the demographic, social, economic and proximate factors associated with the utilization of maternal health care services. The SDGs are known to support reduction in inequalities and ensure health for all populations. In the light of the above, beyond the utilization of maternal health care, also to reach the most disadvantaged group of the women, vis-a-vis the use of maternal care services must be considered to achieve the set goals [26]. The findings in this study showed that women with lower educational level, inaccessibility of the media (newspaper, radio and television), low economic class, rural dwellers amongst others are less likely to utilize maternal healthcare services. This revealed disproportionate share of maternal healthcare services by certain class of people despite of the high demand. The results were in line with previous studies in other countries [27–30].

Though there are interventions to improve coverage of maternal and child health care services in sub-Saharan Africa, the disparity in access and use by several factors such as place of residence, use of media, geographical region, educational attainment, age of women and wealth quintile amongst others has remained persistently high in the two rounds of data utilized [30, 31]. Explaining differentials in accessing maternal and reproductive care services is a critical issue, because several other contributory factors, including distance, cultural beliefs or practices, health care seeking behavior, affordability and need for services must also be considered [31]. The findings of this study were consistent with previous studies that reported that improvement in economic status was connected to better use of maternal health

Table 2 Odds ratios antenatal care visits, skilled birth delivery and contraceptive use for the years 2006 and 2012

Variable	ANC		Facility-based delivery		Postnatal care		Contraceptive use	
	2006	2012	2006	2012	2006	2012	2006	2012
Age								
15–19	1.00	1.00	1.00	1.00	1.00	1.00	1.00	1.00
20–24	0.95 (0.69–1.29)	1.19 (0.93–1.52)	0.95 (0.62–1.47)	0.83 (0.31–2.22)	0.90 (0.61–1.33)	0.89 (0.54–1.48)	1.10 (0.69–1.75)	1.04 (0.85–1.28)
25–29	0.92 (0.68–1.26)	1.25 (0.98–1.58)	1.25 (0.83–1.88)	0.84 (0.32–2.21)	0.83 (0.57–1.21)	1.12 (0.70–1.79)	1.06 (0.67–1.68)	1.19 (0.97–1.47)
30–34	1.07 (0.77–1.49)	1.08 (0.85–1.37)	1.49 (0.96–2.32)	0.67 (0.23–1.91)	0.87 (0.58–1.29)	1.09 (0.67–1.77)	1.10 (0.68–1.77)	1.04 (0.83–1.29)
35–39	1.20 (0.85–1.69)	1.05 (0.82–1.35)	1.81 (1.10–2.97)	1.21 (0.42–3.50)	1.04 (0.67–1.59)	1.25 (0.76–2.04)	1.10 (0.67–1.80)	1.33 (1.06–1.68)
40–44	1.12 (0.76–1.66)	1.08 (0.81–1.43)	3.45 (1.96–6.10)	1.41 (0.48–4.18)	0.70 (0.43–1.15)	1.14 (0.64–2.01)	0.92 (0.56–1.52)	1.31 (1.04–1.65)
45–49	1.07 (0.72–1.59)	1.29 (0.86–1.94)	8.39 (4.74–14.83)	14.5 (3.55–59.41)	0.91 (0.52–1.61)	0.59 (0.25–1.37)	0.55 (0.33–0.93)	0.90 (0.69–1.16)
Region								
Alibori	1.00	1.00	1.00	1.00	1.00	1.00	1.00	1.00
Atacora	1.56 (0.99–2.46)	1.09 (0.73–1.60)	1.68 (0.99–2.82)	1.07 (0.49–2.33)	1.29 (0.70–2.38)	2.72 (1.59–4.66)	1.98 (1.16–3.36)	1.53 (0.79–2.96)
Atlantique	3.14 (2.01–4.92)	0.87 (1.29–2.71)	31.1 (15.64–61.85)	5.37 (2.52–11.41)	0.22 (0.10–0.45)	1.43 (0.89–2.32)	5.18 (3.03–8.86)	0.81 (0.48–1.37)
Borgou	1.69 (1.02–2.80)	0.93 (0.65–1.34)	1.14 (0.65–2.00)	0.97 (0.54–1.72)	0.37 (0.20–0.71)	2.85 (1.71–4.74)	1.63 (0.95–2.81)	1.61 (1.02–2.55)
Collines	2.02 (1.28–3.19)	1.30 (0.87–1.94)	5.63 (2.96–10.69)	3.39 (1.38–8.36)	0.91 (0.47–1.75)	3.77 (2.82–6.24)	5.12 (3.04–8.64)	1.67 (0.96–2.92)
Couffo	1.55 (0.98–2.43)	2.07 (1.39–3.11)	2.64 (1.51–4.63)	1.78 (0.76–4.19)	1.04 (0.52–2.10)	1.29 (0.72–2.32)	1.67 (0.94–2.96)	1.58 (0.95–2.62)
Donga	1.57 (0.97–2.55)	0.92 (0.61–1.39)	1.85 (1.01–3.82)	1.46 (0.61–3.53)	1.80 (1.01–3.21)	1.60 (0.86–3.00)	1.04 (0.59–1.84)	0.47 (0.26–0.84)
Littoral	3.88 (2.24–6.73)	1.49 (0.98–2.26)	7.80 (3.13–19.14)	1.50 (0.46–4.89)	1.29 (0.53–3.13)	2.27 (1.36–3.80)	2.69 (1.57–4.62)	1.32 (0.81–2.17)
Mono	2.32 (1.44–3.72)	2.74 (1.77–4.24)	9.24 (4.46–19.14)	14.75 (4.74–45.88)	1.23 (0.63–2.42)	2.47 (1.41–4.32)	1.55 (0.89–2.72)	0.39 (0.22–0.67)
Quémé	2.60 (1.69–3.99)	2.84 (1.94–4.18)	28.60 (14.52–56.33)	35.33 (4.67–267.4)	0.41 (0.20–0.85)	2.30 (1.46–3.63)	3.00 (1.81–4.96)	0.62 (0.38–0.99)
Plateau	2.07 (1.31–3.29)	0.74 (0.49–1.13)	4.38 (2.46–7.81)	1.38 (0.61–3.12)	0.77 (0.35–1.70)	1.83 (0.76–4.40)	0.98 (0.53–1.81)	1.33 (0.79–2.24)
Zou	2.85 (1.81–4.49)	2.42 (1.64–3.55)	19.49 (10.48–36.24)	8.47 (3.66–19.61)	0.57 (0.28–1.17)	1.03 (0.61–1.73)	1.96 (1.15–3.32)	1.32 (0.78–2.23)
Type of place of residence								
Urban	1.00	1.00	1.00	1.00	1.00	1.00	1.00	1.00
Rural	1.02 (0.86–1.24)	1.01 (0.85–1.19)	0.93 (0.64–1.34)	0.68 (0.42–1.10)	0.82 (0.61–1.10)	0.86 (0.67–1.09)	0.83 (0.70–0.98)	1.17 (0.94–1.47)
Educational attainment								
No formal education	1.00	1.00	1.00	1.00	1.00	1.00	1.00	1.00
Primary	1.29 (1.08–1.53)	1.63 (1.39–1.92)	2.12 (1.56–2.89)	1.97 (1.20–3.26)	1.04 (0.75–1.45)	0.91 (0.68–1.23)	1.42 (1.22–1.65)	1.33 (1.14–1.56)
Secondary	1.28 (0.91–1.79)	2.13 (1.69–2.68)	5.79 (1.89–17.72)	3.40 (1.25–9.24)	1.08 (0.57–2.08)	1.12 (0.75–1.68)	1.95 (1.59–2.38)	1.87 (1.55–2.25)
Higher		2.60 (0.90–7.54)			15.35 (0.95–247.2)	1.16 (0.24–5.55)	1.16 (0.68–1.97)	2.09 (1.35–3.26)

Table 2 Odds ratios antenatal care visits, skilled birth delivery and contraceptive use for the years 2006 and 2012 *(Continued)*

Variable	ANC		Facility-based delivery		Postnatal care		Contraceptive use	
	2006	2012	2006	2012	2006	2012	2006	2012
Religion								
Christianity	1.00	1.00	1.00	1.00	1.00	1.00	1.00	1.00
Islam	0.76 (0.61–0.95)	0.80 (0.67–0.96)	0.60 (0.45–0.81)	0.59 (0.39–0.90)	0.84 (0.55–1.29)	0.87 (0.68–1.12)	0.83 (0.68–1.02)	1.29 (1.08–1.55)
Traditional	0.81 (0.67–0.97)	0.68 (0.57–0.82)	0.48 (0.35–0.64)	0.57 (0.32–1.02)	1.30 (0.97–1.75)	1.07 (0.77–1.49)	0.86 (0.69–1.08)	0.80 (0.63–0.99)
Others	0.80 (0.64–0.98)	0.70 (0.56–0.88)	0.53 (0.39–0.73)	0.56 (0.34–0.92)	1.33 (0.91–1.94)	0.84 (0.58–1.3)	0.71 (0.55–0.92)	0.64 (0.46–0.88)
Read newspaper/magazine	1.19 (0.78–1.82)	0.89 (0.68–1.16)	0.85 (0.37–1.94)	0.62 (0.22–1.76)	1.07 (0.53–2.18)	1.31 (0.83–2.05)	1.46 (1.17–1.81)	0.89 (0.75–1.07)
Listen to radio	1.36 (1.17–1.57)	0.96 (0.84–1.10)	1.38 (1.13–1.70)	1.29 (0.93–1.78)	0.98 (0.76–1.26)	1.06 (0.83–1.36)	1.39 (1.14–1.68)	1.16 (1.01–1.34)
Watch TV	1.39 (1.18–1.63)	1.31 (1.13–1.52)	1.49 (1.13–1.97)	1.69 (1.20–2.37)	1.56 (1.13–2.15)	0.99 (0.79–1.23)	1.28 (1.08–1.52)	1.38 (1.16–1.65)
Wealth index								
Poorest	1.00	1.00	1.00	1.00	1.00	1.00	1.00	1.00
Poorer	1.39 (1.18–1.63)	1.36 (1.15–1.60)	2.02 (1.67–2.45)	1.55 (1.13–2.13)	1.22 (0.95–1.56)	0.82 (0.61–1.10)	1.27 (1.01–1.60)	1.06 (0.83–1.34)
Middle	1.86 (1.58–2.20)	1.78 (1.51–2.11)	2.97 (2.38–3.72)	2.36 (1.63–3.43)	0.95 (0.72–1.25)	0.91 (0.67–1.22)	1.40 (1.11–1.76)	1.19 (0.94–1.51)
Richer	2.64 (2.19–3.17)	2.62 (2.15–3.20)	7.36 (5.31–10.18)	7.14 (4.08–12.49)	1.06 (0.76–1.48)	0.86 (0.61–1.23)	1.48 (1.16–1.87)	1.10 (0.85–1.43)
Richest	5.19 (3.96–6.80)	3.71 (2.78–4.94)	13.04 (7.10–23.95)	21.63 (7.30–64.08)	1.67 (1.09–1.60)	1.16 (0.79–1.70)	2.07 (1.59–2.71)	1.14 (0.85–1.54)
Parity								
1–4	1.00	1.00	1.00	1.00	1.00	1.00	1.00	1.00
> 4	0.71 (0.61–0.82)	0.93 (0.84–1.04)	0.59 (0.48–0.72)	0.78 (0.58–1.04)	1.01 (0.81–1.21)	1.03 (0.84–1.25)	1.48 (1.27–1.71)	1.06 (0.94–1.21)
Women decision making power								
Low	1.00	1.00	1.00	1.00	1.00	1.00	1.00	1.00
Moderate	1.04 (0.91–1.19)	1.02 (0.86–1.21)	0.91 (0.74–1.12)	0.96 (0.70–1.31)	0.97 (0.74–1.27)	0.76 (0.55–1.06)	1.26 (1.10–1.44)	0.97 (0.81–1.18)
High		1.22 (1.01–1.47)		1.47 (1.03–2.10)		1.12 (0.77–1.63)		1.04 (0.85–1.27)
Currently working	1.10 (0.94–1.28)	1.71 (1.49–1.95)	0.69 (0.55–0.86)	2.52 (1.51–4.22)	1.09 (0.78–1.53)	0.87 (0.71–1.07)	0.97 (0.87–1.08)	1.37 (1.21–1.56)
Sex of household head								
Male	1.00	1.00	1.00	1.00	1.00	1.00	1.00	1.00
Female	1.11 (0.92–1.33)	1.09 (0.92–1.30)	1.58 (1.18–2.11)	2.04 (1.14–3.67)	1.11 (0.82–1.51)	1.02 (0.75–1.37)	1.13 (1.00–1.26)	1.12 (0.98–1.28)

N.B. Numbers represent odds ratios. Ref = reference category

services [10]. Again, religious beliefs and residency usually indicate cultural background and influence norms, values and beliefs in relation to women's status, service use and childbirth. Previous studies have reported low levels of maternal healthcare utilization among ethnic minority women in rural areas [32–34]. Also, maternal decision-making power was associated with health care behaviors. Women's empowerment enhance the knowledge and need of health care and awareness of services which can improve through behavior change communication and increase the ability of a woman to have positive health care-seeking behavior. Overall, our study is consistent with the findings from a review of numerous studies in developing countries that women's empowerment is positively associated with the use of maternal health care services [35].

Strengths and limitations

The main strength of this study is that it leverages on nationally representative data collected through a consistent methodology in 2006 and 2011–12. In addition, this is the foremost nationwide analyses that explores antenatal visits, facility-based delivery, postnatal and contraceptive utilization in Benin, and as such could serve as benchmark and stimulus for further nationwide studies on related subjects. Nonetheless, cross sectional data are unable to sufficiently establish causality, again due to self-report method of eliciting information from respondents, there could be possibility of recall bias which could affect the level of utilization of maternal health care services reported in this study.

Conclusion

This study has identified the importance of vital maternal care services and associated socio-demographic, economic and proximate factors disparities against the backdrop of poor maternal health indicators in Benin. The findings showed consistent differentials in the use of key maternal health services, such as ANC visits, facility-based delivery, postnatal care and contraceptive use, in favor of women in urban, educated, high economic status and use of media. Though the study revealed disparities in selected determinants of maternal care services in Benin, however, there are other factors such as environmental conditions, governance, culture, infrastructure and availability of medical equipment and personnel that play vital role in reduction of these differences. Hence, the findings would guide stakeholders in health care system to address the unequal access in health care services. As we strive for universal health coverage, health care interventions, programmes and policies should be strengthened to enhance maternal care services utilization, and tackle the disparities in the utilization of maternal care services, especially for the disadvantaged who live in hard-to-reach rural areas in Benin. The Benin government needs to create strategies that cover both the supply and demand side interventions, specifically to reach the uneducated, living in remote areas with inadequate resources to have access to health care services. Such strategy must go beyond any specific intervention for maternal health care to accommodate a wider developmental agenda and human capital development.

Abbreviations

ANC: Antenatal care; DHS: Demographic Health Survey; IRB: Institutional Review Board; MMR: Maternal Mortality Ratio; SDGs: Sustainable Development Goals; SSA: Sub-Saharan Africa; TBA: Traditional Birth Attendant; USAID: United States Agency for International Development; WHO: World Health Organization

Acknowledgments

The authors thank the MEASURE DHS project for their support and for free access to the original data.

Funding

The authors have no support or funding to report.

Authors' contributions

SY and ME contributed to the study design, the review of literature, and analysis of literature, manuscript conceptualisation and preparation. OU, AA and GB critically reviewed the manuscript for its intellectual content. SY had final responsibility to submit for publication. All authors read and approved the final manuscript.

Competing interests

The authors declare that they have no competing interests.

Author details

[1]School of International Development and Global Studies, University of Ottawa, Ottawa, Canada. [2]Warwick Centre for Applied Health Research and Delivery (WCAHRD), Division of Health Sciences, Warwick Medical School, University of Warwick, Coventry CV4 7AL, UK. [3]Bloomberg School of Public Health, Johns Hopkins University, Baltimore, MD, USA. [4]Department of Epidemiology and Medical Statistics, Faculty of Public Health, College of Medicine, University of Ibadan, Ibadan, Nigeria.

References

1. Yaya S, Bishwajit G, Shah V. Wealth, education and urban–rural inequality and maternal healthcare service usage in Malawi. BMJ Global Health. 2016;1: e000085. https://doi.org/10.1136/ bmjgh-2016-000085.
2. WHO, UNICEF, UNFPA, the World Bank and the United Nations population division estimates. Estimates of maternal mortality ratio (MMR, maternal deaths per 100 000 live births), number of maternal deaths, and lifetime risk, by United Nations MDG region, 2013.
3. Prata N, Passano P, Sreenivas A, Gerdts CE. Maternal mortality in developing countries: challenges in scaling-up priority interventions. Women's health. 2010;6(2):311–27. https://doi.org/10.2217/whe.10.8. PMID: 20187734
4. The World Factbook. Maternal mortality rate. In: Central intelligence agency; 2010.

5. Alvarez JL, Gil R, Hernandez V, Gil A. Factors associated with maternal mortality in sub-Saharan Africa: an ecological study. BMC Public Health. 2009;9:462. https://doi.org/10.1186/1471-2458-9-462. PMID: 20003411
6. Birmeta K, Dibaba Y, Woldeyohannes D. Determinants of maternal health care utilization in Holeta town, Central Ethiopia. BMC Health Serv Res. 2013; 13:256. https://doi.org/10.1186/1472-6963-13-256. PMID: 23822155
7. Tey NP, Lai SL. Correlates of and barriers to the utilization of health services for delivery in South Asia and sub-Saharan Africa. Sci World J. 2013;2013: 423403. https://doi.org/10.1155/2013/423403. PMID: 24288482
8. Zere E, Kirigia JM, Duale S, Akazili J. Inequities in maternal and child health outcomes and interventions in Ghana. BMC Public Health. 2012;12:252. https://doi.org/10.1186/1471-2458-12-252. PMID: 22463465
9. World Health Organization. Trends in maternal mortality: 1990 to 2010. Tech. Rep., WHO, UNICEF, UNFPA and The World Bank Estimates. Geneva, Switzerland: 2012.
10. Ahmed S, Creanga AA, Gillespie DG, Tsui AO. Economic status, education and empowerment: implications for maternal health service utilization in developing countries. PLoS One. 2010;5(6):e11190. https://doi.org/10.1371/journal.pone.0011190. PMID: 20585646
11. Fournier P, Dumont A, Tourigny C, Dunkley G, Drame S. Improved access to comprehensive emergency obstetric care and its effect on institutional maternal mortality in rural Mali. Bulletin of the WHO. 2009;87(1):30–8. PMID: 19197402
12. David-Wayas O, Ugbor IK, Arua M, Nwanosike DU. Analysis of inequality in healthcare utilization among pregnant women in Nigeria: concentration index approach. Int'l J of Asian Social Science. 2017;7(5):424–33.
13. Irwin A, Valentine N, Brown C, Loewenson R, Solar O, Brown H, Koller T, Vega J. The commission on social determinants of health: tackling the social roots of health inequities. PLoS Med. 2006;3:e106.
14. Culyer AJ. Equity - some theory and its policy implications. J Med Ethics. 2001;27:275–83.
15. Gwatkin DR, Bhuiya A, Victora CG. Making health systems more equitable. Lancet. 2004;364:1273–80.
16. Gwatkin D, Rutstein S, Johnson K, Suliman E, Wagstaff A, Amozou A. Initial country-level information about socioeconomic differences in health, nutrition, and population. Washington: The World Bank; 2007.
17. Boerma JT, Bryce J, Kinfu Y, Axelson H, Victora CG. Mind the gap: equity and trends in coverage of maternal, newborn, and child health services in 54 countdown countries. Lancet. 2008;371:1259–67.
18. Victora CG, Wagstaff A, Schellenberg JA, Gwatkin D, Claeson M, Habicht JP. Applying an equity lens to child health and mortality: more of the same is not enough. Lancet. 2003;362(9379):233–41.
19. Qian Y, Gao J, Zhou Z, Yan J, Xu Y, Yang X, et al. An equity analysis of health examination service utilization by women from underdeveloped areas in western China. PLOS ONE. 2017;12(10):e0186837.
20. Benin Demographic and Health Survey, 2006 & 2012.
21. Wanjira C, Mwangi M, Mathenge E, Mbugua G, Ng'ang'a Z. Delivery practices and associated factors among mothers seeking child welfare services in selected health facilities in Nyandarua South District, Kenya. BMC Public Health. 2011;11:360.
22. Adebowale AS, Palamuleni ME. Modern contraceptive use, sex refusal and spousal difference in level of education among married women in Nigeria: are they interrelated? Int'l J of humanities and. Soc Sci. 2014;4(6):217–30.
23. Babalola S, Fatusi A. Determinants of use of maternal health services in Nigeria-looking beyond individual and household factors. BMC Pregnancy Childbirth. 2009;9:43.
24. Idris SH, Sambo MN, Ibrahim MS. Barriers to utilisation of maternal health services in a semiurban community in northern Nigeria: the clients' perspective. Niger Med J. 2013;54(1):27–32.
25. Mpembeni RN, Killewo JZ, Leshabari MT. Use pattern of maternal health services and determinants of skilled care during delivery in southern Tanzania: implications for achievement of MDG-5 targets. BMC Pregnancy and Childbirth. 2007;7(1):1.
26. United Nations. Sustainable development goals. Full report of the Open Working Group of the General Assembly on Sustainable Development Goals 2014. https://sustainabledevelopment.un.org/focussdgs.html.
27. Eyob Z, Doyin O, Joses MK, Mwikisa CN. Inequities in skilled attendance at birth in Namibia: a decomposition analysis. BMC Pregnancy & Childbirth. 2011;11:34.
28. Limwattananon S, Tangcharoensathien V, Prakongsaib P. Equity in maternal and child health in Thailand. Bull World Health Organ. 2010;88:420–7.
29. Daniel F, Chunhuei C. Health care utilization in Ecuador: a multilevel analysis of socio-economic determinants and inequality issues. Health Pol Plann. 2010;25:209–18.
30. Houweling TA, Kunst AE, Huisman M, Mackenbach JP. Using relative and absolute measures for monitoring health inequalities: experiences from cross-national analyses on maternal and child health. Int J Equity Health. 2007;6:15.
31. Houweling TA, Ronsmans C, Campbell OM, Kunst AE. Huge poor-rich inequalities in maternity care: an international comparative study of maternity and child care in developing countries. Bull World Health Organ. 2007;85(10):745–54. PMID: 18038055
32. Long QA, Zhang TH, Xu L, Tang SL, Hemminki E. Utilisation of maternal health care in western rural China under a new rural health insurance system (new co-operative medical system). Tropical Med Int Health. 2010;15:1210–7.
33. Harris A, Zhou Y, Liao H, Barclay L, Zeng WY, Gao Y. Challenges to maternal health care utilization among ethnic minority women in a resource-poor region of Sichuan Province China. Health Pol Plann. 2010;25:311–8.
34. Simkhada B, van Teijlingen ER, Porter M, Simkhada P. Factors affecting the utilization of antenatal care in developing countries: systematic review of the literature. J Adv Nurs. 2008;61:244–60.
35. Pratley P. Associations between quantitative measures of Women's empowerment and access to care and health status for mothers and their children: a systematic Reviewof evidence from the developing world. Soc Sci Med. 2016;169:119–31.

11

Views on and experiences of electronic cigarettes: a qualitative study of women who are pregnant or have recently given birth

Katharine Bowker[1], Sophie Orton[1], Sue Cooper[1], Felix Naughton[2], Rachel Whitemore[1], Sarah Lewis[3], Linda Bauld[4], Lesley Sinclair[4], Tim Coleman[1], Anne Dickinson[1] and Michael Ussher[4,5*]

Abstract

Background: Electronic cigarettes (ECs) are increasingly used for reducing or stopping smoking, with some studies showing positive outcomes. However, little is known about views on ECs during pregnancy or postpartum and previous studies have nearly all been conducted in the US and have methodological limitations, such as not distinguishing between smokers and ex/non-smokers. A greater understanding of this topic will help to inform both clinicians and EC interventions. We elicited views and experiences of ECs among UK pregnant or recently pregnant women.

Methods: We conducted semi-structured telephone interviews, using topic guides, with pregnant or recently pregnant women, who were current or recent ex-smokers. To ensure broad views of ECs were obtained, recruitment was from several geographical locations and via various avenues of recruitment. This included stop smoking services, antenatal and health visitor clinics, a pregnancy website and an informal network. Participants were 15 pregnant and 15 postpartum women, including nine current EC users, 11 ex-users, and 10 never-users. Five women who were interviewed in pregnancy were later interviewed in postpartum to explore if their views had changed. Audio data was transcribed verbatim and framework analysis was applied.

Results: Five main themes emerged: motivations for use (e.g., for stopping or reducing smoking), social stigma (e.g. , avoiding use in public, preferring 'discrete' NRT), using the EC (e.g., mostly used at home); consumer aspects (e.g., limited advice available), and harm perceptions (e.g., viewed as less harmful than smoking; concerns about safety and addiction).

Conclusions: ECs were viewed positively by some pregnant and postpartum women and seen as less harmful than smoking and useful as aids for reducing and stopping smoking. However, due to perceived social stigma, some women feel uncomfortable using ECs in public, especially during pregnancy, and had concerns about safety and nicotine dependence. Health professionals and designers of EC interventions need to provide women with up-to-date and consistent information and advice about safety and dependence, as well as considering the influence of social stigma.

Keywords: Pregnancy, Postpartum, Electronic cigarettes, Qualitative, Interviews

* Correspondence: mussher@sgul.ac.uk
[4]Institute for Social Marketing and UK Centre for Tobacco and Alcohol Studies, University of Stirling, Stirling FK9 4LA, UK
[5]Population Health Research Institute, St George's, University of London, London SW17 0RE, UK
Full list of author information is available at the end of the article

Background

Maternal smoking in pregnancy is the main preventable cause of morbidity and death among women and infants [1, 2]. In high income countries smoking rates in pregnancy tend to be between 10 and 13% [3–5]. Despite nicotine replacement therapy's (NRT) effectiveness for non-pregnant smokers [6], in pregnancy it has been shown to be no more effective than placebo [7]. This is most likely due to low adherence, as well as insufficient dosage because of higher nicotine metabolism in pregnancy [7]. Financial incentives have shown promise for smoking cessation in pregnancy, but there are ethical challenges [8]; for example, there is the possibility that women might falsify their smoking status in order to receive the incentive. Electronic cigarettes (ECs) may have a role to play, as they potentially address both nicotine addiction and the behavioural aspects of smoking.

ECs are increasingly used in many countries, including the US [9], and are the most popular cessation aid in the UK [10]. It has been argued that the potential benefits of ECs probably outweigh harms, and that ECs may have an important role in harm reduction [11–13]. As regards the prevalence of EC use in pregnancy, one recent US study observed that 53% of 103 pregnant smokers reported having tried ECs [14] and a nationally representative US survey found that 29% of 100 pregnant smokers were currently using ECs [15]. The efficacy and safety of using ECs in pregnancy is untested. Nicotine has the potential to show teratogenic effects in the fetus [16], but there is no evidence for this. ECs share a similar pharmacokinetic profile to NRT, which does not appear to have detrimental effects on offspring at birth or 2 years postpartum, compared with placebo [17, 18]. In the UK, it is recommended that pregnant women should not be discouraged from using ECs for stopping smoking if they have struggled to quit without a cessation aid [19]. However, due to lack of evidence on efficacy and safety, in Australia [20] and the US [21] women are advised not to use ECs in pregnancy.

While several studies have investigated views on EC use in pregnancy, these have significant limitations such as the inclusion of women who were neither pregnant nor postpartum [22, 23], investigation of a restricted set of views [22, 24], recruiting from one geographical area [25, 26], and not distinguishing between smokers and ex/non-smokers [24, 27, 28]. Moreover, only one of these studies [25] included postpartum women. In addition, besides one online study [28], they were all conducted in the US. Given these limitations, there are significant knowledge gaps in this area. We attempted to overcome the limitations of previous studies by conducting a UK-based qualitative, in-depth exploration of pregnant and postpartum women's views and experiences of ECs.

Methods

A qualitative descriptive methodology was chosen, allowing an in-depth approach to eliciting a rich description of views and experiences for individual women. This approach also enabled the exploration of differences between individuals. A purposive sampling strategy was adopted to ensure the inclusion of a wide variation of participants to maximise the chances that a full spectrum of views on e-cigarette use in pregnancy were captured. Semi-structured telephone interviews were conducted with 30 UK pregnant or recently pregnant (given birth in last 6 months) women, self-reporting as current smokers (smoked in past 30 days) or recent ex-smokers (stopped smoking in 3 months before pregnancy or after finding out about pregnancy). Women were recruited with various experience of ECs and at different gestations. Following their initial interview, pregnant participants were invited to be re-interviewed within 3 months of the birth, in order to observe if views had changed.

The interview schedule and study materials were reviewed by a Patient and Public Involvement (PPI) representative (ex-smoker and current EC user). We also consulted a Smokers Panel of the UK Centre for Tobacco and Alcohol Studies for advice on the recruitment and research process. Interviews were conducted between October 2015 and October 2016. We used the Consolidated Criteria for Reporting Qualitative Research tool to promote a comprehensive report of the methods and findings [29].

Recruitment and screening procedures

Participants were purposively sampled from the following groups: current EC users (used EC in previous 30 days), ex-users (used EC, but not in last 30 days); from each trimester of pregnancy, and from varying stages within 6 months postpartum. Various sites were used to place recruitment adverts: UK Stop Smoking Services (SSS), hospital antenatal clinics and health visitor clinics in locations across England and Scotland; social media (Facebook pages of the Nottingham Smoking in Pregnancy Research group (www.facebook.com/mumssmokingresearch/) and Tommy's pregnancy charity (https://www.facebook.com/tommys/) and the PPI representative's Twitter account); an advert on the pregnancy website Mumsnet (www.mumsnet.com); and through informal networks. Women attending SSS or clinics were informed of the study by a researcher or stop smoking advisor and contact details of those interested were sent to a researcher.

Participant consent

Women selected for interview were sent a participant information sheet. Approximately 1 week later, a researcher telephoned to seek verbal informed consent to participate; pregnant women were asked for consent to contact them again postpartum. Women were ineligible if they could not understand the study procedure sufficiently or were under 16 years. Background questions included: age, ethnicity, gestation, smoking status, whether living with a partner, age left full-time education and employment. Ex and current EC users were asked about the frequency of EC use: (i) EC used daily (intensive users); (ii) ECs used regularly but not daily (intermittent users); (iii) ECs only used once or twice, or occasionally (triers).

Interviews

Two experienced, female researchers conducted the interviews (KB: PhD, midwife, non-smoker and SO: PhD, health psychologist, non-smoker). The interviewers introduced themselves as researchers working at the University of Nottingham. Interviews were audio recorded. Data were transcribed verbatim by a transcriber external to the research team. Interviewees received a £15 shopping voucher. This payment was not offered on recruitment adverts.

Interview questions were adapted from previous topic guides related to ECs for smokers [30–33], with pregnancy-specific questions added. The main topics were: patterns of EC use (including motivations for using ECs), perceived social norms, views on ECs compared with cigarettes and NRT, views on support with using ECs and on legislation and advertising (see Additional files 1, 2, 3, 4, 5 and 6). Interview questions differed slightly according to participant's experience of ECs. After interviewing 30 participants, and conducting initial coding, we reflected on whether data saturation had been reached. For those pregnant women who were interviewed a second time, during postpartum, we covered the same topics as in pregnancy and focussed on changes in views and experiences since the first interview. For the latter interviews, we interviewed all the women who were willing and we did not attempt to reach data saturation.

Analysis

The framework method of thematic analysis was used to manage, summarize and analyse the data [34]. Researchers produced a set of framework matrices according to interviewees level of experience of ECs and whether they were pregnant or postpartum; thus, in total, there were six matrices (i.e., pregnant/current EC user, pregnant/ex-user, pregnant/never user, postpartum/current user, postpartum/ex-user, postpartum/never user). This enabled researchers to gain insight into the views and experiences of each participant, while also identifying any differences between participants according to their experience of ECs. Interviews from women who were interviewed twice (pregnancy and postpartum) were compared to explore if views had changed. The analysis was both inductive, from the accounts (experiences and views) of participants, and deductive, through being informed by existing literature as reflected in the study objectives and the topics chosen for the interviews.

First, KB and SO independently read and open coded all the transcripts line by line, referring to any notes made during the interviews. Also, in order to gain familiarity with the dataset, these two researchers listened to all the recordings. These researchers then met to discuss their respective codes and agree the codes and define code categories representing conceptually related codes that together formed a 'working' analytical framework. The transcripts were then independently coded a third time by either MU, FN, SC, LB or RW (all non-smokers), using the working framework and noting any codes that deviated from the framework. All the researchers then discussed possible refinements to the codes and categories. The revised analytical framework was then applied to each transcript to attach the final codes and to identify particularly meaningful extracts of text to be transferred to an Excel spreadsheet, consisting of one row per participant and a column per code. The matrix was then reviewed by KB and SO, with discussion with the entire team, to identify, label and refine the themes which best explained the data. To increase the integrity of the findings, attention was given to deviant cases. NVivo 11 software was used to assist with coding and analysis.

Results

One hundred twenty-three women were eligible and interested in participating in the study; 30 (26%) were contactable and consented to an interview. Participants were recruited from: SSS (Glasgow ($n = 4$), Leicester ($n = 7$), London ($n = 2$)), Nottinghamshire antenatal clinic ($n = 4$) and health visitor clinics ($n = 10$), Tommy's Facebook ($n = 2$), and informally ($n = 1$).

There were nine current-EC users, 11 ex-users and 10 never-users; 16 smoked and 14 were ex-smokers (see Table 1). Seven of the nine current EC users were dual users of cigarettes and ECs. Participants were aged 21 to 38 years, the majority were white British, lived with a partner, did not attend formal education beyond 18 years and were employed. Among the 15 pregnant women, three were in the first trimester (≤ 12 weeks gestation), seven in the second trimester (13 to 26 weeks), and five in the third (27–40 weeks). Fifteen women were postpartum: six were 0–3 months postpartum and nine were 4–6 months. Ten pregnant women gave consent to be re-interviewed postpartum and, of those, five were interviewed and five were uncontactable. Two of the participants changed their smoking/EC status by the second

Table 1 Characteristics of participants

ID	Smoking status	EC status	EC level of use	Age range	Weeks' gestation/ months postpartum	Living with partner	Age left Education	Ethnicity	Employed	Interviewed second time Smoking status and EC
1	ex-smoker	ex-user	trier	30–39	37 weeks	yes	17	white British	yes	No change: smoker/ex EC user
2	ex-smoker	ex-user	trier	30–39	37 weeks	yes	16	white British	yes	
3	ex-smoker	never user	n/a	30–39	5 months postpartum	yes	21	Asian	yes	
4	ex-smoker	ex-user	trier	20–29	36 weeks	yes	18	white British	yes	
5	smoker	current user	intermittent	20–29	6 months postpartum	yes	18	white British	yes	
6	smoker	current user	intermittent	30–39	10 weeks	yes	26	white British	yes	
7	smoker	current user	intensive	20–29	4 months postpartum	yes	16	white British	yes	
8	smoker	current user	intensive	20–29	25 weeks	yes	19	white British	yes	
9	smoker	ex-user	intensive	20–29	27 weeks	no	16	white British	no	No change: smoker/ ex EC user
10	ex-smoker	current user	intensive	20–29	11 weeks	no	still in education	white British	yes	
11	smoker	never user	n/a	30–39	33 weeks	yes	18	white British	yes	
12	smoker	ex-user	intermittent	30–39	19 weeks	no	16	white British	no	
13	ex-smoker	never user	n/a	30–39	19 weeks	yes	16	white British	no	
14	ex-smoker	ex-user	trier	20–29	16 weeks	yes	17	white British	no	No change: ex-smoker/ ex EC user
15	smoker	never user	n/a	30–39	19 weeks	no	16	white British	yes	
16	ex-smoker	ex-user	trier	20–29	35 weeks	no	18	white British	yes	
17	smoker	never user	n/a	20–29	12 weeks	no	15	White/ black Caribbean	yes	Change: smoker/ ex EC user (trier)
18	smoker	ex-user	intensive	20–29	4 months postpartum	yes	16	white British	yes	
19	ex-smoker	current user	intermittent	20–29	21 weeks	yes	16	white British	yes	Change: Smoker/ current EC user
20	smoker	never user	n/a	20–29	4 months postpartum	no	15	white British	no	
21	ex-smoker	never user	n/a	20–29	4 months postpartum	yes	17	white British	yes	
22	smoker	current user	intermittent	20–29	1 month postpartum	no	23	black Caribbean	yes	
23	ex-smoker	ex-user	trier	20–29	< 1 month postpartum	yes	16	white British	yes	
24	smoker	current user	intensive	30–39	5 months postpartum	yes	22	white Asian	yes	
25	smoker	never user	n/a	20–29	3 months postpartum	yes	16	white British	yes	
26	smoker		intensive			yes	15	white British	yes	

Table 1 Characteristics of participants *(Continued)*

ID	Smoking status	EC status	EC level of use	Age range	Weeks' gestation/ months postpartum	Living with partner	Age left Education	Ethnicity	Employed	Interviewed second time Smoking status and EC
		current user		20–29	3 months postpartum					
27	ex-smoker	ex-user	trier	20–29	4 months postpartum	yes	21	white British	yes	
28	ex-smoker	never user	n/a	20–29	3 months postpartum	no	21	White/ black Caribbean	yes	
29	ex-smoker	never user	n/a	20–29	< 1 month postpartum	yes	21	white British	yes	
30	smoker	ex-user	trier	20–29	4 months postpartum	yes	21	white British	yes	

interview; one smoker/never EC user tried an EC since the interview and an ex-smoker/current EC user had returned to smoking. Interviews lasted for a mean (SD) 29 (8.7) minutes (range 18 to 53 min). We considered that data saturation and been reached following the initial 30 interviews.

The initial codes were very similar for each level of experience of using ECs as well as for pregnancy and postpartum women, except that aspects related to triggers for use and experiences of use were not relevant for never users. Therefore, it was decided that a common analytical framework would be developed, while noting any divergence for particular sub-groups of participants. The framework included six categories: social factors, general experience and usage, patterns of usage, comparison of ECs and NRT, perceived benefits of ECs and negative views on ECs; nested under these categories were a total of 32 codes (see Additional file 7). Review of the matrices, through discussion between the entire team, suggested that five main themes offered the best explanation of the data: motivations to use ECs, social stigma, using the EC, consumer aspects, and harm perceptions. The process of defining and labelling the themes was influenced by both the study objectives and by new concepts identified inductively from the data. Any differences in views according to level of experience of ECs or between pregnant and postpartum women are highlighted below. When pregnant women were interviewed for a second time at postpartum their views appeared unchanged except regarding the perceived stigma of ECs (see 'Social Stigma' theme).

Motivations for use

Most women were motivated to quit smoking; some felt that ECs could help them quit and dual users of ECs and cigarettes said they felt that ECs helped them to reduce their smoking.

> *'I tried them but at the time* [prior to pregnancy] *I didn't really have the motivation to stop properly but then, as I say, when I fell pregnant this time the first thing I did was buy an electronic cigarette'.*
>
> ***(06 antenatal smoker and current EC user)***

The majority indicated that they believed ECs were a less harmful alternative to smoking during pregnancy, reducing foetal exposure to toxins. Most women were aware that ECs usually contained nicotine but were unaware of other ingredients. Some said that ECs would reduce smoke odours on their clothes, in their home and on their children. A few felt ECs were safer than cigarettes for second-hand smoke exposure.

> *'it* [EC] *doesn't pass on second-hand smoke, because even if the baby was close-by, which I wouldn't have a baby close-by, it wouldn't be dangerous'.*
>
> **(19 antenatal ex-smoker and current EC user)**

Most interviewees felt ECs were a cheaper alternative to smoking. A few women were motivated to use an EC based on cost alone. In terms of what first triggered women to use ECs, some women were introduced to ECs, and encouraged to quit using ECs, by family and friends. A few tried ECs after recommendations from a health professional. Others reported experimenting out of curiosity, often on the *'Spur of the moment'* **(09 antenatal ex-smoker and ex-EC user)** and these women generally reported they were not ready to quit, so didn't pursue the EC.

> *'They* [family] *were a lot happier about me using that* [EC] *than obviously smoking. My Mum actually bought me the e-cigarette and she never ever bought me cigarettes in my life'.*
>
> ***(08 antenatal smoker and current EC user)***

A few women, having quit smoking, said they were more likely to use NRT than ECs if they relapsed, primarily due to the potential for ECs to steer them back to smoking, as a result of the similarity to smoking. Some 'never' and ex-users believed NRT would better support a quit attempt than ECs as regards 'weaning off' nicotine.

Social stigma

Most women expressed feeling uncomfortable (both actual and perceived experience) about using ECs in public during pregnancy and, for some, also in postpartum, especially when with children. The women said they felt that they would be judged and perceived as a bad mother. Two women who were interviewed again after pregnancy indicated they felt more comfortable about the idea of using ECs after the pregnancy, believing that there was less public judgement and less risk to the baby at this time. Some women also expressed a strong belief that it was socially unacceptable for a pregnant woman to smoke or vape in public.

> *'If I was pregnant I would feel embarrassed because I think it looks disgusting. If I'm honest, pregnant women drinking or smoking any type of fags, cigar, electronic fags, I don't think it looks very nice, so I wouldn't do it pregnant in public. Afterwards I wouldn't be bothered. I suppose it depends if I had the baby with me in a pushchair I wouldn't be too keen on the idea.'*
>
> ***(04 antenatal ex-smoker and ex-EC user)***

Compared with cigarette smoking, some felt it was more socially acceptable to use an EC and felt empathetic towards pregnant women using ECs as they could relate to the struggles of cessation. A few mentioned that a benefit of NRT is that it can be administered discreetly in public.

Using the EC (EC current users/ex-users only)

Regarding the context of where the EC was used, EC 'triers' reported vaping with friends and family, often in the home environment. Regular users generally reported vaping in similar environments as for smoking, often the home, workplace or car. A few said that, similarly to smoking, they avoided using ECs around their children.

Some said they were attracted by ECs as they replicated and substituted smoking, especially in terms of inhaling and blowing vapour and the hand-to-mouth action. One woman, who had struggled to quit using NRT, said she found that ECs helped her as they assisted with both the addiction and behavioural aspects of smoking. However, some ex-users indicated they felt ECs were too much of a reminder of smoking but, compared with a cigarette, didn't provide the same satisfaction and often required use over longer periods in order to alleviate cravings.

> *'One thing I missed when I have quit smoking is inhaling the smoke, so when I used an e-cigarette obviously you've got that kind of experience of inhaling the vapour. It was too much, it was too similar to having a cigarette, so it made me miss it even more.'*
>
> ***(01 antenatal ex-smoker and ex-EC user)***

Some women reported negative first experiences of ECs; others felt side effects reduced as they adapted. One woman compared her initial experience to learning to smoke.

Consumer aspects

Among EC users/ex-users there was a general preference for smaller and lighter ECs; one woman reported she liked the convenience of it fitting in her handbag. Most participants were aware of the variety of flavours and some were aware of various nicotine strengths. To economise, a few women purchased the cheapest EC; however, they also felt the price of ECs reflected their value, with more expensive devices being more user-friendly. Women tended to either choose an EC impulsively, based on cost, or based on the advice of friends/family. Many had not received instructions about their device from the retailer or on the EC packaging, leaving some feeling uninformed.

> *'When you are pregnant you want to know....how is the best way to use it* [EC] *to help you stop....you literally had to go and buy it like a loaf of bread'.*
>
> ***(07 postpartum smoker and current EC user)***

Rather than receiving information about ECs from retailers, women generally said they would prefer to receive information from a health professional or through National Health Service leaflets or websites.

Harm perceptions

Never-users, in particular, and some ex-users, said they felt there was a lack of information available about the safety of ECs, which led to fears. In order to make an informed decision about whether to use ECs, they said they needed further information and advice, preferably from health professionals.

> *'Everyone just says 'oh there's only five chemicals in an e-cigarette, while there's 4000 in a cigarette' but my concern was those five chemicals that are in the e-cigarette'.*

(18 postpartum smoker and ex-EC user)

Women were asked whether they thought ECs should be made available on prescription and many felt it was important to first establish their safety. One smoker and never user said that she would require the government to provide assurance on their safety in pregnancy before she would consider using one.

'Yeah and I think obviously if there was some sort of government stamp on it or you know you don't buy toys without having something, you don't buy anything without, even the bad stuff you know, you buy a packet of cigarettes and the government have put what it can do to you on it, with all the pictures. Whereas there's nothing is there? There's no nothing, no good, no bad, no nothing.'

(15 antenatal smoker and never user)

Some women indicated they felt more confident about NRT because the health service clearly advocated it, whereas they had received conflicting advice from health professionals about using ECs. Concerns about the safety of ECs were heightened by negative media reports, referring to malfunctioning devices, links to cancer or other health harms. A couple of women were concerned that ECs were becoming a fashion accessory, and one woman reported ECs had appealed to her young nephew.

Several women were worried that vaping might increase their consumption of nicotine compared with smoking:

'Obviously with a cigarette you can only smoke it for so long till it's finished, but with an e-cigarette you can smoke for as long as you want to. So sometimes, I guess, I was taking in more than the usual nicotine intake that I would have done with a cigarette.'

(01 antenatal ex-smoker and ex-EC user)

'So my friends that have used them they're constantly in their mouth whereas a cigarette, you have a cigarette and then you don't have another one for, say, three hours.'

(13 antenatal ex-smoker never user)

Discussion

This study explored in-depth views surrounding EC use in both pregnancy and postpartum, identified five main themes, and gained important new insights that are specific to this population. Some pregnant and postpartum women viewed ECs as less harmful than smoking and as aids for reducing and stopping smoking. However, due to perceived social stigma, some felt uncomfortable using ECs in public, especially during pregnancy. They also had concerns about safety and nicotine dependence, requesting more consistent information from health professionals. Some expressed a preference for NRT over ECs; they felt that NRT was both consistently sanctioned by health professionals and could be used more discretely than ECs.

Strengths of this study include the use of a broad-based topic guide and a series of individual interviews to capture the views of UK women with varying experience of ECs. Additionally, we recruited women from a number of UK regions and recruitment sites. Together, this approach increases the likelihood of capturing a diverse set of views. The use of framework analysis ensured data analysis was transparent and enabled all members of the research team to contribute.

There were also limitations. Telephone rather than face-to-face interviews were used; we were therefore unable to gather potentially important contextual information about the participant's environment. However, considering both the wide geographical spread of the participants and that pregnancy is a busy time with many antenatal appointments, telephone interviews were considered the most practicable option. As regards reflexivity, there is the potential for unconscious, or even conscious, bias as this research was conducted in a UK research and policy climate in which ECs have largely been advocated as a less harmful alternative to smoking [11]. As with most qualitative research [35], the intention of the study was not to ensure the findings are fully representative of the wider population; although, the ethnic and education characteristics of women (i.e., mostly white ethnicity and not receiving formal education beyond 18 years) suggest that they are fairly typical of women who smoke in pregnancy [3]. Our intention was, purposively, to capture potential diversity around the phenomenon of views on and experiences of ECs during pregnancy and postpartum. Thus, as we purposively sampled for both level of experience with ECs and pregnancy versus postpartum, there was great heterogeneity in the characteristics of the sample. This can make it difficult to draw overall conclusions. Despite this, except for instances where experiences were irrelevant to the 'never-users' sub-group (e.g., regarding triggers for using ECs), the findings were very similar for the different sub-groups.

As with smokers in general [33], there were mixed findings concerning women's experiences of using ECs; some favoured ECs because they mimicked smoking, while, conversely, others didn't like ECs as they reminded them of smoking. Again, as found in the general population [36], most women were interested in using ECs either to stop smoking or to reduce their smoking with dual use of ECs and cigarettes. The majority (seven of nine) of the current EC users were dual users of ECs and cigarettes and these women said they felt that ECs helped them to reduce their smoking. Outside of pregnancy, 45% of British EC users report dual use [36]. The results of a recent nationally representative US survey suggest that rates of dual use may be higher in pregnancy than outside for pregnancy: 79% of 34 pregnant women using ECS were currently still smoking and the remaining 21% were ex-smokers [15]. Dual use of NRT and cigarettes is also common during pregnancy [37]. Dual use may increase attempts to stop smoking [12, 38], although it is unclear whether this increases cessation [39]. Among smokers in general, dual use is likely to maintain similar levels of carcinogens and toxicants as smoking [14], although it is not known if this is also the case in pregnancy.

Interestingly, many of the women said that they began using ECs spontaneously, 'on the spur of the moment'. This may need to be considered in public health policy as ECs are increasingly widely used and available, and pregnant women may be frequently exposed to them and readily triggered to experiment with them.

This is the first study to report that, due to perceived social stigma, some women would avoid using ECs in public while pregnant or with an infant. Similar to US findings [26], others felt that using an EC was less stigmatising than smoking and would feel empathetic towards pregnant women using ECs, as they understood the difficulties of cessation. The presence of perceived social stigma contrasts with non-pregnant populations, where ECs are largely viewed as sociable and enjoyable [31, 39, 40], but is consistent with the strong social stigma felt by pregnant smokers [41–43] and with negative public perceptions of smoking in pregnancy [44]. Moreover, a US survey observed that most people view ECs as being as harmful, if not more harmful, as smoking during pregnancy [45]. Pregnant women hide their smoking [43] and, similarly, we observed that women often preferred vaping at home and in other places where they usually smoked. Moreover, there was no indication that women vaped with others or shared their ECs. These women may be responding to the societal focus on maternal responsibility and the notion of the 'bad mother', in relation to health threats to the fetus, which can serve to marginalise and stigmatise women [46]. Related to this, due to its discrete nature, some women favoured NRT over ECs; clinicians may need to be sensitive to this preference and EC manufacturers might want to consider producing more discrete devices that are not perceived to give a 'bad' impression. A further, related, new finding is that a few women felt it was more socially acceptable to use an EC after having a baby, compared with pregnancy, as they felt there was less stigma and less harm for the baby. Thus, ECs may be suitable for preventing return to smoking in the postpartum period, although it has also been observed that women who use ECs in pregnancy may be at risk of resuming smoking after the birth [26].

Consistent with US research among pregnant women [22, 25, 26, 47], many considered ECs to be safer than cigarettes during pregnancy and around infants. They also had concerns about harm and felt that health professionals needed to provide more consistent safety information. There were also worries that ECs continue or even increase nicotine addiction. Among non-pregnant smokers, laboratory analysis suggests it is unlikely vapers would consume more nicotine than when smoking, as they self-titrate to satisfy their cravings [48, 49]. The women's need for more safety information may be partly alleviated by recent UK guidance to help healthcare professionals to advise pregnant women about ECs [19]. This guidance states the likely relative harms of ECs versus smoking and advises that NRT is the recommended option in pregnancy but that women should not be discouraged from using ECs if they help them to stay smoke free. Together, these findings highlight the urgent need for studies investigating EC toxicants and carcinogens for mother and fetus, similar to studies conducted with non-pregnant smokers [13].

Conclusions

ECs were viewed positively by some pregnant and postpartum women and seen as less harmful than smoking and useful as aids for reducing and stopping smoking. However, due to perceived social stigma, some women feel uncomfortable using ECs in public, especially during pregnancy, and had concerns about safety and nicotine dependence. These findings highlight the need for both health professionals and designers of EC interventions to provide women with up-to-date and consistent information and advice, as well as considering the influence of social stigma. There remains a need for investigations of any harms of ECs for the mother and fetus and of the effectiveness of these devices for helping women to reduce and stop smoking during pregnancy and postpartum.

Additional files

Additional file 1: Coding framework mind map. Brief description of the data A mind-map figure, showing the six categories and 32 codes making up the coding framework.

Additional file 2: Topic Guide pregnant users or used. Brief description of the data: Topic guide for women who are pregnant and are currently using ECs or have previously used them.

Additional file 3: Topic Guide pregnant never used. Brief description of the data: Topic guide for women who are pregnant and have never used ECs.

Additional file 4: Topic Guide postpartum users or used. Brief description of the data: Topic guide for women who are postpartum and are currently using ECs or have previously used them.

Additional file 5: Topic Guide postpartum never used. Brief description of the data: Topic guide for women who are postpartum and have never used ECs.

Additional file 6: Topic Guide Follow up used. Brief description of the data: Topic guide for women for postpartum follow-up interview who in first interview (during pregnancy) said that they were currently using ECs or had previously used them.

Additional file 7: Topic Guide Follow up never used. Brief description of the data: Topic guide for women for postpartum follow-up interview who in first interview (during pregnancy) said that they had never used ECs.

Abbreviations

EC: Electronic cigarette; NRT: Nicotine replacement therapy

Acknowledgements

We thank all the women who volunteered for the study and readily shared their experiences and views.

Funding

This work was supported by a grant from Cancer Research UK, Tobacco Advisory Group (reference C8641/A20490). The funders had no role in in the design of the study or in the collection, analysis, and interpretation of data or in writing the manuscript. Professor Coleman is a National Institute for Health Research (NIHR) Senior Investigator.

Authors' contributions

MU led the application for funding, with all co-authors acting as co-applicants. MU, KB, TC, SC, LS, SL and FN devised and designed the study. MU and KB jointly managed the study. KB and MU drafted the topic guides, with assistance from TC, SC, LS, SL and FN, and drafts were commented on by all the co-authors. KB, SO, RW and AD recruited participants to the study. KB and SO conducted the interviews. The analysis was led by KB with a major contribution from SO. MU, FN, SC, LB and RW also assisted with the analysis. MU, KB, SO, TC, SC, LS, SL, LB and FN interpreted the findings. KB and MU drafted the manuscript with assistance from TC, SC, SL, LS and FN. All authors commented on draft manuscripts, and read and approved the final manuscript. All authors are accountable for all aspects of the work in ensuring that questions related to the accuracy or integrity of any part of the work where appropriately investigated and resolved.

Competing interests

SC is a member of the editorial board (as an Associate Editor) of this journal. The other authors declare that they have no competing interests

Author details

[1]NIHR School for Primary Care Research and UK Centre for Tobacco and Alcohol Studies, Division of Primary Care, School of Medicine, University of Nottingham, Nottingham NG7 2RD, UK. [2]School of Health Sciences, University of East Anglia, Edith Cavell Building, Norwich NR4 7TJ, UK. [3]Division of Epidemiology and Public Health and UK Centre for Tobacco and Alcohol Studies and, University of Nottingham, Clinical Sciences Building 2, Nottingham City Hospital, Hucknall Road, Nottingham NG5 1PB, UK. [4]Institute for Social Marketing and UK Centre for Tobacco and Alcohol Studies, University of Stirling, Stirling FK9 4LA, UK. [5]Population Health Research Institute, St George's, University of London, London SW17 0RE, UK.

References

1. Kallen K. The impact of maternal smoking during pregnancy on delivery outcome. Eur J Pub Health. 2001;11:329–33.
2. Salihu HM, Wilson RE. Epidemiology of prenatal smoking and perinatal outcomes. Early Hum Dev. 2007;83:713–20.
3. Lifestyles Statistics Team Health and Social Care Information Centre. Statistics on Women's Smoking Status at Time of Delivery: England April 2015 to March 2016. 2016. https://digital.nhs.uk/data-and-information/publications/statistical/statistics-on-women-s-smoking-status-at-time-of-delivery-england Accessed 29th Apr 2018.
4. Ford C, Greenhalgh EM, Winstanley MH. Pregnancy and smoking. In: Scollo MM, Winstanley MH, editors. Tobacco in Australia: Facts and issues. Melbourne: Cancer council Victoria; 2015. http://www.tobaccoinaustralia.org.au/3-7-pregnancy-and-smoking.
5. Centers for Disease Control and Prevention. Pregnancy Risk Assessment Monitoring System (PRAMS), 2011. https://www.cdc.gov/prams/pramstat/index.html Accessed 7th Dec 2017.
6. Stead LF, Perera R, Bullen C, Mant D, Hartmann-Boyce J, Cahill K, et al. Nicotine replacement therapy for smoking cessation. Cochrane Database Syst Rev. 2012;11:CD000146.
7. Coleman T, Chamberlain C, Davey MA, Cooper SE, Leonardi-Bee J. Pharmacological interventions for promoting smoking cessation during pregnancy. Cochrane Database Syst Rev. 2015;12:CD010078.
8. Tappin D, Bauld L, Purves D, Boyd K, Sinclair L, MacAskill S, et al. Financial incentives for smoking cessation in pregnancy: randomised controlled trial. BMJ. 2015;350:h134.
9. Delnevo CD, Giovenco DP, Steinberg MB, Villanti AC, Pearson JL, Niaura RS, et al. Patterns of electronic cigarette use among adults in the United States. Nicotine Tob Res. 2016;18:715–9.
10. West RH, McNeill A, Brown J, Arnott D. Electronic cigarettes: what we know so far, 2015. http://www.smokinginengland.info/reports/ Accessed 7th Dec 2017.
11. McNeil AB, Brose LS, Calder R, Bauld L, Robson D (2018). Evidence review of e-cigarettes and heated tobacco products. London: Public Health England. https://www.gov.uk/government/publications/e-cigarettes-and-heated-tobacco-products-evidence-review/evidence-review-of-e-cigarettes-and-heated-tobacco-products-2018-executive-summary Accessed 29th Apr 2018.
12. Royal College of Physicians. Nicotine without smoke: Tobacco harm reduction. 2016. https://www.rcplondon.ac.uk/projects/outputs/nicotine-without-smoke-tobacco-harm-reduction-0 Accessed 29th Apr 2018.
13. Shahab L, Goniewicz ML, Blount BC, Brown J, McNeill A, Alwis KU, et al. Nicotine, carcinogen, and toxin exposure in long-term E-cigarette and nicotine replacement therapy users: a cross-sectional study. Ann Intern Med. 2017;166:390–400.
14. Oncken C, Ricci KA, Kuo CL, Domelas E, Kranzler HR, Sankey HZ. Correlates of electronic cigarette use before and during pregnancy. Nicotine Tob Res. 2016;19:585–90.
15. Kurti AN, Redner R, Lopez AA, Keith DR, Villanti AC, Stanton CA, et al. Tobacco and nicotine delivery product use in a national sample of pregnant women. Prev Med. 2017;S0091–7435:30277–3.
16. Dempsey DA, Benowitz NL. Risks and benefits of nicotine to aid smoking cessation in pregnancy. Drug Saf. 2001;24:277–322.
17. Coleman T, Cooper S, Thornton JG, Grainge MJ, Watts K, Britton J, et al. A randomized trial of nicotine-replacement therapy patches in pregnancy. N Engl J Med. 2012;366:808–18.
18. Cooper S, Taggar J, Lewis S, Marlow N, Dickinson A, Whitemore R. Effect of nicotine patches in pregnancy on infant and maternal outcomes at 2 years: follow-up from the randomised, double-blind, placebo-controlled SNAP trial. Lancet Respir Med. 2014;2:728–37.
19. Smoking in Pregnancy Challenge Group. Use of electronic cigarettes in pregnancy: A guide for midwives and other healthcare professionals. 2016. http://smokefreeaction.org.uk/wp-content/uploads/2017/06/eCigSIP.pdf Accessed 7th Dec 2017.
20. Australian Medical Association. Tobacco Smoking and E-cigarettes - The AMA position, 2015 https://ama.com.au/position-statement/tobacco-smoking-and-e-cigarettes-2015.Accessed 7th Dec 2017.
21. American Congress of Obstetricians and gynecologists. New Fact Sheet on E-Cigarettes. 2015. https://www.acog.org/About-ACOG/ACOG-Departments/Tobacco-%2DAlcohol-%2Dand-Substance-Abuse/Tobacco/New-Fact-Sheet-on-E-Cigarettes Accessed 7th Dec 2017.
22. England LJ, Tong VT, Koblitz A, Kish-Doto J, Lynch MM, Southwell BG. Perceptions of emerging tobacco products and nicotine replacement therapy among pregnant women and women planning a pregnancy. Prev Med Rep. 2016;4:481–5.

23. Ashford K, Wiggins A, Butler K, Ickes M, Rayens MK, Hahn E. E-cigarette use and perceived harm among women of childbearing age who reported tobacco use during the past year. Nurs Res. 2016;65:408–14.
24. Wagner NJ, Camerota M, Propper C. Prevalence and perceptions of electronic cigarette use during pregnancy. Matern Child Health J. 2017; 21:1655–61.
25. Fallin A, Miller A, Assef S, Ashford K. Perceptions of electronic cigarettes among Medicaid-eligible pregnant and postpartum women. J Obstet Gynecol Neonatal Nurs. 2016;45:320–5.
26. Kahr MK, Padgett S, Shope CD, Griffin EN, Xie SS, Gonzalez PJ, et al. A qualitative assessment of the perceived risks of electronic cigarette and hookah use in pregnancy. BMC Public Health. 2015;15:1273.
27. Mark KS, Farquhar B, Chisolm MS, Coleman-Cowger VH, Terplan M. Knowledge, attitudes, and practice of electronic cigarette use among pregnant women. J Addict Med. 2015;9:266–72.
28. Wigginton B, Gartner C, Rowlands IJ. Is it safe to vape? Analyzing online forums discussing E-cigarette use during pregnancy. Womens Health Issues. 2017;27:93–9.
29. Tong A, Sainsbury P, Craig J. Consolidated criteria for reporting qualitative research (COREQ): a 32-item checklist for interviews and focus groups. Int J Qual Health Care. 2007;19:349–57.
30. Dockrell M, Morrison R, Bauld L, McNeill A. E-cigarettes: prevalence and attitudes in great Britain. Nicotine Tob Res. 2013;15:1737–44.
31. McQueen A, Tower S, Sumner W. Interviews with "vapers": implications for future research with electronic cigarettes. Nicotine Tob Res. 2011;13:860–7.
32. Peters RJ Jr, Meshack A, Lin MT, Hill M, Abughosh S. The social norms and beliefs of teenage male electronic cigarette use. J Ethn Subst Abus. 2013;12: 300–7.
33. Rooke C, Cunningham-Burley S, Amos A. Smokers' and ex-smokers' understanding of electronic cigarettes: a qualitative study. Tob Control. 2016;25(e1):e60–6.
34. Gale NK, Heath G, Cameron E, Rashid S, Redwood S. Using the framework method for the analysis of qualitative data in multi-disciplinary health research. BMC Med Res Methodol. 2013;13:117.
35. Mays N, Rigour PC, qualitative r. BMJ. 1995;311:109–12.
36. Action on Smoking and Health (ASH). Use of electronic cigarettes (vapourisers) among adults in Great Britain, May 2017. http://ash.org.uk/information-and-resources/fact-sheets/use-of-e-cigarettes-among-adults-in-great-britain-2017/ Accessed 7th Dec 2017.
37. Bowker K, Campbell KA, Coleman T, Lewis S, Naughton F, Cooper S. Understanding pregnant Smokers' adherence to nicotine replacement therapy during a quit attempt: a qualitative study. Nicotine Tob Res. 2016; 18:906–12.
38. Pasquereau A, Guignard R, Andler R, Nguyen-Thanh V. Electronic cigarettes, quit attempts and smoking cessation: a 6-month follow-up. Addiction. 2017; 112:1620–8.
39. Wadsworth E, Neale J, McNeill A, Hitchman SC. How and why do smokers start using E-cigarettes? Qualitative study of vapers in London, UK. Int J Environ Res Public Health. 2016;13:E661.
40. Cooper M, Harrell MB, Perry CL. Comparing young adults to older adults in e-cigarette perceptions and motivations for use: implications for health communication. Health Educ Res. 2016;31:429–38.
41. Wigginton BL, Lee C. A story of stigma: Australian women's accounts of smoking during pregnancy. Crit Pub Health. 2012;23:466–81.
42. Bull L, Burke R, Walsh S, Whitehead E. Social attitudes towards smoking in pregnancy in east surrey: a qualitative study of smokers, former smokers and non-smokers. J Neonatal Nurs. 2007;13:100e106.
43. Wigginton BL, LaFrance MN. How do women manage the spoiled identity of a 'pregnant smoker'? An analysis of discursive silencing in women's accounts. Feminism Psychol. 2016;26:30–51.
44. Wigginton B, Lee C. Stigma and hostility towards pregnant smokers: does individuating information reduce the effect? Psychol Health. 2013;28:862–73.
45. Nguyen KH, Tong VT, Marynak KL, King BA. US Adults' perceptions of the harmful effects during pregnancy of using electronic vapor products versus smoking cigarettes, styles survey, 2015. Prev Chronic Dis. 2016;22:E175.
46. Bell K, McNaughton D, Salmon A. Medicine, morality and mothering: public health discourses on foetal alcohol exposure, smoking around children and childhood over nutrition. Critical Public Health. 2009;19:2.
47. Rowa-Dewar N, Amos A. Disadvantaged Parents' engagement with a National Secondhand Smoke in the home mass media campaign: a qualitative study. Int J Environ Res Public Health. 2016;13:E901.
48. Dawkins LE, Kimber CF, Doig M, Feyerabend C, Corcoran O. Self-titration by experienced e-cigarette users: blood nicotine delivery and subjective effects. Psychopharmacology. 2016;233:2933–41.
49. Ramoa CP, Hiler MM, Spindle TR, Lopez AA, Karaoghlanian N, Lipato T, et al. Electronic cigarette nicotine delivery can exceed that of combustible cigarettes: a preliminary report. Tob Control. 2016;25(e1):e6–9.

12

Optimal profile limits for maternal mortality rate (MMR) in South Sudan

Gabriel Makuei*, Mali Abdollahian and Kaye Marion

Abstract

Background: Reducing Maternal Mortality Rate (MMR) is considered by the international community as one of the eight Millennium Development Goals. Based on previous studies, Skilled Assistant at Birth (SAB), General Fertility Rate (GFR) and Gross Domestic Product (GDP) have been identified as the most significant predictors of MMR in South Sudan.

This paper aims for the first time to develop profile limits for the MMR in terms of significant predictors SAB, GFR, and GDP. The paper provides the optimal values of SAB and GFR for a given MMR level.

Methods: Logarithmic multi- regression model is used to model MMR in terms of SAB, GFR and GDP. Data from 1986 to 2015 collected from Juba Teaching Hospital was used to develop the model for predicting MMR. Optimization procedures are deployed to attain the optimal level of SAB and GFR for a given MMR level. MATLAB was used to conduct the optimization procedures. The optimized values were then used to develop lower and upper profile limits for yearly MMR, SAB and GFR.

Results: The statistical analysis shows that increasing SAB by 1.22% per year would decrease MMR by 1.4% (95% CI (0.4–5%)) decreasing GFR by 1.22% per year would decrease MMR by 1.8% (95% CI (0.5–6.26%)).

The results also indicate that to achieve the UN recommended MMR levels of minimum 70 and maximum 140 by 2030, the government should simultaneously reduce GFR from the current value of 175 to 97 and 75, increase SAB from the current value of 19 to 50 and 76.

Conclusions: This study for the first time has deployed optimization procedures to develop lower and upper yearly profile limits for maternal mortality rate targeting the UN recommended lower and upper MMR levels by 2030. The MMR profile limits have been accompanied by the profile limits for optimal yearly values of SAB and GFR levels. Having the optimal level of predictors that significantly influence the maternal mortality rate can effectively aid the government and international organizations to make informed evidence-based decisions on resources allocation and intervention plans to reduce the risk of maternal death.

Keywords: Profile limits, Optimisation, Maternal mortality rate, Ln multi-regression, South Sudan

Background

Improving maternal health and reducing related mortality has been the key concern of the international community as one of the Eight Millennium Development Goals (MDG) [1]. Maternal health is a major global development challenge particularly in Africa which accounts for about half of the world's maternal deaths, with little or no progress towards reduction of maternal mortality. Factors associated with maternal mortality in sub-Saharan Africa (SSA) include prenatal care coverage and skilled attendance at delivery. Kruk, et al., (2010) investigated the impact of the community perceptions on the quality of care provided by the local health system on pregnant women's decisions to deliver in a clinic. They suggest that improving the quality of care at first level clinics may assist the efforts to increase facility delivery in sub-Saharan Africa [2]. However, there are other contributing factors including socio-economic factors, macro-economic factors and physiological factors. South Sudan has about 1147 health care facilities that function to serve

* Correspondence: s3097012@student.rmit.edu.au; G.makuei@student.rmit.edu.au
School of Science (Mathematical and Geospatial Sciences), College of Science, Engineering, and Health, RMIT University, GPO BOX 2476, Melbourne, VIC 3001, Australia

population of around 13 million. Out of these facilities, only 37 are hospitals. Ill-equipped buildings with poor hygiene are the common feature of these primary health care units. Chronic shortage of health care professional staff at all levels is demonstrated by 1.5 doctors and two nurses per 100,000 people (National Bureau of Statistic [3]' Report, (2013, 2014, 2015), and World Health Organization, (2014) [4]. All the above factors affect the total health care system and in particular the high maternal mortality rate problem.

The maternal mortality rate (MMR) in South Sudan is one of the highest in the world [3, 5, 6]. The risk of a pregnant woman dying is as high as one in seven. In Africa overall the risk of a pregnant woman dying is one in 16, in contrast with Asia (1 in 105), Europe (1 in 1895) and in North America (1 in 3750), [4, 7, 8], [9]. Thus, there is an urgent need for evidence-based intervention to significantly reduce mortality rate in South Sudan.

The data released by WHO, UNICEF, UNFPA, World Bank and the United Nations Division, [4] shows that even though the maternal mortality rate in South Sudan has decreased from 1000 to 730 per 100,000 live births between 2005 to 2015, it is still one of the highest in the world. Combining this with the high fertility rates in the country gives the probability of an average reproductive South Sudanese woman (12–49 years of age) dying during pregnancy to be 14.3% [10]. Therefore, understanding the trends in MMR and factors significant to MMR would be vital for developing health care systems that can ensure safe delivery.

The World Health Organization and USAID (2015) have recommended that all countries with high MMR level should aim to reduce MMR to the minimum of 70 and the maximum of 140 by 2030 [7].

This paper only investigates the impact of the most influential economic factors on the non-HIV MMR in South Sudan [11]. The authors have identified the most economical influential factors for MMR in South Sudan [10]: The Skilled Attendants at Births (SAB), the General Fertility Rate (GFR) and the Gross Domestic Product (GDP). The MMR is expressed as the annual number of maternal deaths per 100,000 live births. The SAB is the annual percentage of Skilled Attendants at Birth; the GFR is expressed as the annual percentage of live births per 1000 women of reproductive age (ages of 12 to 49 years) in a population. The GDP is expressed in US Dollars (USD). The relevant data for this research was collected for the period from January 1986 to October 2015 from Juba Teaching Hospital (JTH) which is one of the major health care referral centres in South Sudan. The hospital is a 580-bed facility located in the capital city. Additional data was collected from other reliable sources such as: Reproductive Health Department from Ministry of Health (MoH), National Bureau of Statistics NBS Report [12], the South Sudan 2009 National Baseline Household Survey Report, South Sudan Household Health Survey [13], Census of Population and Housing [14], and United Nations' organizations and their partners (e.g. WHO, UNAID, UNICEF, UNDP).

The findings show that Generals Fertility Rate (GFR) is the most influential factor in increasing the maternal death (MDs) followed by skilled attendant at birth (SAB) and the Gross Domestic Product (GDP). MMR decreases when SAB increases and the GFR decreases.

In their comprehensive discussions regarding strategies to reduce MMR, the Campbell, Graham, and Lancet Maternal Survival Series Steering Group [15] stressed the intra-partum care, which includes different types of skilled assistants at birth. Use of contraception to reduce the fertility rate is also mentioned though considered less important. However, the viability of both methods is positive for South Sudan.

According to the data from Juba Teaching Hospital (JTH) any efforts to increase SAB through increasing the number of trained attendants either directly or indirectly would affect the GFR and the GDP. According to the current statistics, only 20% births are attended by skilled assistants [3]. This indicates the need to increase the SAB and decrease the GFR levels. For more rapid impact on MMR, however, the programme of training birth attendants at village and community levels needs to be accelerated and this involves considerable funding.

Currently, the GFR in South Sudan is very high at around five children per mother (6.9 in 2014 cited by the Population Reference Bureau, 2016) [16] which is double the global average of 2.5%. Decrease in GFR has a much longer term effect in reducing MMR, however, contraceptive use has only reached 4% of the population compared to 62% globally [16]. Consequently, there is scope for improvement in this respect; yet this also involves substantial funding. However, acceleration in reducing GFR involves substantial funding to provide improved and affordable health care access to pregnant women. Although increase in GDP would increase MMR, because of the cultural practice of polygamy, the country needs economic growth as a fundamental requirement to provide improved and affordable health care access to pregnant women.

The only likely strategy in the current environment is to increase SAB while decreasing GFR in order to reduce MMR. The importance of attending to socio-economic factors to reduce MMR was highlighted in recent Indian research by Rai, and Tulchinsky (2015) [17]. Decreased fertility rate will decrease the number of births and thus reduce the number of SAB required. Consequently large scale effort to use birth control methods and increase trained birth attendants at village and community levels needs to be implemented.

In this paper we use the logarithmic multi-regression model suggested by Makuei et al. [10] to estimate MMR based on SAB, GFR and GDP. The mathematical optimization is then used to obtain the optimal values of SAB and GFR (when GDP is kept constant) for a given level of MMR. This study for the first time aims to develop yearly lower and upper profile limits for the MMR expressed in terms of significant predicators SAB, GFR and GDP using real data collected from the resources outlined above. The MMR profile limits are then accompanied by yearly optimal profile limits of SAB and GFR to achieve the recommended UN MMR levels by 2030. The optimal profile limits provide a quantitative guide-line for the government and partners in terms of yearly SAB and GFR targets in order to reduce MMR to the level recommended by the UN agencies [4].

Based on the previous study, Log Linear Regression can model maternal deaths more accurately compared with Poisson regression [10]. Thus, Log Linear Regression model has been developed and is used for optimization purpose. A reliable model that can estimate the maternal deaths and the optimized values of its corresponding predictors will assist the government to make an inform decision on resource allocation and lacking resources in order to reduce the domestic MMR.

The results of our analysis show that increasing SAB rapidly to the highest level is possible. Under this condition, a slow increase in GFR will not increase MMR too much above the UN maximum recommended level of 140. On the other hand, considering that the GFR in South Sudan is already at almost the highest level, it is more likely that it will decrease with increased education, income levels and awareness.

Methods

This section outlines the data collection tasks, prediction model for MMR, mathematical optimization and development of linear profile limits for MMR in terms of its significant predictors.

Data collection

The research has used 30 years of data (1986–2015) to carry out the statistical analysis. The data was collected from the Department of Statistics at the Juba Teaching Hospital (JTH), Reproductive Health Department from Ministry of Health (MoH) [3] National Bureau of Statistics NBS Report [12], the South Sudan 2009 National Baseline Household Survey Report, South Sudan Household Health Survey [13], Census of Population and Housing [14], and the United Nations' Organizations and their partners (e.g. WHO, UNAID, UNICEF, UNDP).

The yearly data included the number of non-HIV +/AIDS maternal deaths, yearly SAB, GDP and yearly GFR. The data on GDP was mainly obtained from National Bureau of Statistics (NBS) Yearly' Report, World Health Organization (WHO), UNICEF, the World Bank and the United Nations Population Division [12].

Prediction model for MMR

Several models for predicting MMR based on different predictors were developed by Makuei, et al. [10]. We used randomly selected two third of the Yearly Data to build the models. The models were then used to predict the remaining ten years' data. The mean errors and the standard error of the mean (SE Mean) were used to compare the efficacy of the models. The analysis was carried out using Microsoft Excel, R and Minitab version 17 statistical soft-ware.

The following two models were the predictive models best describing MMR (based on their respective mean error and SE Mean):

Log Regression Equation, $R^2 = 77.11\%$

$$Log\ (Non\text{–}HIV/AIDS) = \text{-}20.8\text{-}8.30\ Log\ (SAB) + 8.10\ Log\ (GFR) + 5.12\ Log\ (GDP) \quad (1)$$

Poisson Regression Equation, $R^2 = 79.75\%$.
Non-HIV+/AIDS MDs Rate Per 1000 = exp.(Y')

$$Y' = 4.227\text{–}0.3819\ SAB + 0.03237\ GFR + 0.002902\ GDP \quad (2)$$

Since mean errors and SE Mean for the Log Linear Regression is much less than Poisson Regression, we can conclude that Log linear regression outperforms Poisson regression in predicting the MMR for South Sudan.

In this paper we deployed Ln-regression and used 30 years of data to develop the following optimal prediction model for MMR.

$$\text{Ln}\ (\text{MMR}) = -10\text{–}1.73 * \text{Ln}\ (\text{SAB}) + 2.83 * \text{Ln}\ (\text{GFR}) + 0.943 * \text{Ln}\ (\text{GDP}) \quad (3)$$

Equation (3) indicates that one unit change in Ln (SAB) will decrease Ln (MMR) by 1.73 units while one unit change in Ln (GFR) and Ln (GDP) will increase Ln (MMR) by 2.83 and 0.943 respectively. As the relationships are logarithmic, the effect on actual values of MMR, in terms of maternal death per 100,000 live births, will be several times higher.

Compared to the decrease in MMR which can be brought about by increasing Ln (SAB), the increasing effect of Ln (GFR) on Ln (MMR) is much higher (1.64 times) than that of Ln (SAB). Meanwhile, the effect that one unit change in Ln (GDP) has on Ln (MMR) is (0.55 times) less than that of Ln (SAB).

This result on GDP is aligned with the finding by the authors in [32] who investigated the relationship between MMR and GDP in 79 developing countries and concluded that per capital GDP was one of the most significant predictor (– 0.83) for MMR. Similarly in China, Feng XL et al. observed that log (GDP) per capita was a determinant of crude MMR with the adjusted rate ratio of 0.85–0.86 compared to a crude ratio of 0.66 [18] . In their study Du et al. noted that reduction of MMR over the period of 1996–2009 in Guizhou province of China was negatively related to GDP [19] . In our study, due to lack of the yearly GDP data in South Sudan, the GDP value was held constant at the average GDP over the period of 1986–2015 (Ln (GDP) =7.480, or GDP = 1772).

Optimization is often used to optimize and observe optimal values, patterns and structures in data over time. In this analysis we used MATLAB, Excel Solver, R, and Minitab 17. They have been used to conduct optimization procedures and obtain optimal values for the predictors SAB and GFR for a given value of MMR. The optimized values were then used to develop and plot lower and upper profile limits for the MMR, SAB and GFR to achieve the UN recommended lower and upper MMR limits of between 70 and 140.

Mathematical optimization

In mathematics, computer science, and operation research, mathematical optimization is the selection of a best value from some set of available alternatives. An optimization problem consists of minimizing or maximizing a real function systematically by choosing input values for its individual variables from within an allowed domain. In addition to that, optimization includes.

Finding the best available values of some objective function given a defined domain or input including a variety of various types of constrains.

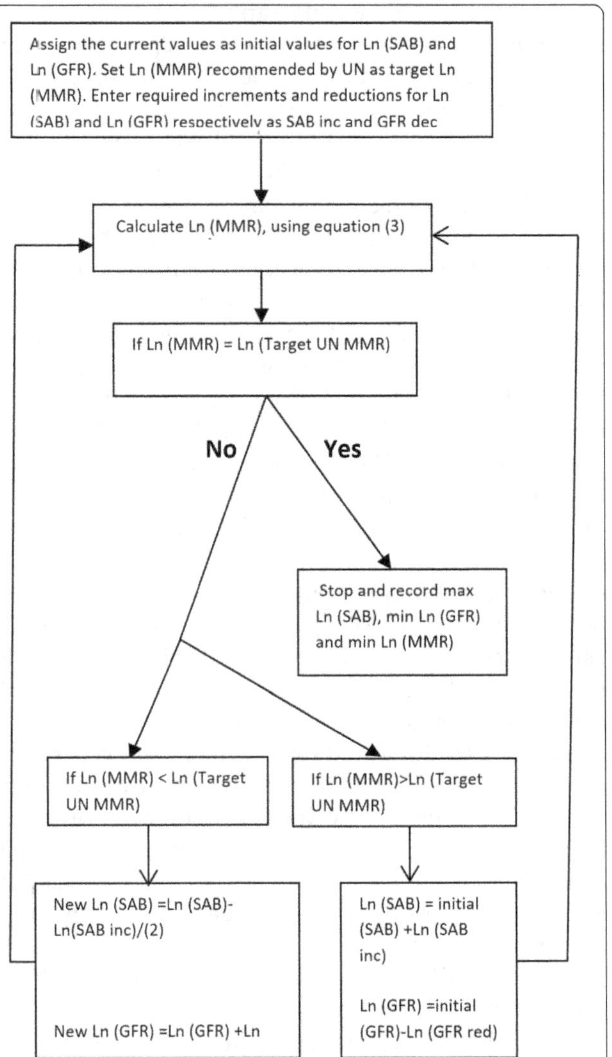

Fig. 1 Calculation optimal max Ln (SAB) and min Ln (GFR) values for a given MMR level

Optimization using solver package and MATLAB

Solver is part of a collection of commands to determine the minimum or maximum value of one cell by changing the values of other cells. With Solver, an optimal (minima or maxima) value could be found for the objective cell, subject to constraints or limits on the values of the predictors. In this study Ln (SAB) and Ln (GFR) were optimized for given values of Ln (MMR) while keeping Ln (GDP) constant at 7.480 or GDP = 1772 which is the average of Ln (GDP) over the period that data were collected. The results from solver are then confirmed with the results of the algorithm developed in MATLAB. Optimization procedures to attain optimal max Ln (SAB) and min Ln (GFR) values for a given Ln (MMR) level is outlined in the algorithm presented in Fig. 1 below.

Linear profile limits

Profile monitoring systems assist and help to identify factors related to an observed phenomenon, assess the effect of changing any factor/s on the event and predict the behaviour of the phenomenon under different situations. In many situations the quality and performance of a process may be better characterized and summarized by relationship between the response (dependent) variable and one or more explanatory (independent) variables referred to as profile [20].

The general parametric linear profile model relating the explanatory variables X_{1i}, X_{2i}, X_{3i} ..., X_{pi} to the response Y_{ij}, is presented by.

$$Y_{ij} = A_{0j} + A_{1j}X_{1i} + ..., +A_{pj} + \varepsilon_{ij}, i = 1, 2, 3, ..., n, \quad j = 1, 2, 3, ..., k$$

where A_{1j} (l = 0,1,2, ..., p) is the regression coefficient. The pair observation (X_{li}, Y_{ij}) is obtained in the jth random sample, where X_{li} is the ith design point (i = 1,2,3,

..., n) for the lth explanatory variable (l = 1.2,3, ..., p). It is assumed that the errors ε_{ijs} are independent, identically distributed (i.i. d.) variables with mean zero and variance $\sigma^2{}_j$, when the process is in control.

Profile monitoring is used to understand and to check the stability of this relationship over time [21].

Recently many practitioners and researchers have used profile monitoring as a new sub-area of statistical process control exploring the application of profile monitoring in different disciplines and in real life [22–24]. The application of profile monitoring is often focussed on processes with multiple quality characteristics and has also been extended to detect clusters of disease incident and used in public health surveillance [25–32].

In this study, profile monitoring will be used to monitor maternal mortality rate (MMR) in South Sudan and assess its variation influenced by SAB and GFR.

Development of profile limits

In this paper, MATLAB, Minitab, R and Excel Solver are used to obtain optimal values of Ln (SAB) and Ln (GFR) for a given value of Ln (MMR) while keeping Ln (GDP) constants at 7.480 (GDP = 1772) which is the average of Ln (GDP) over the period that the data were collected.

Furthermore, to generate the lower and upper profile control limits for Ln (MMR), the proposed predictive models presented in eq. (3) and the target minimum and maximum levels of MMR proposed by the UN agencies; MMR = 70 and MMR = 140 have been used. It was recommended that these limits should be achieved by 2030. The current MMR in South Sudan is about 730 deaths per 100,000.

The statistical analysis shows that increasing SAB by 1.22% per year would decrease MMR by 1.4% (95% CI (0.4–5%)) while decreasing GFR by 1.22% per year would decrease MMR by 1.8% (95% CI (0.5–6.26%)).

The following steps were taken to generate the lower and upper profile limits for yearly target values of SAB and GFR in order to reduce MMR to the target minimum and maximum levels recommended by UN agencies.

Step 1 To achieve MMR = 140 (the maximum recommended by the UN) from the current value of 730 by 2030, the government should reduce MMR by (approximately) 39 deaths per year (or Ln (MMR) by 0.11 per year). Therefore, the optimization program was deployed to obtain the optimal sets of Ln (SAB) and Ln (GFR) for a given Ln (MMR) with the starting value of Ln (730). The Ln (MMR) was then reduced by 0.11, year by year. The results in terms of Ln function and numerical values are presented in Tables 1 and 2. The profile limits are presented in Figs. 1, 2, 3 and 4. It should be noted that the constraint on Ln (SAB) is that, it should be greater than the existing maximum (Ln (SAB) = 3.178), as our aim is to increase SAB year by year. While the constraint on Ln (GFR) was to be smaller than the existing current minimum value of 5.024, its value should be further decreased. The results presented in the first 3 columns of Table 2 show that to decrease MMR from 730 to 140 by the year 2030, the government should increase SAB from the current value of 19 to 50 while the value of GFR should be decreased from the current value of 175 to 97. The five years break-up values are highlighted in Table 2. Thus, for the year 2020, South Sudan should target to have MMR decreased from the current value of 730 to 421 by simultaneously increasing SAB from 19 to 26 and deceasing GFR from 175 to 144. By the year 2025 the country should target to have MMR declined from the present value of 730 to 243 by simultaneously increasing SAB from 19 to 36 and decreasing GFR from 175 to 118. Moreover, by the year 2030, the government and stakeholders should target to have MMR decreased from the current value of 730 to 140 by increasing SAB from 19 to 50 and decreasing GFR from 175 to 97.

Step 2 To attain MMR = 70 (the minimum recommended by the UN) from the current value of 730 by 2030, step one was followed except that the target value was changed from 140 to 70 and the decrease in Ln (MMR) was 0.156 per year. The optimization results in terms of Ln function and numerical values are presented in Tables 1 and 2. The last three columns of Table 2 show that to achieve MMR of 70 by the year 2030, the authorities in South Sudan should reduce GFR from 175 to 75 while increasing SAB from the current value of 19 to 76. The target statistics for 2020 would be MMR = 334 with SAB being increased to 30 and GFR reduced to 133. By the year 2025 the government and partners should target to have MMR decreased from the present value of 730 to 153, by simultaneously increasing SAB from 19 to 47 and decreasing GFR from 175 to 101. Therefore, developing health policies that target MMR, the SAB and GFR profile limits out lined in Table 2 would ensure the successful accomplishment of the UN target maternal mortality rate proposal.

The optimization results presented in Table 2 and Fig. 2 show that if it is desired to reduce MMR to 140 by 2030, we should decrease Ln (MMR) by 0.11 units annually (MMR by 39 units). This will be achieved by

Table 1 Shows error analysis for independent variables of SAB, GFR and GDP

Model	Mean Errors	SE Mean
Log Linear regression (1)	*0.008*	*0.171*
Poisson regression (2)	*−216*	*316*

Table 2 Optimal values of Ln (SAB) and Ln (GFR) for given Ln (MMR)

Years	MMR Target 140			MMR Target 70		
	Min values of Ln (MMR), changing by 0.11, per a year	Max values of Ln (SAB)	Min values of Ln (GFR)	Min values of Ln (MMR) changing by 0.156	Max values of Ln (SAB)	Min values of Ln (GFR)
2015	6.59	2.95	5.16	6.59	2.95	5.16
2016	6.48	3.01	5.12	6.44	3.04	5.11
2017	6.37	3.08	5.09	6.28	3.13	5.05
2018	6.26	3.14	5.05	6.12	3.22	5.00
2019	6.15	3.21	5.01	5.97	3.31	4.94
2020	6.04	3.27	4.97	5.81	3.40	4.89
2021	5.93	3.33	4.93	5.66	3.49	4.83
2022	5.82	3.40	4.99	5.50	3.58	4.78
2023	5.71	3.46	4.85	5.34	3.67	4.72
2024	5.60	3.52	4.81	5.19	3.76	4.67
2025	5.49	3.59	4.77	5.03	3.85	4.61
2026	5.38	3.65	4.74	4.87	3.94	4.56
2027	5.27	3.71	4.70	4.72	4.03	4.50
2028	5.16	3.78	4.66	4.56	4.12	4.45
2029	5.05	3.84	4.62	4.41	4.22	4.39
2030	4.94	3.91	4.58	4.25	4.33	4.31

The target MMR for 2030 is 140 in the first three columns and 70 in the last three columns

simultaneously increasing the value of Ln (SAB) by 0.06 units and reducing Ln (GFR) by 0.04 units. In contrast to achieve MMR of 70, we should decrease Ln (MMR) by 0.156, per year. This requires concurrently increasing Ln (SAB) by 0.09 and decreasing Ln (GFR) by 0.06, per year.

The optimization results presented in Table 3 and Fig. 3 show that to achieve the UN target of 140 by 2030, we should simultaneously increase the value of SAB to 50 and reduce the value of GFR to 97. While to achieve MMR of 70, we should simultaneously increase SAB to 76 and decrease GFR to 75.

The target MMR for 2030 is 140.

The target MMR for 2030 is 70.

Figure 4a and b visually show that to achieve minimum MMR we must reduce GRF to its minimum value while increasing SAB to it maximum value. Figure 4b shows sharper reduction in MMR requires deeper increase and decrease in SAB and GFR values respectively.

Discussion

Reducing the maternal mortality rate has been the main concern of the global health agenda over the last two decades. It has been documented that 74–98% of maternal deaths can be averted even in the lowest income nations [33–38]. According to Chou et al. & Yi et al. improving maternal health and reducing related mortality have been the key concern of the international community as one of the eight Millennium Development Goals (MDG 5) [32, 39]. Maternal mortality is a complex problem requiring complex intervention. It challenges the key performers in resource limited countries to acknowledge the problem and scale up the means and advocated measures to address this problem. The maternal mortality rate in South Sudan is one of the highest in the world. Based on previous studies, authors have identified the Skilled Assistant at Birth (SAB), the General Fertility Rate (GFR) and per capita the Gross Domestic Product (GDP) as the most significant predictors of MMR [10].

The study has deployed mathematical optimization methods and for the first time has developed the optimal lower and upper profile limits for MMR, SAB and GFR. Table 3 provides the yearly optimal values of these variables and can effectively aid the government to achieve the target maternal mortality rate recommended by UN agencies by 2030. The following discussion compares the findings from this research to other similar research, and also seeks to identify the best options for South Sudan to reduce MMR.

Sab

WHO has defined the term skilled assistant and listed the essential and additional skills required for the expected duties. Although at individual level, skilled assistance can be beneficial, at the population level, evidence is weak. The authors proposed a model which can reduce MMR by 16–33% through primary and secondary prevention of four major complications of pregnancy

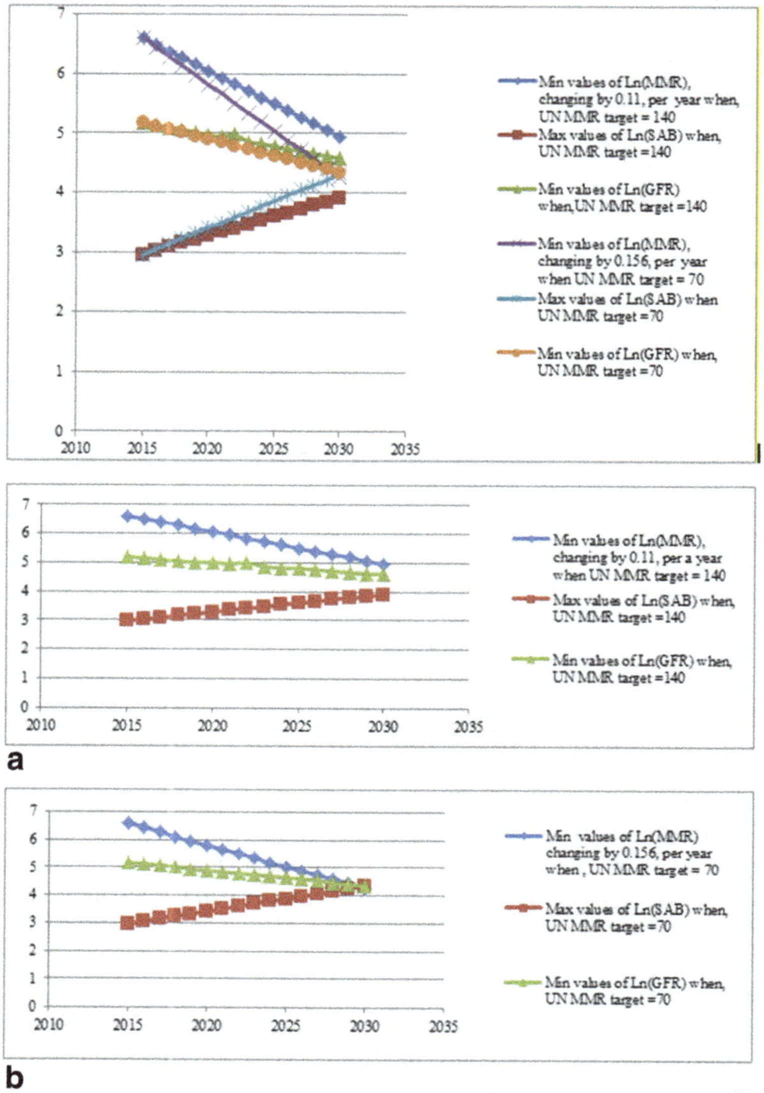

Fig. 2 Lower and upper profile limits for Ln (MMR), Ln (SAB) and Ln (GFR). **a** Profile limits for Ln (MMR), Ln (SAB) and LN (GFR). The target MMR for 2030 is 140. **b** Profile limits for Ln (MMR), Ln (SAB) and LN (GFR). The target MMR for 2030 is 70

and delivery. Skilled assistant can reduce mortality rate as well as morbidities. Timely access to quality care and professional staff are also important in the implementation of skilled assistance. In Pakistan, traditional birth attendants are assisting deliveries, but MMR remains high. Training the traditional attendants and then deploying them for assisted deliveries and increasing access to emergency care were found to be very effective [40]. Improved quality of primary care through professional midwifery combined with referral care at hospitals takes less time to reduce MMR significantly. As exemplified by the experiences in some developing countries, the time taken to reduce MMR from 400 to 200 is around 9–12 years, from 200 to 100 is about 7–9 years and for 100 to 50 is 4–8 years [41]. Graham et al., [42] point out that increasing skilled assistance can take time and significant resources and funds. Politics play a critical role in the agenda setting in health affairs; therefore, understanding the priorities of the political agenda in health is vital [43]. Any improvement in the SAB can be influenced by political will. The ingredients of implementing methods to increase SAB in any country are useful for adaption into South Sudan also. The authors have also identified SAB as one of the most influential factors for MMR in South Sudan [10]. Our analysis shows that GFR is the most influential factor in increasing the MMR followed by the SAB and GDP. The South Sudan current statistics shows that only 20% births are attended by skilled assistants [3].

GFR

In a review of international data, Stover and Ross 2010 [44] found that using contraceptives and family planning

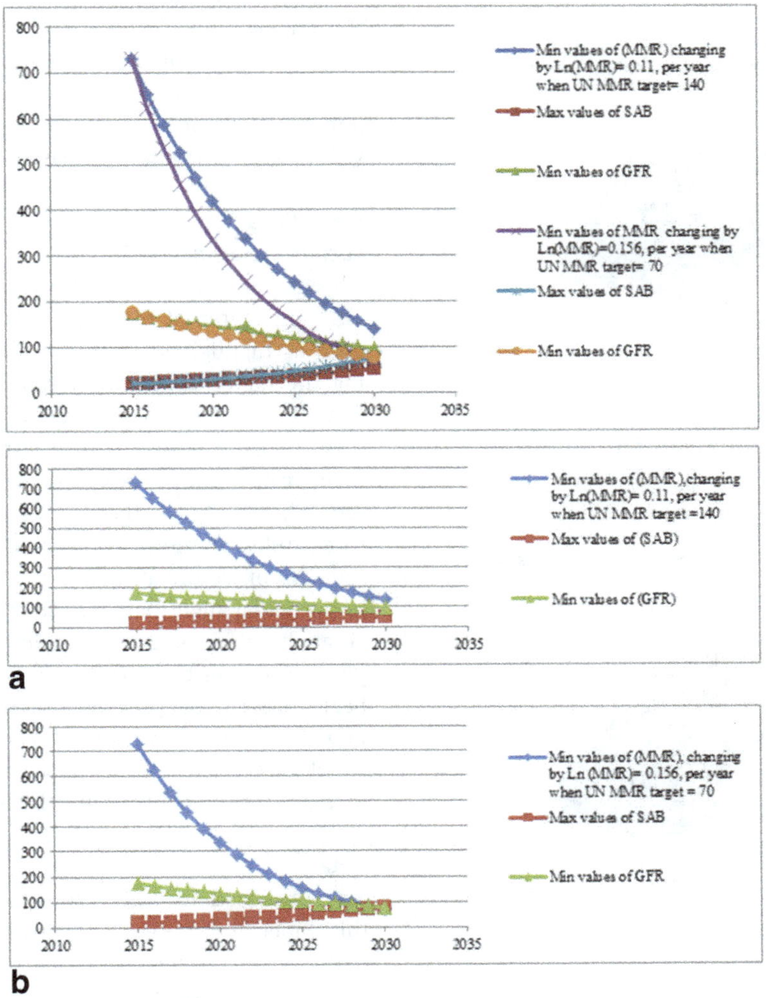

Fig. 3 The lower and upper profile limits for MMR, SAB and GFR. Figure 3a: Profile limits for the numerical values of MMR, SAB and GFR. The target MMR for 2030 is 140. Fig. 3b: Profile limits for the numerical values of MMR, SAB and GFR. The target MMR for 2030 is 70

reduced MMR by about one million between 1990 and 2005. This was due to the effect of contraceptives on fertility rates, especially in developing countries. Transition from low to high levels of contraceptive use can reduce the country's MMR by 450 per 100,000 live births. These observations justify the use of contraceptives to reduce GFR in South Sudan. Reduction of unsafe abortion led to significant reduction in MMR in Uruguay between 2001 and 2015, according to the findings of Briozzo 2016 [45]. Thus, abortion as a fertility reduction method among pregnant women is risky. Our study also shows that GFR is the most influential factor in increasing the MMR.

Other methods to reduce MMR

Mbaruku and Bergström [46] have reported a variety of strategies that resulted in reducing MMR from 933 to 186 per 100,000 live births during 1984–91 in Tanzania. Low cost strategies combined with local problem solving methods show that it is possible for developing countries, like South Sudan, to achieve significant reduction in MMR level.

Lassi and Bhutta (2015) in a review stressed community-based integrated packages of care for both mothers and new-born babies to help reduce MMR along-with neonatal mortality [47].

Best option

Clear evidence on reduction of MMR by the use of contraceptives was provided in the review of data on 172 countries by Ahmed et al. [48]. Using predictive models, they estimated that 342,203 women died of maternal causes in 2008. Contraceptive use prevented death of another 272,040 (44%) deaths. If unmet needs of contraceptive use were satisfied, another 104,000 maternal deaths could be prevented every year. The basic model of the authors for estimation of MMR is.

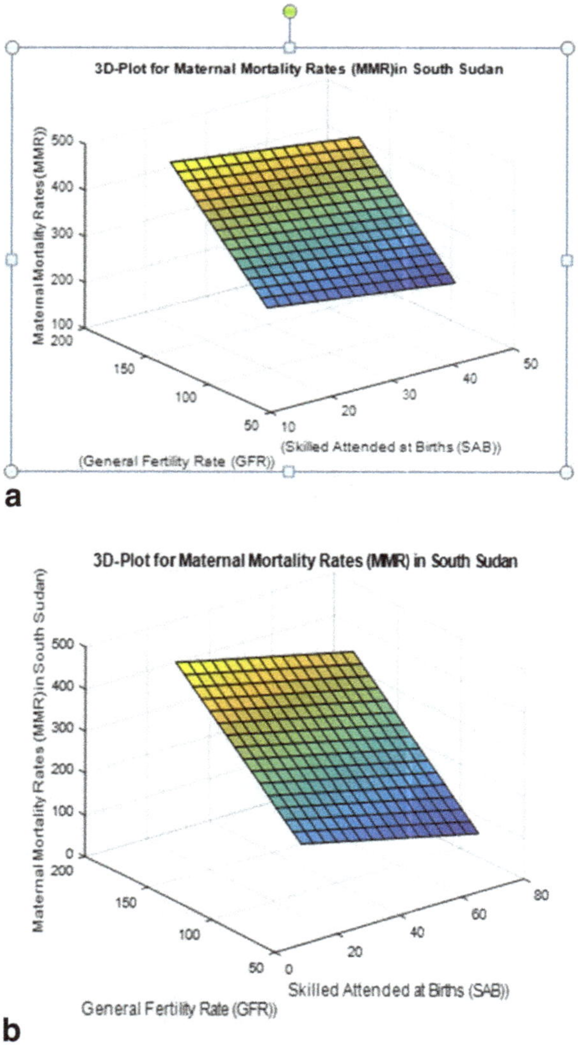

Fig. 4 a Three dimensional Surface Plot of MMR values vs SAB and GFR for target MMR 140. **b** Three dimensional Surface Plot of MMR values vs SAB and GFR for target MMR 70

$$\text{Log (PMDFi)} = \beta_0 + \beta_1 \log(\text{GDP}_i) + \beta_2 \log(\text{GFR}_i) + \beta_3 \text{SAB}_i + \alpha^c{}_{j[i]} + \alpha^R k_{[i]} + \log(1 - a_i) + \varepsilon_i$$

This is similar to the model used in this paper.

In the above equation, PMDF is the proportion of maternal deaths among all deaths of reproductive-age women (15–49 years) in year i, country j, and geographical region k. While α^c and α^R are random intercepts for country j in geographical region k, respectively, a_i is the proportion of death due to AIDS among the women of reproductive age, and ε_i is the error term. The GDP was adjusted according to purchasing power parity in 2005. But they have modified the equation for predicting MMR for contraceptive use.

In conclusion, the outlined research in other countries shows that increase in SAB and decrease in GFR can reduce MMR. These are consistent with the findings of this paper.

Based on the above discussion it appears that initiatives to increase SAB and reduce GFR are vitally important for reducing MMR. However, in a short run, reducing GFR is relatively easier than increasing SAB.

Limitations

Factors impacting MMR

This paper investigates the impact of SAB, GFR and GDP on maternal mortality rate in South Sudan. However, as highlighted in the introduction, factors impacting the maternal mortality rate include socio-economic factors, macro-economic factors and physiological factors [1]. Lack of access to health care facilities is also a major factor due to lack of roads and transportation system [7, 10]. More than 50% of the population walks three miles or more to the nearest primary health care unit. All of factors affect the total health care system and in particular high maternal mortality rate problem. Kruk et al. have investigated the impact of the community perceptions on the quality of care provided by the local health system on pregnant woman's decision to deliver in a clinic. They have suggested that improving the quality of care at first level clinics may assist the efforts to increase facility delivery in sub-Saharan Africa [2].

Data

The proposed Ln-linear regression model deployed in this paper and the constraints on SAB and GFR used to develop the profiles are based on 30 years of manually recorded data obtained from the sources listed under "data collection". The authors acknowledge that some of these data may be an estimate rather than the true values. Although this may result in underestimate/overestimate of the profiles, it is unlikely to impact on the validity of the analyses. Furthermore, our results on the impact of GFR, SAB and GDP on MMR in South Sudan are aligned with that of other researchers (as highlighted in the discussion section).

Conclusions

This study for the first time has deployed optimisation procedures to develop yearly lower and upper profile limits for maternal mortality rate (MMR), targeting the UN recommended lower and upper MMR levels by 2030. The MMR profile limits have been accompanied in by the profile limits for optimal yearly values of SAB and GFR levels. Studies on predictors of logarithmic multi-regression models provided distinct evidence that increasing Skilled Attendant at Birth (SAB) and decreasing General Fertility Rate (GFR) while leaving the Gross Domestic Product (GDP) constant at 1772, can reduce the Maternal Mortality Rate in South Sudan by 2030 to

Table 3 Optimal values of SAB and GFR for a given MMR when GDP) is constant at 1772

Years	MMR Target 140			MMR Target 70		
	Min values of MMR changing by Ln (MMR) = 0.11, per a year	Max values of SAB	Min values of GFR	Min values of MMR changing by Ln (MMR) = 0.156, per a year	Max values of SAB	Min values of GFR
2015	730	19	175	730	19	175
2016	654	20	168	625	21	165
2017	586	22	162	534	23	156
2018	525	23	155	457	25	148
2019	470	25	150	391	27	140
2020	421	26	144	334	30	133
2021	377	28	138	286	33	125
2022	338	30	146	244	36	119
2023	302	32	128	209	39	112
2024	271	34	123	179	43	106
2025	243	36	118	153	47	101
2026	217	39	114	131	52	95
2027	195	41	110	112	57	90
2028	175	44	105	96	62	85
2029	156	47	101	82	68	81
2030	140	50	97	70	76	75

The target MMR for 2030 is 140 in the first three columns and 70 in the last three columns

the limits proposed by the UN agencies (WHO, USAID, UNICEF & World Bank, 2015) and beyond. The statistical analysis shows that increasing SAB by 1.22% per year would decrease MMR by 1.4%. [95% CI (0.4–5%)] while decreasing GFR by 1.22% per year would decrease MMR by 1.8% [95% CI (0.5% - 6.26], when the GDP is held constant.

The comparison of the findings of this study to other similar studies suggests that reducing GFR is more effective and achievable than increasing SAB when aiming to reduce MMR.

The optimal profile limits provide a quantitative guide-line for the government and partners in terms of yearly SAB and GFR target in order to reduce MMR to the level recommended by the UN. The outcomes of this study can effectively aid authorities to make informed evidence-based intervention decisions on resources allocation to reduce the MMR.

Abbreviations

AIDs: Acquired Immune Deficiency Syndrome (AIDs); GDP: Gross Domestic Product (GDP); GFR: General Fertility Rate (GFR); HIV^+: Human Immunodeficiency Virus; Inc.: increment (See Fig. 1); Ln: Logarithmic of natural number; MATLAB: Matrix Laboratory is multi-paradigm numerical computing environment and fourth- generation programming language; MDG: Millennium Development Goals; MDs: Maternal Deaths; Minitab: Statistical analysis software; MMR: Maternal Mortality Rate; R: Multi-paradigm numerical computing environment and generation of computer programming language; Red: reduction (See Fig. 1); SAB: Skilled Attendance at Births; SSA: Sub-Saharan Africa (a region in Africa); UNICEF: United Nations International Children's Emergency Fund; USAID: United States Agency for International Development; USD: United States Dollar; WHO: World Health Organisation

Acknowledgements

The authors would like to thank WHO (World Health Organisation), and UNICEF (United Nations International Children's Emergency Fund), South Sudan Country Offices and South Sudan National Bureau of Statistics (NBS) and Juba Teaching Hospital for providing the dataset. The authors appreciate the Australian Government for financially supporting this study through Australian Government Research Training Program Scholarship. We also express our gratitude to the Higher Degree by Research (HDR), RMIT University for financial support, Melbourne, Australia. Furthermore, our appreciation and thank to the RMIT University Learning Centre for their language advisory review in particular Dr. Ken Manson. The contents are solely the responsibility of the authors and don't necessarily represent the official views of the supporting offices.

Funding

The research was funded by the Federal Government of Australia, through Australian Government Research Training Program Scholarship and RMIT University, Higher Degree Research (HDR). The funder didn't play a significant role in the planning of the study and collection, analysis and interpretation of data and writing the manuscript.

Authors' contributions

GM designed study, conducted data collection, literature review, performed data analysis, interpretation of data and drafted the manuscript. MA and KM involved in the designed research, literature review, performed data analysis, proofreading and modification of the whole paper. All authors (GM, MA and KM), reviewed and approved the final version of the paper.

Authors' information

G. Makuei is a PhD candidate at RMIT University, Melbourne, Australia and was a lecturer for statistics and operation research courses at DR John Garang University of Science and Technology from 2010 to 2012, Bor, South Sudan. Mali Abdollahian and Kaye Marion are both senior lecturers and lecturers at RMIT University, School of Science, Melbourne, Australia.

Competing interests

The authors declare that they have no competing interests.

References

1. Alkema L, Chou D, Hogan D, Zhang S, Moller AB, Gemmill A, Fat DM, Boerma T, Temmerman M, Mathers C, et al. Global, regional, and national levels and trends in maternal mortality between 1990 and 2015, with scenario-based projections to 2030: a systematic analysis by the UN maternal mortality estimation inter-agency group. Lancet. 2016;387(10017): 462–74.
2. Kruk ME, Rockers PC, Mbaruku G, Paczkowski MM, Galea S. Community and health system factors associated with facility delivery in rural Tanzania: a multilevel analysis. Health Policy. 2010;97(2–3):209–16.
3. (NBS) MoHMaNBoS. The Republic of South Sudan: The Sudan Household Health Survey 2010. South Sudan: (NBS) MoHMaNBoS. Juba; 2014.
4. Trends in Maternal Mortality: 1990 to 2015: estimates by WHO, UNICEF, UNFPA, World Bank Group and the United Nations Division.
5. Rau A. Reducing maternity mortality rate in South Sudan. In: Borgen; 2015.
6. South Sudan: Maternal and Child Health in South Sudan.
7. Ending Preventable Maternal Mortality: USAID Maternal Health Vision for Action Evidence for Strategic Approches.
8. WHO U, UNFPA, World Bank Groun and the United Nations Population Division. Meauring Maternal Mortality, key facts. In: Geneva Foundation for Medical Education and Research. vol. Fact sheet No 348, vol. 20. Geneva 27, Switzerland: World Heath Organization (WHO); 2016.
9. Risk - Lifetime Risk of Death in Childbearing.
10. Makuei G, Abdollahian M, Marion K. Modeling maternal mortality rate in South Sudan. Int'l Conf Information and Knowledge Engineering. 2016;107-112:6.
11. WHO. Fact Sheet. Geneva: Worl Health Organization: Worl Health Oraganization (WHO); 2008.
12. (NBS) NBoS. SOUTH SUDAN STATISTICAL YEAR BOOK 2015. In: 2015 SYB. m; 2015.
13. National Bureau of Statistics NBS. Census of Population and Housing (the NBS, 2008), Southern Sudan. Juba, South Sudan: National Bureau of Statistic Office; 2008.
14. National Bureau of Statistics SS. The South Sudan National Baseline Household Survey' 2009 Report. Juba Southern Sudan: Statistics NBo. National Bureau of Statistics' Office; 2009.
15. Campbell OM, Graham WJ, steering g LMSS. Strategies for reducing maternal mortality: getting on with what works. Lancet. 2006;368(9543): 1284–99.
16. World Highlights.
17. Rai RK, Tulchinsky TH. Addressing the sluggish progress in reducing maternal mortality in India. Asia Pac J Public Health. 2015;27(2):NP1161–9.
18. Feng XL, Zhu J, Zhang L, Song L, Hipgrave D, Guo S, Ronsmans C, Guo Y, Yang Q. Socio-economic disparities in maternal mortality in China between 1996 and 2006. BJOG. 2010;117(12):1527–36.
19. Du Q, Lian W, Naess O, Bjertness E, Kumar BN, Shi SH. The trends in maternal mortality between 1996 and 2009 in Guizhou, China: ethnic differences and associated factors. J Huazhong Univ Sci Technolog Med Sci. 2015;35(1):140–6.
20. Yin H, Zhao Y, Zhang Y, Zhang H, Xu L, Zou Z, Yang W, Cheng J, Zhou Y. Genome-wide analysis of the expression profile of Saccharomyces cerevisiae in response to treatment with the plant isoflavone, wighteone, as a potential antifungal agent. Biotechnol Lett. 2006;28(2):99–105.
21. Kang S, Ren D, Xiao G, Daris K, Buck L, Enyenihi AA, Zubarev R, Bondarenko PV, Deshpande R. Cell line profiling to improve monoclonal antibody production. Biotechnol Bioeng. 2014;111(4):748–60.
22. Gupta SK, Bansal D, Malhi P, Das R. Developmental profile in children with iron deficiency anemia and its changes after therapeutic iron supplementation. Indian J Pediatr. 2010;77(4):375–9.
23. Gupta S. Profile monitoring-control chart schemes for monitoring linear and low order polynomial profiles. In: A Dissertation Presented in Partial Fulfillment of the Requirements for the Degree Doctor of Philosopy. Arizona: Arizona State University; 2010.
24. Hosseinifard SZ. Monitoring and performance analysis of regression profiles. This thesis is submitted in total fulfillment of the requirements for the degree of Doctor of Philosophy. Melbourne, Victoria, Australia: RMIT University; 2012.
25. Woodall WH. Current research on profile monitoring. SciELO Brasil. 2007; 17(3):420–5.
26. Grigg OA, Farewell VT. A risk-adjusted sets method for monitoring adverse medical outcomes. Stat Med. 2004;23(10):1593–602.
27. Grigg OA, Farewell VT, Spiegelhalter DJ. Use of risk-adjusted CUSUM and RSPRT charts for monitoring in medical contexts. Stat Methods Med Res. 2003;12(2):147–70.
28. Chopra M, Daviaud E, Pattinson R, Fonn S, Lawn JE. Saving the lives of South Africa's mothers, babies, and children: can the health system deliver? Lancet. 2009;374(9692):835–46.
29. Woodall J, Dixey R, South J. Control and choice in English prisons: developing health-promoting prisons. Health Promot Int. 2014;29(3):474–82.
30. Montgomery AL, Fadel S, Kumar R, Bondy S, Moineddin R, Jha P. The effect of health-facility admission and skilled birth attendant coverage on maternal survival in India: a case-control analysis. PLoS One. 2014;9(6): e95696.
31. Montgomery AL, Ram U, Kumar R, Jha P, Million Death Study C. Maternal mortality in India: causes and healthcare service use based on a nationally representative survey. PLoS One. 2014;9(1):e83331.
32. Chou D, Tuncalp O, Firoz T, Barreix M, Filippi V, von Dadelszen P, van den Broek N, Cecatti JG, Say L, Maternal Morbidity Working G. Constructing maternal morbidity - towards a standard tool to measure and monitor maternal health beyond mortality. BMC pregnancy and childbirth. 2016;16:45.
33. Bale JRS, B J, Lucas AO. Improving birth outcomes: meeting the Challange in the developing world. Washington: The National Academy Press; 2003.
34. Prual A. Reducing maternal mortality in developing countries: theory and practice. Medecine tropicale : revue du Corps de sante colonial. 2004;64(6): 569–75.
35. Prual A, Bouvier-Colle MH, de Bernis L, Breart G. Severe maternal morbidity from direct obstetric causes in West Africa: incidence and case fatality rates. Bull World Health Organ. 2000;78(5):593–602.
36. Prual A, De Bernis L, El Joud DO. Potential role of prenatal care in reducing maternal and perinatal mortality in sub-Saharan Africa. Journal de gynecologie, obstetrique et biologie de la reproduction. 2002;31(1):90–9.
37. Prual A, Gamatie Y, Djakounda M, Huguet D. Traditional uvulectomy in Niger: a public health problem? Soc Sci Med. 1994;39(8):1077–82.
38. Prual A, Huguet D, Garbin O, Rabe G. Severe obstetric morbidity of the third trimester, delivery and early puerperium in Niamey (Niger). Afr J Reprod Health. 1998;2(1):10–9.
39. Yi S, Tuot S, Chhoun P, Pal K, Ngin C, Choub SC, Brody C. Improving prevention and care for HIV and sexually transmitted infections among men who have sex with men in Cambodia: the sustainable action against HIV and AIDS in communities (SAHACOM). BMC Health Serv Res. 2016;16(1):599.
40. Jokhio AH, Winter HR, Cheng KK. An intervention involving traditional birth attendants and perinatal and maternal mortality in Pakistan. N Engl J Med. 2005;352(20):2091–9.
41. Van Lerberghe W, De Brouwere V. Reducing maternal mortality in a context of poverty. Safe motherhood strategies: a review of the evidence. 2001;17:1–5.
42. Graham WJ, Bell JS, Bullough CH. Can skilled attendance at delivery reduce maternal mortality in developing countries. Safe motherhood strategies: a review of the evidence. 2001;17:97–130.
43. Jat TR, Deo PR, Goicolea I, Hurtig AK, San Sebastian M. The emergence of maternal health as a political priority in Madhya Pradesh, India: a qualitative study. BMC pregnancy and childbirth. 2013;13:181.

44. Stover J, Ross J. How increased contraceptive use has reduced maternal mortality. Matern Child Health J. 2010;14(5):687–95.
45. Briozzo L. From risk and harm reduction to decriminalizing abortion: the Uruguayan model for women's rights. Int J Gynaecol Obstet. 2016;134(Suppl 1):S3–6.
46. Mbaruku G, Bergstrom S. Reducing maternal mortality in Kigoma, Tanzania. Health Policy Plan. 1995;10(1):71–8.
47. Lassi ZS, Bhutta ZA. Community-based intervention packages for reducing maternal and neonatal morbidity and mortality and improving neonatal outcomes. Cochrane Database Syst Rev. 2015;(3) CD007754
48. Ahmed S, Li Q, Liu L, Tsui AO. Maternal deaths averted by contraceptive use: an analysis of 172 countries. Lancet. 2012;380(9837):111–25.

13

Correlates of the Women's Development Army strategy implementation strength with household reproductive, maternal, newborn and child healthcare practices

Zufan Abera Damtew[1*], Ali Mehryar Karim[2], Chala Tesfaye Chekagn[1], Nebreed Fesseha Zemichael[2], Bantalem Yihun[2], Barbara A. Willey[3] and Wuleta Betemariam[2]

Abstract

Background: To address the shortfall in human resources for health, Ethiopia launched the Health Extension Program (HEP) in 2004, establishing a health post with two female health extension workers (HEWs) in every *kebele* (community). In 2011, the Women's Development Army (WDA) strategy was added, using networks of neighboring women to increase the efficiency of HEWs in reaching every household, with one WDA team leader for every 30 households. Through the strategy, women in the community, in partnership with HEWs, share and learn about health practices and empower one another. This study assessed the association between the WDA strategy implementation strength and household reproductive, maternal, newborn and child health care behaviors and practices.

Methods: Using cross-sectional household surveys and community-level contextual data from 423 kebeles representing 145 rural districts, an internal comparison group design was applied to assess whether HEP outreach activity and household-level care practices were better in kebeles with a higher WDA density. The density of active WDA leaders was considered as WDA strategy implementation strength; higher WDA density in a kebele indicating relatively high implementation strength. Based on this, kebeles were classified as higher, moderate, or lower. Multilevel logit models, adjusted for respondents' individual, household and contextual characteristics, were used to assess the associations of WDA strategy implementation strength with outcome indicators of interest.

Results: Average numbers of households per active WDA team leader in the 25th, 50th and 75th percentiles of the kebeles studied were respectively 41, 50 and 73. WDA density was associated with better service for six of 13 indicators considered ($p < 0.05$). For example, kebeles with one active WDA team leader for up to 40 households (higher category) had respectively 7 (95% CI, 2, 13), 11 (5, 17) and 9 (1, 17) percentage-points higher contraceptive prevalence rate, coverage of four or more antenatal care visits, and coverage of institutional deliveries respectively, compared with kebeles with one active WDA team leader for 60 or more households (lower category).

Conclusion: Higher WDA strategy implementation strength was associated with better health care behaviors and practices, suggesting that the WDA strategy supported HEWs in improving health care services delivery.

Keywords: Ethiopia, Community health workers, Health extension workers, Women's development Army, RMNCH

* Correspondence: zufana2003@yahoo.com
[1]Federal Ministry of Health of Ethiopia, Health Extension and Primary Health Service Directorate, Sudan Street, Addis Ababa, Ethiopia
Full list of author information is available at the end of the article

Background

Despite progress over the last two decades, improvements in maternal and newborn survival have not been felt equally across the globe, and low and middle-income countries continue to be disproportionately affected, experiencing 99% of maternal deaths [1], with 66% in Sub-Saharan African countries [2]. Furthermore, within countries, mortality is higher among women and newborns living in rural areas, and among those from poorer communities [3]. Ethiopia reported a neonatal mortality rate of 28 per 1000 live births [4] and a maternal mortality ratio of 353 per 100,000 live births in 2015 [1]. Although these represent declines of 38 and 43% respectively from 2003 levels [5], maternal mortality in Ethiopia remains over 20 times higher than in European countries [1]. The majority of maternal and newborn deaths worldwide could be prevented by providing quality antenatal, delivery, postpartum and postnatal care [1]. Estimates for Ethiopia suggest improved uptake of professional care, but access remains well below levels required, with 32% of pregnant women having the recommended four antenatal care (ANC) visits, 28% skilled attendance at delivery and 17% of mothers having a postpartum check within two days of delivery [6, 7]. Furthermore, marked inequalities exist, for example data from the 2016 Ethiopia Demographic and Health Survey (DHS) show that although 80% of women living in urban areas experienced skilled attendance at delivery, only 21% of pregnant women living in rural areas did so [7].

Reasons for low access to quality services are multi-faceted; however, challenges of insufficiently skilled health workers and inequitable distribution of the health workforce play a role [8]. This is especially the case in countries like Ethiopia, where a large population live in rural areas with low health worker per population density. In total, over 80% of the population of Ethiopia live in rural areas [9]. The ratio of available health workers (including: doctors, health officers, nurses and midwives) is 7 per 10,000 population [9], far below the World Health Organization-recommended minimum threshold of 23 per 10,000 population required to provide basic health coverage [10]. Numerous countries have responded to this growing challenge with the creation and deployment of community health workers, an alternative health worker cadre who can deal effectively with common health problems and improve access to services [11, 12].

Community health workers can contribute to maternal health and child survival through basic curative care and preventive services, and act as a conduit to professional care [13, 14]. The incorporation of community health workers has a long history in public health, and national-scale programs exist in a number of low and middle-income countries. For example, in the late 1970s the Ghanaian Ministry of Health introduced substantial numbers of community or village health workers aimed at implementing primary health care strategies [15]. In 1982, Indonesia deployed village health volunteers, selected and paid by local communities. Their activities included family planning, health education, growth monitoring, nutrition support, immunization and treatment, particularly of diarrheal diseases [16]. In 1988, the Female Community Health Volunteer Program was established by the Nepalese Government and covers most of the country, with over 48,000 volunteers [17]. In 1994, Pakistan implemented the Lady Health Worker Program as part of a national strategy to reduce poverty and improve health by bringing health services to the doorsteps of underserved communities [18].

The effectiveness of such community health worker programs for delivering disease preventive and basic curative services has generally been positive, and in some contexts contributed to declines in maternal, infant and child mortality, although the extent and quality of the evidence available for low and middle-income countries is limited [19, 20]. A recent systematic review from Gilmore and McAulifee reported on the effectiveness of community health worker programs with a focus on preventative strategies to improve reproductive, maternal, newborn and child health (RMNCH) in 10 low and middle-income countries [21]. Based on 17 studies, the authors concluded that, although additional evidence for some strategies was needed, common packages included health education, breastfeeding promotion, essential newborn care and psychosocial support, and that strategies promoting mother-performed behaviors (e.g. skin-to-skin contact for thermal care) were especially effective.

In Ethiopia, the Health Extension Program (HEP) is a community-based health service delivery system, launched in 2004 to provide equitable access to promotive, preventive and limited curative health interventions, with emphasis to the needs of the majority, less-privileged, rural population [22]. In each *kebele*, (community) a health post was established, staffed by two salaried female Health Extension Workers (HEWs) who had graduated from high school and undergone one year's training. The Ethiopian Federal Ministry of Health's HEP aims to provide primary health services through one HEW for every 2500 people. Since its inception, over 40,000 HEWs have been deployed in rural, pastoral and urban areas, and more than 16,500 health posts have been built across the country to provide and manage primary health care [23]. The HEP provides 16 health service packages categorized in four essential health components: hygiene and environmental health services (e.g. encouraging the construction and use of latrines), family health services (e.g. antenatal care (ANC)), disease prevention and control (e.g. malaria prevention and control), and health education and communication (Additional file 1: Table S1). The design of the HEP packages was based on analysis of the major health problems and disease burdens of the population. Recently, additional services were included, particularly for children and women, such as Integrated Community-Based Case Management, Community-Based Newborn Care, and the provision of long-acting family planning methods.

The HEP has brought impressive results: large reductions in maternal and child mortality, and morbidity and mortality by major communicable diseases, through providing basic health services and bridging the gap between the community and health facilities [9]. However, to enhance these efforts and improve geographical penetration and equity, in 2011 the Ethiopian Government introduced a complementary initiative, the Women's Development Army (WDA) strategy, also known as the Health Development Army. WDA members are organized by their neighborhood and are commonly called "one-to-five" networks (denoting one leader and five member households). Based on the neighborhood, five or six "one-to-five" networks are grouped into a women's development team that comprises 25 to 30 households, called "one-to-30" (denoting one team leader to about 30 member households) (Fig. 1). The WDA is a systematic, organized, inclusive and collaborative movement of neighboring households. The WDA leaders of the 1-to-5 networks receive initial training from a HEW, with technical support from the health center staff, on the 16 key health packages, which form the core of the HEP. Under the guidance of HEWs and community leaders, all community members participate, teach and learn from each other and take practical actions to improve the health of individuals, families and the community. The WDA team leaders support the HEWs by mobilizing the community to take up key health services, disseminating essential health messages to the communities, practicing key health actions and collecting health information on community members eligible for health services. This approach helps to increase community engagement and health seeking behavior.

The activities of community health workers are expected to lead to enhanced demand for care and improved home-based practices. For example, enhanced demand for ANC and facility-based delivery care; improved home-based maternal and newborn care practices, such as thermal care; enhanced frequency and timing of postpartum home visits; and increased coverage of immunization [14].

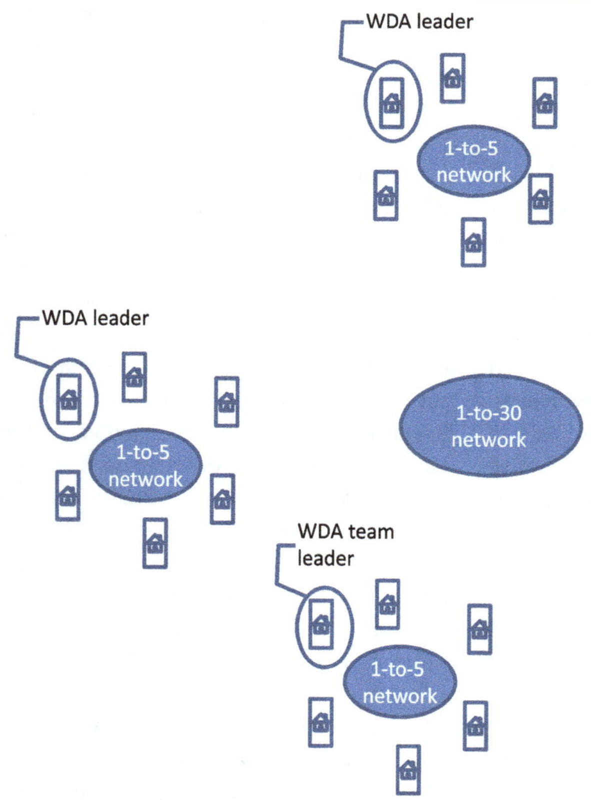

Fig. 1 The Women's Development Army 1–30 network. The Women's Development Army 1–30 network is organised in the community, with five participating neighboring households creating a women's development team, and groups of five or six teams brought together as a network, under one leader

This paper is the first of a series of four investigating innovations designed to support the HEP and the WDA strategy, to improve maternal and newborn health in Ethiopia. The other three papers consider Community-Based Data for Decision-Making [24], the use of a Participatory Community Quality Improvement strategy [25], and a Family Conversation strategy [26]. The WDA strategy has been reported to enhance the demand and access of the community to the health services [23, 27], but there is a lack of evidence isolating the contribution of the WDA strategy in enhancing maternal and child health care outcomes. This study therefore aimed to examine the relationship between the density of active one-to-30 network leaders and uptake of RMNCH services in 145 rural districts, in four regions of Ethiopia. Although the WDA are taking part in a variety of developmental activities, including the implementation of the HEP more widely, the focus of this study is on the contribution of the WDA and HEWs to improving maternal, neonatal and child health.

Methods

Settings

Administratively, Ethiopia is composed of nine regional states: Tigray, Afar, Amhara, Oromia, Somali, Southern Nation Nationalities and Peoples' (SNNP) Region, Benishangul-Gumuz, Gambella, and Harari; and the city administrative councils of Dire Dawa and Addis Ababa. Projections from the 2007 population and housing census estimate the total population in 2017 to be more than 95 million, with the majority of the population (over 80%) residing in rural areas [28]. The availability of health workers — doctors, health officers, nurses and midwives — to population ratio is 0.7 per 1000 population, far behind the minimum threshold of 2.3 doctors, nurses and midwives to 1000 population ratio required to ensure high coverage with essential health interventions [29]. This study was conducted in four most populous regions of Ethiopia: Oromia, Amhara, Tigray and SNNP. According to the Centeral Statistical Agency population projection, these four regions account 86% of the total population. Including health posts, 18,107 health facilities are providing services in these regions [30].

The WDA strategy was introduced in 2011 with the objective of supporting the HEP to reach households and communities with actionable messages. Since 2008, the Last Ten Kilometers project (L10 K) has also been supporting the HEP. In partnership with 12 local civil society organizations, L10 K has been implementing innovative community-based strategies primarily aimed at improving utilization of high impact maternal, newborn, and child health services through strengthening the HEP and the WDA strategy. Details of the L10 K intervention strategies are provided in Additional files 1, 2 and 3.

Study design

Since the WDA strategy was implemented across the four most populous regions of Ethiopia; Amhara, Oromia, SNNP and Tigray, using a conventional intervention comparison group design was not possible. Instead, we constructed an internal comparison group by taking advantage of the natural variability in the intensity of WDA strategy implementation across 423 kebeles. Accordingly, we assessed whether HEP outreach activity and household RMNCH care behaviors and practices were better in kebeles with comparatively better implementation of the WDA strategy with active WDA leaders.

Study participants and data collection

We used data from a cross-sectional household and health post survey, conducted from December 2014 to January 2015 (Additional file 1). The survey was a two-stage cluster survey, stratified by region and program domain, in 145 *woredas* (districts), of which 115 were in the L10 K project intervention (L10 K Platform) area and 30 were not. We used data from three target groups: i) family planning information from women aged 15 to 49 years; ii) maternal and newborn health information from women with children 0 to 11 months of age; and iii) childhood immunization information from women with children 12 to 23 months of age. At the first stage, kebeles were selected as primary sampling units with probability proportional to their estimated population sizes, stratified by region and by whether or not they were in the L10 K Platform area. At the second stage, the 30 by seven cluster survey strategy, commonly used for monitoring the coverage of childhood immunization services, was adapted to obtain information from the three target groups [31]. In brief, the first household was selected from the middle of the kebele and then every fifth household was visited, moving away from the center, and all the women in that household were interviewed if they were within the target population. If a woman aged 15 to 49 had a child between 0 to 11 months of age, she was interviewed for the women of reproductive age questionnaire and for the questionnaire for women with children aged 0 to 11 months. After completion of the quota for women of reproductive age in a kebele, the interviewers focused on completing interviews for the other target groups. The desired quota for each target group was 12 respondents.

The household survey instruments were translated into the three major local languages (Amharic, Oromifa, and Tigrigna). In the SNNP region, which has 11 additional languages, the interviewers translated from

Amharic while administering the questionnaires. Verbal consent was sought and documented by the interviewer. If the respondent was under 18 years old, consent was sought from her husband, parents or guardian. As it was expected that most of the respondents could not read or write, written consent was not sought. Ethical clearance was obtained from the Institutional Review Boards of the respective Regional Health Bureaus and of JSI Research & Training Institute, Inc.

Information on the WDA strategy implementation strength and other contextual factors of a kebele was obtained from health post records and HEW interviews. For this purpose, the health post in the selected kebele was visited and a HEW in the selected health post was interviewed. If more than one HEW was present, they were interviewed together, after seeking their written consent. In the few cases where there was more than one health post in a kebele, one was randomly selected for the HEW interview and the household interviews were conducted from within the administrative boundaries of the selected health post.

Outcomes of interest

Thirteen indicators were considered as the outcomes of interest. These were grouped into two broad categories: (1) HEP outreach activity indicators, which were measured among unique respondents from all three target groups of women; and (2) RMNCH care practice indicators. The latter were sub-categorized into (i) family planning, which was measured among respondents of reproductive age who were in union; (ii) maternal and newborn health, which included care behavior and practices during the most recent pregnancy as reported by women with children in their first year of life; and (iii) childhood immunization, which was measured among women with children age 12 to 23 months. The definitions of the indicators are given in Table 1.

Independent variables

The independent variable of interest was the WDA density, a measure of the WDA strategy implementation strength. For each kebele, it was defined as the ratio of the number of households in the kebele per active WDA team leader. Active WDA team leaders were those who were recorded by the HEW as having met with her and discussed RMNCH issues within the WDA team leaders' network during the three months preceding the survey. To facilitate the interpretation of the findings, the kebeles were categorized into three groups of WDA strategy implementation strength: higher, moderate and lower. None of the sampled kebeles had one active WDA team leader for every 30 households as expected by the program. Thus, a higher cut-off point of 40 or less households per active WDA team leader was used to define higher WDA density. Kebeles with less than half the expected WDA density (more than 60 households per active WDA team leader) were categorized as having lower WDA density; while those with between 40 and 60 households per active WDA team leader were categorized as having moderate WDA density. Accordingly, 25% (104), 41% (173) and 35% (146) of the kebeles were categorized as having higher, moderate and lower WDA density respectively.

The independent variables considered in the regression analysis were the individual, household and contextual characteristics of the respondents. The individual-level factors were age, education, marital status and parity; the household-level factors were wealth quintile and distance of the respondent's household from the nearest health facility; and the contextual factors were HEW to population ratio of the kebele, administrative region and presence of the L10 K Platform.

We included HEW to population ratio of the kebele to account for variations in the input of the HEP across kebeles. As indicated earlier, HEWs are mentors of WDA members; as such, we do not assume that effects of the WDA strategy implementation strength on RMNCH care behaviors and practices are independent of HEWs' efforts.

The wealth index score was constructed for each household with a principal components analysis of the household possessions (electricity, watch, radio, television, mobile phone, telephone, refrigerator, table, chair, bed, electric stove and kerosene lamp), and household characteristics (type of latrine and water source). The households were ranked according to the wealth score and then divided into five quintiles [32].

Sample size

The household survey obtained data from 14,049 women in 478 kebeles (Additional file 1); however, the analysis was restricted to the data obtained from 12,381 women in 423 kebeles for which measures of both WDA density and HEW to population ratios were available. Of the 12,381 unique women that were included in this study, 26% (3166) were respondents for at least two of the three target groups; 44% (5397) of respondents were women of reproductive age; 41% (5081) of respondents were women with children aged 0 to 11 months; and 41% (5088) of respondents to the questionnaire were women with children aged 12 to 23 months.

Statistical analysis

Stata 14.2 was used for statistical analysis [33]. First, whether the individual and household level characteristics of the 2668 respondents from the 55 kebeles that were excluded from the analysis were different from those that were included was assessed using Pearson's

Table 1 Definition of Health Extension Program outreach activity and RMNCH care practice indicators

Indicator	Definition
(1) HEP outreach activity	
Households with latrine	The percentage of households with functioning latrine
Households visited by HEW	The percentage of respondents whose households were visited by HEWs to discuss about health related issues within six months prior to the survey
Households with family health card	The percentage of respondents whose households have Family Health Card. Distributed by HEWs to all women of reproductive age in a household, the cards are used as a tool to provide health education, such as promoting maternal, newborn and child health
(2) RMNCH care practices	
(i) Family planning	
Contraceptive prevalence rate	The percentage of married (or in union) women of reproductive age and/or their partners who were using any method of contraception to delay or avoid getting pregnant during the survey
(ii) Maternal and newborn health	
Received four or more ANC visits	The percentage of women who went to a health facility for antenatal care at least four times during last pregnancy
Neonatal tetanus protected childbirth	The percentage of women whose last childbirth was protected against neonatal tetanus
Delivery at health facility	The percentage of women who gave their last childbirth at a health facility
Early PNC	The percentage of women who were visited by HEWs at home for PNC or newborn care within 48 h of last childbirth
Practiced clean cord care for their newborn	The percentage of women without skilled birth attendance, who cut the umbilical cord of their last newborn with a sterile instrument, tied the cut end of the cord with sterile thread, and applied nothing to the cut end of the umbilical cord
Practiced thermal care for their newborn	The percentage of women without skilled birth attendance, who dried and wrapped their last newborn immediately after birth, delayed bathing the newborn by six hours or more, and always maintained skin-to-skin contact with the baby
Immediate breastfeeding	The percentage of women without skilled birth attendance, but who initiated breastfeeding the newborn immediately after birth
(iii) Childhood immunization	
Children received all vaccines	The percentage of children between 12 and 23 months who received all childhood vaccines
Dropout	The percentage of children between 12 and 23 months who dropped out between Penta 1 and Penta 3 vaccines

ANC Antenatal care, *HEP* Health Extension Program, *HEW* Health extension worker, *PNC* Postnatal care, *RMNCH* Reproductive, maternal, newborn and child health

chi-squared statistics adjusted for survey design effect. Similar tests were done to assess whether the individual, household and contextual characteristics of the respondents were associated with WDA strategy implementation strength to examine possible program placement bias (such as whether kebeles with higher WDA densities were associated with other kebele-level factors that influenced the outcomes of interest).

Multilevel analysis using kebele-level random effects logistic regression models were used to assess the associations between WDA strategy implementation strength categories and the outcomes of interest. Stata's *'xtlogit'* command was used for the purpose. The models were adjusted for survey design and individual, household and contextual characteristics of the respondents. To assess the contribution of the respondents' characteristics to the model, they were grouped into individual, household and contextual factors. First, the model with all the three groups of independent variables was estimated. Then, the statistical significances of each of the three groups were assessed one by one, using likelihood ratio test. If a particular group was not statistically significant at $p < 0.05$, it was dropped. The goodness-of-fit of the models were assessed using the global Wald's statistics, likelihood ratio test of the kebele-level random effects, and sensitivity of the quadrature approximation that was used to estimate the models. Once the final model was identified for each outcome, Stata's post-estimation 'margins' command was applied to obtain the adjusted estimates of the outcome of interest indicators according to the WDA density categories, holding the kebele-level random effects constant. Then, the percentage-point differences of the adjusted estimates between moderate and lower WDA density and between higher and lower WDA density, with its 95% confidence intervals, were estimated using nonlinear combinations of estimators.

Statistical significance of the associations between exposure and the outcomes of interests were concluded if the 95% confidence intervals of the percentage-point differences did not overlap the value zero.

Results

The community health structure of Ethiopia comprises the HEP, with HEWs supported by the WDA [9, 23, 27]. The sample characteristics of the 2668 respondents from the 55 kebeles that were excluded from the analysis were not statistically significantly different from those that were included ($p > 0.1$; analysis not shown).

The average number of households per active WDA leader in the 25th, 50th and 75th percentiles of the kebeles in the study area were 41, 50 and 73 respectively (analysis not shown). Table 2 describes the sample characteristics of unique respondents and their association with WDA density categories. Nearly half (47%) of the respondents were aged 25 to 34 years; most (60%) could not read; 93% were married; most (59%) had three or more children; more than half (54%) lived within 30 min of a health facility; 84% lived in the L10 K intervention area. About 44% of respondents were from kebeles where fewer than 2500 people received services from one HEW (in line with Ethiopian Federal Ministry of Health guidelines), whereas around 45% were from kebeles where one HEW was serving 2500 to 5000 people, and the remaining 11% were from kebeles where one HEW was serving more than 5000 people. Interestingly, women in the lowest wealth quintile were more likely to be resident in kebeles with higher WDA density ($p < 0.05$). In total, 27% of women in the lowest wealth quintile were resident in a kebele with higher WDA density compared with 14% of women in the highest wealth quintile.

Among the sample characteristics, wealth quintile, religion and administrative regions were statistically significantly associated with WDA density ($p < 0.05$), indicating the possibility of program placement bias (Table 2). The majority (51%) of the respondents from kebeles with higher WDA density were from the lowest two wealth quintiles; indicating that WDA strategy implementation strength was pro poor. The proportion of respondents from Amhara region was comparatively high in kebeles with higher WDA density (46%), compared to from moderate (26%) or lower (24%) density kebeles. A similar trend was observed in respondents from Tigray region; while the opposite was observed in respondents from Oromia and SNNP regions. The proportion of respondents who were Orthodox Christians was higher in higher WDA density kebeles (75%) than those from moderate (55%) or lower WDA density (50%) kebeles. The association between religion and WDA density was not surprising since almost all the respondents from Tigray (97%) and Amhara (99%) regions were Orthodox Christians (analysis not shown).

Multilevel logit models were estimated to assess the associations between the WDA density categories and the outcomes of interest. The coefficients of the multilevel models and their goodness-of-fit statistics (global Wald's statistics) are provided in an additional table (Additional file 4). All three groups of respondents' characteristics were statistically significant ($p < 0.05$) in all the final models. The kebele-level random-effects was statistically significant ($p < 0.001$) for all the models estimated; thus indicating the appropriateness of the multilevel analysis.

Adjusted estimates of the outcomes of interest indicators according to the WDA density category were estimated from the multi-level models and presented in Table 3. The percentage-point differences of the adjusted estimates between moderate and lower WDA density and between higher and lower WDA density categories, with 95% confidence intervals, are also presented. The analyses indicate that all three HEP outreach activities' indicators were higher in kebeles where the WDA density was in the higher category (Table 3). Households with a latrine were respectively 12 (95% Confidence Interval: 7, 16) and 14 (95% CI: 9, 18) percentage-points higher in moderate and higher WDA density areas compared with lower WDA density areas. Similarly, households visited by HEWs were 7 (95% CI: 3, 11) and 9 (95% CI: 4, 14) percentage-points higher in moderate and higher WDA density areas compared with lower WDA density areas. While households with Family Health Cards were 11 (95% CI: 6, 16) percentage-points higher in higher WDA density areas compared with lower WDA density areas.

Density of WDAs, which can be viewed as penetration of the HEP, was also associated with three measures of uptake of services among women: contraceptive prevalence rate, four or more ANC visits and institutional delivery. Respectively, these were 7, 11 and 9 percentage-points higher ($p < .05$) among respondents from higher WDA density areas, compared with those from lower WDA density areas. Although clean cord care was also associated with WDA density, the association was not in the expected direction. We found no evidence that WDA strategy implementation strength was associated with childhood immunization, neonatal tetanus protected childbirth, thermal care, immediate breastfeeding or early postnatal care (PNC).

Discussion

Many countries have produced and deployed community health workers as an alternative health workforce to overcome the critical shortage of health staff [14, 34]. The community health structure of Ethiopia comprises the HEP, with HEWs supported by the WDA [9, 23, 27].

Table 2 Percentage distribution of the sample characteristics by WDA density

Characteristics	Category	WDA density			Total	*p-value
		Lower	Moderate	Higher		
Age group	15–19	9	9	9	9	0.574
	20–24	22	23	23	22	
	25–34	46	49	46	47	
	35–49	23	20	22	22	
Education	Cannot read	60	58	62	60	0.336
	Primary	22	22	23	22	
	Higher	18	20	16	18	
Marital status	Other	6	7	7	7	0.319
	Married/in union	94	93	93	93	
Number of children	0	4	5	4	5	0.151
	1	21	20	24	22	
	2	15	15	15	15	
	3	13	14	15	14	
	4+	46	45	42	45	
Wealth quintile	Lowest	18	18	27	20	0.008
	Second	19	19	24	20	
	Middle	20	21	18	20	
	Fourth	22	20	19	20	
	Highest	22	22	14	20	
Distance to any health facility	< 30 min	52	55	55	54	0.493
	30 to 59 min	33	28	31	30	
	1+ hours	16	17	14	16	
Religion	Orthodox	50	55	75	58	0.005
	Protestant	26	17	12	19	
	Muslim	24	27	13	22	
	Other	1	2	0	1	
Region	Tigray	12	17	25	18	< 0.001
	Amhara	24	26	46	30	
	Oromia	26	25	21	25	
	SNNP	38	31	9	28	
L10 K area	No	17	12	22	16	0.115
	Yes	83	88	78	84	
HEW density (population per HEW in *kebele*)	2499	39	44	49	44	0.690
	2500 to 3499	30	29	26	29	
	3500 to 4999	15	17	17	16	
	5000+	16	10	8	12	
Women of reproductive sample	No	56	55	57	56	0.305
	Yes	44	45	43	44	
Women with children 0 to 11 months sample	No	59	60	58	59	0.205
	Yes	41	40	42	41	
Women with children 12 to 23 months sample	No	59	60	59	59	0.076
	Yes	41	40	42	41	
Number of *kebele*		147	173	103	423	
Number of respondents		4249	5135	2997	12,381	

HEW Health extension worker, *SNNP* Southern Nations, Nationalities and Peoples, *WDA* Women's Development Army

**p*-values are for the chi-square statistics testing the null hypothesis that the sample characteristics are similar between the different levels of WDA density categories

Table 3 Adjusted estimates of the outcome indicators by WDA density

HEP outreach activities and RMNCH indicators	Total (%)	WDA density			%-points difference (95% CI)	
		Lower (%)	Moderate (%)	Higher (%)	Moderate and Lower	Higher and Lower
HEP outreach activity						
Households with latrine	78	70	81	83	12 (7, 16)	14 (9, 18)
Household visits by HEWs	49	44	51	53	7 (3, 11)	9 (4, 14)
Household with Family Health Card	54	49	53	60	4 (−0, 9)	11 (6, 16)
Family planning						
Contraceptive prevalence Rate	48	44	48	52	4 (−1, 8)	7 (2, 13)
Maternal and newborn						
ANC 4+	51	44	54	55	10 (5, 15)	11 (5, 17)
Neonatal tetanus Protected childbirth	68	65	68	64	3 (−2, 7)	-1 (−6, 4)
Institutional deliveries	56	50	53	59	4 (−3, 11)	9 (1, 17)
Early PNC	9	8	9	9	1 (−1, 3)	1 (−1, 3)
Clean cord care	33	30	24	38	-6 (−12, 1)	8 (0, 16)
Thermal care	42	35	36	41	1 (−6, 8)	5 (−2, 13)
Immediate breastfeeding	70	62	63	65	1 (−6, 7)	3 (−5, 10)
Childhood immunization						
Fully vaccinated	65	62	66	65	4 (−1, 10)	3 (−4, 10)
Dropout between Penta 1 and Penta 3	11	13	10	12	-3 (−6, 0)	−2 (−6, 2)

ANC + 4 Received four or more antenatal care visits, *HEP* Health Extension Program, *HEWs* Health extension workers, *PNC* Postnatal care, *WDA* Women's Development Army

The density of the WDA was associated with wealth quintile, suggesting that while WDA density is not as high as desired in all areas, the distribution of higher density WDA appears to be pro-poor. McColloum et al., in a recent systematic review reported that community health worker programs were equitable, including in terms of socio-economic position and geographical location, based on their review of 34 community health worker interventions from all regions of the world [35].

The findings of this study showed that, the contraceptive prevalence rate was positively associated with higher WDA strategy implementation strength, among this sample of mainly married women. The contraceptive prevalence rate among currently married women has increased in Ethiopia from 8 to 36% in the last sixteen years [7, 36], and the Health Sector Transformation Plan target set for the year 2020 is 55%. Our results suggest that the WDA strategy can help to reach that target.

In this study, four or more ANC visits had an overall prevalence of 51%, that was again higher in high WDA density areas. This overall prevalence is higher than the current national average (32%) [7]. Repeated ANC attendance is one of the most important indicators that shows the quality of health services, hence additional effort is required for this service to excel. Repeated ANC visits, at least four during pregnancy, provide opportunities for reaching pregnant women with a number of interventions at different stages of pregnancy [9, 37]. A Cochrane review of community-based services for maternal care from 2010, reported similar findings of increased access to ANC where community health workers were present, across a variety of settings [38].

Institutional delivery in this survey was 56% overall and more elevated in areas with higher WDA density. Overall, institutional delivery was higher in our study population when compared with the Ethiopia Demographic Health Survey (DHS) 2016 report, which showed 28% [7]. Currently, Ethiopia is experiencing an unprecedented acceleration in institutional delivery, following many years of little change despite being a priority focus for the Federal Ministry of Health. For instance, reports for three consecutive Ethiopia DHS, 2010, 2014 and 2016, showed a rise in institutional deliveries from 10, to 15%, to 28%, respectively. This increase is likely to be a multi-faceted process, including the government's efforts and investments under a national movement with the logo "No mother should die while giving life", amplified by community involvement through the WDA. In their systematic review, Gilmore and McAulifee suggest that increased contact points with community health workers may have an increased impact [21]. Increased density of the WDA may facilitate penetration of public health messages and work towards message saturation [39]. However, the performance is still far behind the Health Sector Transformation Plan institutional delivery target of 90% by the year 2020. For institutional delivery to be effective, it is essential to understand the factors that influence individuals and households to utilize institutions for delivery and develop effective interventions to promote respectful care in this context [40, 41].

The findings of this study showed immunization coverage is relatively high (65%), albeit far behind the Health Sector Transformation Plan target (95%). We found no evidence of association of the Expanded Program of Immunization with WDA density. This may be because the Expanded Program of Immunization started in Ethiopia over thirty years ago and is well established throughout the country. Client perceptions are shaped by cultural values, previous experiences, perceptions of the role of the health system and interactions with providers [42].

Interestingly, we found no evidence of an influence of WDA density on immediately initiating breastfeeding or thermal care ($p > 0.05$). Other community health worker programs have reported improvements in thermal care [43] and breastfeeding [44], and improving these essential life-saving interventions [9] requires more attention and further improvement.

Only 9% mothers in our study received early PNC, which is much lower than the 2016 Ethiopia DHS report (17%) [7]. Early PNC was low across all levels of WDA density. Given that the highest number of maternal deaths occur during labor, delivery and in the first few days after delivery, there is a critical need for good quality care during these periods [9, 45]. Different studies [46, 47] and consecutive Ethiopia DHS have also reported low PNC service coverage, suggesting the need for immediate action. Similar challenges in achieving adequate PNC coverage have been reported in other countries. For instance, a study analyzing data from 30 surveys conducted between 1999 and 2004, showed substantial increases worldwide in the use of ANC services, but wide gaps between ANC and delivery care and even more so between delivery care and PNC [37]. Recent data from Morocco (2016) [48], showed that the proportion of women who attended a postnatal consultation was only 30%. A meta-analysis conducted by Langlois et al. indicates that the use of PNC remains highly inequitable according to socioeconomic status, education and geographical access to health facilities [49]. There is a need to identify constraining factors on both the demand and supply sides and find appropriate solutions for improving coverage [41, 46, 47].

Analyzing the findings of our study across the continuum of care, the contraceptive prevalence rate, four or more ANC visits and skilled delivery were higher in areas with higher or moderate WDA density than in areas with low WDA density. Latrine coverage was also high in these areas, and improving hygiene and sanitation, including latrine coverage, plays a key role in the improvement of maternal and child health. The findings of this study showed that 54% had a Family Health Card, the communication tool used by HEWs to promote knowledge and behavior change. In line with this, Gilmore and McAuliffe's systematic review also described the vital role of community health workers in facilitating the implementation of the continuum of care, acting as a bridge between the community and health facility [21].

The WDA strategy is an integral part of the HEP, thus WDA density can be seen as the penetration of the HEP. Consistent with the strategy, we found that kebeles with higher WDA implementation strength were associated with better outcomes. The WDA provides an effective platform to engage the community to bring significant practical and attitudinal change. As the HEP outreach activities reflect the performance of the HEWs, the observed effects of WDA density on the reproductive, maternal and newborn health indicators in this study are the combination of the performances of the HEWs and the active WDAs.

In sum, our study shows that strategies to train and deploy community health workers show great promise in increasing access to treatment and care of mothers and children.

Limitations

There are several limitations to the study. First, due to the cross-sectional nature of the study, there remains temporal ambiguity between program exposure (WDA density) and the outcomes of interest. The WDA strategy implementation strength represented the situation of the WDA program during the three months before the survey. Thus, the assumption of the analysis is that the WDA strategy implementation strength remained the same when the outcomes of interest (for example, women seeking four or more ANC visits) took place. However, this may not have been the case. Second, the effect of WDA strategy implementation strength on the outcomes of interest may be biased due to confounding. Third, the generalizability of the study is limited to the 145 districts from which data were obtained. Fourth, the 30 by seven survey sampling method can be criticized because the interviewers may avoid hard-to-reach areas and non-responders are not revisited [31]. To minimize the bias the interviewers moved away from the center of the kebele towards the periphery to select subsequent households for interview; which was closely monitored by survey supervisors. Nonetheless, it is likely that some of the service utilization indicators could still be over-estimated. In addition, this study employed a quantitative survey method, hence, the data collected were not sufficient to make a detailed analysis to understand complex issues, for example the reasons for low PNC service uptake.

Conclusion

Many studies conducted both nationwide and in selected regions of Ethiopia, have assessed the performance of HEWs and the WDA for improving RMNCH, yet the question of the density of active WDA leaders has not been addressed. This work analyzed the correlation of density (number) of active WDA leaders and uptake of RMNCH services in selected indicators. Most of the RMNCH indicators showed better results in areas with higher WDA strategy implementation strength areas than in areas with lower implementation strength. Several studies, including United Nations reports, have described how community health workers have contributed to improved access and uptake of health services, including RMNCH, in different contexts, especially for underserved populations in low and middle-income countries [14, 34].

The WDA initiative, through ensuring that every Ethiopian household is reached and involved in active participatory learning and sharing of experiences, aims to bring about transformational change in health behaviors and outcomes [23, 24]. Previous studies and official reports have shown that there have been major improvements in the health system since the introduction of the WDA implementation strategy [9, 23, 27, 47]. The present study also shows that a higher density of active WDA members has intensified the undertaking of HEWs to advance the implementation of RMNCH services, which is one of the four main components of HEP packages and a key priority of the country.

The lessons gained from this study may be important for other countries that have similar working setups. The need of further research on the effect of WDA density, such as, the challenges to achieving the 'higher' density of active WDA members, may help in accelerating WDA strategy implementation strength.

Additional files

Additional file 1: Community-based strategies to improve maternal and newborn health in Ethiopia. Background to the Health Extension Program and the intervention strategies introduced under the L10 K project.

Additional file 2: Figure S1. Intervention timeline. An implementation timeline for L10 K's strategies.

Additional file 3: Figure S2. L10 K survey domain and strategy. A map showing woredas implementing the various program strategies. (PDF 541 kb)

Additional file 4: Kebele-level random effects logit model coefficients predicting the outcomes of interest and goodness-of-fit statistics. The coefficients of the multilevel models and their goodness-of-fit statistics (global Wald's statistics).

Abbreviations

ANC: Antenatal care; DHS: Demographic Health Survey; HEP: Health Extension Program; HEW: Health Extension Worker; L10 K: Last 10 Kilometers Project; PNC: Postnatal Care; RMNCH: Reproductive Maternal Neonatal and Child Health; SNNP: Southern Nations, Nationalities and Peoples; WDA: Women's Development Army

Acknowledgements

We would like to acknowledge the study participants and the health sector staff who gave their time to the study. We are also grateful to the data collection team, and our sincere gratitude goes to Krystyna Makowiecka for her constructive comments. The authors declare that this paper embodies only their own work and all the sources used are indicated or acknowledged by means of a complete reference list.

Funding

Funding for the study and for publication was provided by the Bill & Melinda Gates Foundation.

Authors' contributions

WB and AK conceived the study. AK planned and carried out data analysis. BW contributed to drafting the manuscript. ZD, WB and AK wrote the first draft. NF and BY contributed to the design and implementation of the field surveys. CT and BY critically reviewed the manuscript for key content and BW proofread it. ZD prepared the final manuscript and all authors read and approved it.

Competing interests

The authors declare that they have no competing interests.

Author details

[1]Federal Ministry of Health of Ethiopia, Health Extension and Primary Health Service Directorate, Sudan Street, Addis Ababa, Ethiopia. [2]Last 10 Kilometers Project (L10K) 2020, JSI Research & Training Institute, Inc, Bole Sub-City, Kebele 03/05, Hs #, 2111 Addis Ababa, Ethiopia. [3]Department of Infectious Disease Epidemiology, Faculty of Epidemiology and Population Health, London School of Hygiene and Tropical Medicine, Keppel Street, London WC1E 7HT, UK.

References

1. World Health Organization. Trends in Maternal Mortality: 1990 to 2015 Estimates by WHO, UNICEF, UNFPA, World Bank Group and the United Nations Population Division 2015. http://www.who.int/reproductivehealth/publications/monitoring/maternal-mortality-2015/en/. Accessed 24 Feb 2017.
2. Alkema L, Chou D, Hogan D, Zhang S, Moller AB, Gemmill A, et al. Global, regional, and national levels and trends in maternal mortality between 1990 and 2015, with scenario-based projections to 2030: a systematic analysis by the UN maternal mortality estimation inter-agency group. Lancet. 2016; https://doi.org/10.1016/s0140-6736(15)00838-7.
3. van de Poel E, O'Donnell O, van Doorslaer E. What explains the rural-urban gap in infant mortality: household or community characteristics? Demography. 2009;46(4):827–50.
4. UNICEF, World Health Organization, World Bank, United Nations DESA/population division. Levels & Trends in child mortality. Report 2015. Estimates developed by the UN inter-agency Group for Child Mortality Estimation. New York: UNICEF; 2015. http://www.who.int/maternal_child_adolescent/documents/levels_trends_child_mortality_2015/en/. Accessed 15 Feb 2017.
5. Mullan Z. Transforming health care in Ethiopia. Lancet Glob Health. 2016; https://doi.org/10.1016/S2214-109X(15)00300-9.
6. World Health Organization, UNICEF. A decade of Tracking Progress for Maternal, Newborn, and Child Survival: 2015 Final Report. Geneva: World Health Organization; 2015. http://countdown2030.org/documents/2015Report/Countdown_to_2015_final_report.pdf. Accessed 15 Feb 2017.

7. Central Statistical Agency (CSA) Ethiopia, ICF. Ethiopia Demographic and Health Survey 2016: Key Indicators Report. Addis Ababa, Ethiopia, and Rockville, Maryland, USA. CSA and ICF; 2016. https://dhsprogram.com/pubs/pdf/PR81/PR81.pdf. Accessed 14 Feb 2017.
8. Haines A, Sanders D, Lehmann U, Rowe AK, Lawn JE, Jan S, Walker DG, Bhutta Z. Achieving child survival goals: potential contribution of community health workers. Lancet. 2007;369:2121–31.
9. Federal Ministry of Health. National Newborn and child Survival Strategy in Ethiopia: 2015–2020. Addis Ababa: FMOH; 2015. https://www.medbox.org/national-strategy-for-newborn-and-child-survival-in-ethiopia-201516-201920.pdf. Accessed 6 Aug 2018.
10. World Health Organisation. A universal truth: No health without a workforce. Geneva: WHO. 2013. http://www.who.int/workforcealliance/knowledge/resources/hrhreport2013/en/. Accessed 23 Feb 2017.
11. Frenk J, Chen L, Bhutta ZA, Cohen J, Crisp N, Evans T, et al. Health professionals for a new century: transforming education to strengthen health systems in an interdependent world. Lancet. 2010; https://doi.org/10.1016/S0140-6736(10)61854-5.
12. Christopher JB, Le May A, Lewin S, Ross DA. Thirty years after Alma-Ata: a systematic review of the impact of community health workers delivering curative interventions against malaria, pneumonia and diarrhoea on child mortality and morbidity in sub-Saharan Africa. Hum Resour Health. 2011; https://doi.org/10.1186/1478-4491-9-27.
13. Lehmann U, Sanders D. Community health workers: what do we know about them. The state of the evidence on programmes, activities, costs and impact on health outcomes of using community health workers. Geneva: WHO. 2007. http://www.chwcentral.org/community-health-workers-what-do-we-know-about-them-state-evidence-programmes-activities-costs-and. Accessed 27 Feb 2017.
14. World Health Organization. The world health report: 2006: Working together for health 2006. http://www.who.int/whr/2006/en/. Accessed 24 Feb 2017.
15. Morrow RH. A primary health care strategy for Ghana. In: Morley D, Rohde JE, Williams G, editors. Practising health for all. Oxford: Oxford University Press; 1983. p. 272–99.
16. Yahya SRR. Indonesia: implementation of the health-for-all strategy. In: Tarimo EAC, editor. Achieving health for all by the year 2000. Geneva: WHO; 1990. p. 133–50.
17. Glenton C, Scheel IB, Pradhan S, Lewin S, Hodgins S, Shrestha V. The female community health volunteer programme in Nepal: decision makers' perceptions of volunteerism, payment and other incentives. Soc Sci Med. 2010; https://doi.org/10.1016/j.socscimed.2010.02.034.
18. Hafeez A, Mohamud BK, Shiekh MR, Shah SAI, Jooma R. Lady health workers programme in Pakistan: challenges, achievements and the way forward. J Pak Med Assoc. 2011;61:210. http://www.jpma.org.pk/PdfDownload/2633.pdf. Accessed 6 Aug 2018
19. Bhutta ZA, Lassi ZS, Pariyo G, Huicho L. Global experience of community health workers for delivery of health related millennium development goals: a systematic review, country case studies, and recommendations for integration into national health systems. Global Health Workforce Alliance. 2010; http://www.who.int/workforcealliance/knowledge/publications/CHW_FullReport_2010.pdf?ua=1. Accessed 3 Mar 2017
20. Lewin S, Munabi-Babigumira S, Glenton C, Daniels K, Bosch-Capblanch X, van Wyk BE, et al. Lay health workers in primary and community health care for maternal and child health and the management of infectious diseases. Cochrane Library. 2010; https://doi.org/10.1002/14651858.CD004015.pub3.
21. Gilmore B, McAuliffe E. Effectiveness of community health workers delivering preventive interventions for maternal and child health in low-and middle-income countries: a systematic review. BMC Public Health. 2013; https://doi.org/10.1186/1471-2458-13-847.
22. Banteyerga H. Ethiopia's health extension program: improving health through community involvement. MEDICC Rev. 2011;13:46–9.
23. Admasu K, Balcha T, Ghebreyesus TA. Pro-poor pathway towards universal health coverage: lessons from Ethiopia. J Glob Health. 2016; https://doi.org/10.7189/jogh.06.010305.
24. Karim AM, Fesseha Zemichael N, Shigute T, Emaway Altaye D, Dagnew S, Solomon F, et al. Effects of a community-based data for decision-making intervention on maternal and newborn health care practices in Ethiopia: a dose-response study. BMC Pregnancy Childbirth. 2018;18(Suppl 1) https://doi.org/10.1186/s12884-018-1976-x.
25. Wereta T, Betemariam W, Karim AM, Fesseha Zemichael N, Dagnew S, Wanboru A, et al. Effects of a participatory community quality improvement strategy on improving household and provider health care behaviors and practices: a propensity score analysis. BMC Pregnancy Childbirth. 2018; 18(Suppl 1) https://doi.org/10.1186/s12884-018-1977-9.
26. Emaway Altaye D, Karim AM, Betemariam W, Fesseha Zemichael N, Shigute T, Scheelbeek P. Effects of family conversation on health care practices in Ethiopia: a propensity score matched analysis. BMC Pregnancy Childbirth. 2018; 18(Suppl 1) https://doi.org/10.1186/s12884-018-1978-8.
27. Damtew ZA, Chekagn CT, Moges AS. The Health Extension Program of Ethiopia: Strengthening the Community Platform. Harvard Health Policy Rev. 2016; http://www.hhpronline.org/articles/2016/12/17/the-health-extension-program-of-ethiopia. Accessed 26 Jan 2017
28. Central Statistical Agency (CSA) [Ethiopia]. Population Projection of Ethiopia for all regions at Woreda level from 2014-2017. Addis Ababa: CSA; 2013.
29. Federal Ministry of Health of Ethiopia (FMOH). Human resources for health strategic plan (2009-2020). Addis Ababa, Ethiopia: FmoH, 2009.
30. Federal Ministry of Health of Ethiopia (FMOH). Health & health related indicators: 2009 EFY (2016/2017). Addis Ababa: FMoH; 2017.
31. Lemeshow S, Robinson D. Surveys to measure programme coverage and impact: a review of the methodology used by the expanded programme on immunization. World Health Stat Q. 1985;38:65–75.
32. Filmer D, Pritchett LH. Estimating wealth effects without expenditure data--or tears: an application to educational enrollments in states of India. Demography. 2001;38:115–32.
33. StataCorp. Stata Longitudinal-Data/Panel-Data Reference Manual Release 14. College Station, Texas: StataCorp LP; 2015.
34. World Health Organization. Crisis in Human Resources for Health in African Region. African Health Monitor. 2007;7:10–15.
35. McCollum R, Gomez W, Theobald S, Taegtmeyer M. How equitable are community health worker programmes and which programme features influence equity of community health worker services? A systematic review. BMC Public Health. 2016; https://doi.org/10.1186/s12889-016-3043-8.
36. Central Statistical Authority [Ethiopia], ORC Macro. Ethiopia Demographic and Health Survey 2000. Addis Ababa, Ethiopia, Calverton, Maryland, USA: Central Statistical Authority and ORC Macro; 2000. http://www.dhsprogram.com/pubs/pdf/FR118/FR118.pdf. Accessed 19 Mar 2017
37. Lincetto O, Mothebesoane-Anoh S, Gomez P, Munjanja S. Antenatal care. In: Opportunities for Africa's newborns: Practical data, policy and programmatic support for newborn care in Africa; 2006. p. 51–62. http://www.who.int/pmnch/media/publications/oanfullreport.pdf. Accessed 17 Mar 2017.
38. Lassi ZS, Haider BA, Bhutta ZA. Community-based intervention packages for reducing maternal and neonatal morbidity and mortality and improving neonatal outcomes. Cochrane Library. 2010; https://doi.org/10.1002/14651858.CD007754.pub2.
39. Murray J, Remes P, Ilboudo R, Belem M, Salouka S, Snell W, et al. The saturation+ approach to behavior change: case study of a child survival radio campaign in Burkina Faso. Glob Health Sci Pract. 2015;3:544–56.
40. Rosen HE, Lynam PF, Carr C, Reis V, Ricca J, Bazant ES, et al. Direct observation of respectful maternity care in five countries: a cross-sectional study of health facilities in East and Southern Africa. BMC Pregnancy Childbirth. 2015; https://doi.org/10.1186/s12884-015-0728-4.
41. Griffiths P, Stephenson R. Understanding users'perspectives of barriers to maternal health care use in Maharashtra, India. J Biosocial Sci. 2001;33:339–59.
42. Lantis K, Green CP, Joyce S. Providers and quality of care. New perspectives on quality of care: no. 3. New York: Population Council; 2002. http://www.prb.org/pdf/NewPerspQOC-Provdrs.pdf. Accessed: 2 Apr 2017
43. Bhutta ZA, Ali S, Cousens S, Ali TM, Haider BA, Rizvi A, et al. Interventions to address maternal, newborn, and child survival: what difference can integrated primary health care strategies make? Lancet. 2008; https://doi.org/10.1016/S0140-6736(08)61407-5.
44. Bhutta ZA, Darmstadt GL, Hasan BS, Haws RA. Community-based interventions for improving perinatal and neonatal health outcomes in developing countries: a review of the evidence. Pediatrics. 2005; 115(Supplement 2):519–617.

45. Arba MA, Darebo TD, Koyira MM. Institutional delivery service utilization among women from rural districts of Wolaita and Dawro zones, southern Ethiopia; a community based cross-sectional study. PLoS One. 2016; https://doi.org/10.1371/journal.pone.0151082.
46. Wolelie A, Aychiluhm M, Awoke W. Institutional delivery service utilization and associated factors in Banja District, Awie zone, Amhara regional sate, Ethiopia. Open J Epidemiol. 2014;4:30–5.
47. Elkhoudri N, Baali A, Amor H. Postnatal care: levels and determinants in Morocco. Iran J Public Health. 2017;46:242–8.
48. Langlois EV, Miszkurka M, Zunzunegui MV, Ghaffar A, Ziegler D, Karp I. Inequities in postnatal care in low- and middle-income countries: a systematic review and meta-analysis. Bull World Health Organ. 2015; https://doi.org/10.2471/blt.14.140996.

14

Cost analysis of implementing mHealth intervention for maternal, newborn & child health care through community health workers: assessment of ReMIND program in Uttar Pradesh, India

Shankar Prinja*, Aditi Gupta, Pankaj Bahuguna and Ruby Nimesh

Abstract

Background: The main intervention under ReMiND program consisted of a mobile health application which was used by community health volunteers, called ASHAs, for counselling pregnant women and nursing mothers. This program was implemented in two rural blocks in Uttar Pradesh state of India with an overall aim to increase quality of health care, thereby increasing utilization of maternal & child health services. The aim of the study was to assess annual & unit cost of ReMiND program and its scale up in UP state.

Method and materials: Economic costing was done from the health system and patient's perspectives. All resources used during designing & planning phase i.e., development of application; and implementation of the intervention, were quantified and valued. Capital costs were annualised, after assessing their average number of years for which a product could be used and accounting for its depreciation. Shared or joint costs were apportioned for the time value a resource was utilized under intervention. Annual cost of implementing ReMiND in two blocks of UP along and unit cost per pregnant woman were estimated. Scale-up cost for implementing the intervention in entire state was calculated under two scenarios – first, if no extra human resource were employed; and second, if the state government adopted the same pattern of human resource as employed under this program.

Results: The annual cost for rolling out ReMiND in two blocks of district Kaushambi was INR 12.1 million (US $ 191,894). The annualised start-up cost constituted 9% of overall cost while rest of cost was attributed to implementation of the intervention. The health system program costs in ReMiND were estimated to be INR 31.4 (US $ 0.49) per capita per year and INR 1294 (US $ 20.5) per registered women. The per capita incremental cost of scale up of intervention in UP state was estimated to be INR 4.39 (US $ 0.07) when no additional supervisory staffs were added.

Conclusion: The cost of scale up of ReMiND in Uttar Pradesh is 6% of annual budget for 'reproductive and child health' line item under state budget, and hence appears to be financially sustainable.

Keywords: mHealth, Health system cost, Costing analysis, Maternal and child health, Community health volunteers

* Correspondence: shankarprinja@gmail.com
School of Public Health, Post Graduate Institute of Medical Education and Research, Sector-12, Chandigarh 160012, India

Background

Despite the rapid improvement in maternal, newborn and child health (MNCH) indicators in India, many districts in the country still face high maternal and infant mortalities [1]. On the basis of a composite health index indicator, Government of India (GOI) identified 184 high priority districts across 29 states for focused integrated planning and monitoring of reproductive, maternal, newborn, child and adolescent health care program (RMNCH+A) [2]. District Kaushambi in Uttar Pradesh (UP) state is a high priority district with high maternal mortality ratio (MMR) of 283 per 100,000 live births and infant mortality rate (IMR) of 82 per 1000 live births [3] which are way above the national and state averages of 178 & 258 MMR and 40 & 68 IMR respectively [3]. Most of these maternal and newborn deaths are preventable if a continuum of care is followed right from pregnancy to newborn care. This includes whole spectrum of services including utilization of antenatal care, institutional delivery, early initiation of breastfeeding, essential newborn care, early recognition and referral of maternal and newborn complications with timely access to quality healthcare [4]. In order to strengthen the service provision, National Rural Health Mission (NRHM) was introduced in 2005 to augment primary health care and build capacity of community health workers (CHW) in remote areas to deliver affordable, equitable and accessible care [5]. With this aim, concept of Accredited Social Health Activist (ASHA) was envisaged. These are local women who serve as first contact between public health system and communities. ASHA as a cadre were included in the health system with intent to fulfil three roles i.e., creating awareness among communities for health issues, facilitating access to healthcare services, and as a provider for a limited range of basic health services. They help in addressing community health needs and generating demand for health service utilisation. This huge human resource of 890,000 ASHAs in the country holds immense potential and perform range of services such as mobilizing community for antenatal services during pregnancy, institutional delivery, identification and referral for maternal & newborn complications, home-based postnatal care, universal immunization, prevention of water-borne & other communicable diseases, and nutrition & sanitation [6]. With a minimal educational qualification of high school, ASHAs are provided on job training in various modules as specified by GOI [7, 8]. Various studies have been conducted to determine the effectiveness and functionality of ASHA workers in India. A study conducted in eight states of India highlighted that 75% pregnant women received services from ASHAs across all the states which included whole range of services from antenatal care, accompanying for institutional delivery, immunization etc. [9]. Findings of the 10th Common Review Mission also highlighted that coverage of antenatal care, institutional delivery and immunization services have improved in 16 states of India, which were also attributed to the role of ASHA workers [10]. Another study found that ASHA workers were valued, as service providers by rural communities in creating awareness and behaviour change towards maternal and child care [11]. However, many studies highlighted that the quality and pace of trainings provided to ASHA workers after recruitment were inadequate and service provisioning by ASHA was largely limited to health education and referral. Thus, a need for regular and refresher trainings were realised for improving ASHAs' performance [12]. A review of the home-based care highlighted that skill retention and thus quality of care provided by ASHA could be improved by either conducting periodic refresher trainings or by using information technology, or using audio visual teaching aids that are more interactive and engaging [13]. These job aids are likely to improve retention of information and make ASHAs communication effective [13].

Mobile technology based health solutions are increasingly being utilized in health sector in low and middle income countries to strengthen skills of CHWs. Mobile Health (mHealth) as defined by World Health Organization (WHO) is an area of electronic health that provides health services and information via mobile technologies such as mobile phones and personal digital assistants [14]. For instance, mHealth application has been used for improving maternal and child health indicators in Ethiopia [15], as web based mobile applicable modules for treatment and follow up of malaria cases along Thai-Myanmar border and for community case management of malaria in Saraya, Senegal [16, 17], as diagnostic and management tool in diabetes [18] and as a cardiovascular risk assessment tool in Nyanga district of Cape town [19]. Similarly, one mobile based application was implemented as ReMiND (Reducing Maternal and Newborn Deaths) program in routine health care service delivery through ASHA workers in two blocks of district Kaushambi in UP state. The overall aim of this intervention was to increase the quality of counselling provided by ASHAs with the help of mobile application as an audio visual aid, thereby increasing utilization of MCH services.

However, a global survey done by WHO highlighted the lack of cost effectiveness data as one of major barrier in justifying implementation of mHealth services. It reported that only 13 out of the 112 countries have ever evaluated cost effectiveness of their mHealth programs [20]. Also, a recent systematic review from India highlighted the lack of sufficient evidence on cost effectiveness of mHealth interventions [21]. In order to fill this gap in evidence base, we undertook a study to evaluate the impact of ReMiND program on utilization of MNCH services & its cost effectiveness. In this paper, we specifically report the cost of ReMiND program in district Kaushambi.Also, we estimated the scale up cost of this program in Uttar Pradesh state which is relevant from the fiscal planning point of view.

Methods

Study setting & background

The ReMiND program was undertaken in district Kaushambi which is one of the high priority districts of Uttar Pradesh. Ninety two percent of its 1.6 million population resides in rural areas [22]. The female literacy rate of district is 52.7% in contrast to state average of 63.9% [3]. The district MMR of 283 deaths per 100,000 live births, was 25 and 105 points higher than the state and national averages respectively [3]. The coverage of full antenatal care checkups; haemoglobin and ultrasound test during routine ANC of pregnant women were 5%, 11.3% & 10.7% respectively [3]. Nearly 60% women in the district delivered in health facilities, while 46.9% children had full course of primary immunization during infancy [3].

To improve these maternal and child health indicators, a mHealth program named ReMiND was introduced in two community development blocks namely, Manjhanpur and Mooratganj, of district Kaushambi in year 2012. It resulted from collaborative work of two Non- Government Organizations (NGOs) i.e. Catholic Relief Services (CRS) & Vatsalya; and a social technology innovator, Dimagi. The main focus of the program was to improve the counselling skills of ASHA workers with the help of mHealth application. The detailed description of mHealth application under ReMiND program, its study setting, objectives and methodology are available as a published literature [23].

The preplanning phase of the program started with ten ASHA workers who were trained for piloting an early pregnancy checklist in March 2011. Subsequently, 111 ASHAs from Manjhanpur block were trained in August 2012 followed by training of 148 ASHAs of Mooratganj block in March 2013. These 259 ASHAs were provided Java based phones and trained on use of mobile application to register and counsel women for various MNCH services. The application had a built-in algorithm in the form of five modules which were used to advice and counsel registered women on the complete continuum of care; right from registration and antenatal care to, postnatal & newborn care as per individualized needs and requirements [24]. The data entered by ASHAs were received at Dimagi's online cloud server. Commcare is an open source, mobile platform that enables non-technical users to build mobile applications for their frontline programs across numerous sectors reducing the need for paper based data collection. The data in variety of formats like multiple choice questions, dates, images, videos, global positioning system (GPS) coordinates can be collected through simple mobile interfaces. The data can be collected in offline mode and is sent automatically to the server on regaining internet connectivity. Thus, it can be widely used in rural areas of India which may not have good internet connectivity. Data about pregnant women were restricted and were only accessible to few authenticated users from the program with valid username and password. The data were de-identified before analysis and no reports generated by Dimagi using commcare included information about individual pregnant women. The ASHA supervisors, also called Sector facilitators, used this data to monitor the timeliness and frequency of antenatal and postnatal home care visits by ASHAs to discuss their performance in monthly meetings at block level [24].

Data collection

Economic costing was done from the health system and patient's perspectives to estimate the annual and per-capita cost of implementing the ReMiND program. The cost of resources spent under three time heads were obtained – preplanning phase extending from October 2010 to March 2012, start-up phase from April 2012 to July 2012, and implementation phase from August 2012 to August 2015.

We collected data from all the agencies involved in the program namely, i.e. CRS, Vatsalya, Dimagi and health department of district Kaushambi from May to October, 2015. Cost data was collected from different sources such as financial records, program budget, audit reports, agreements, etc. Data was collected from country office of Dimagi & CRS in New Delhi, state office of CRS in Lucknow and health department in district Kaushambi for health systems costs. Since CRS funded Vatsalya for implementing ReMiND program, the records for latter's expenses were also obtained from CRS. The details about the expenditure on development and maintenance of the software were obtained from Dimagi. Maintenance cost of application included any technical assistance from the designers of the application including assistance on bug fixing and update. Along with this, costs on housing, serving, and maintaining files on the cloud, also called 'hosting service charge', were also obtained from Dimagi. All the cost data were obtained in US dollars, which were converted to Indian Rupees using exchange rates for the respective years. Research costs for two evaluations done during the program namely; baseline study in 2012–13 and mid-term evaluations in 2014 were excluded from the analysis.

Intervention costing methodology

The present analysis determines the cost of ReMiND program from both the health system and patient's perspective separately. The health system costs were stratified based on the agencies which incurred the cost (i.e. developmental partners & government health system) and nature of cost (start-up capital cost and recurrent cost). The recurrent cost in turn is stratified into cost on program implementation by development partners, cost of monitoring & supervision by government officials and the cost of providing services as a result of increased demand in public health system. The scale-up costs were estimated from the health system perspective alone. In addition to the health system cost, we also measured out of pocket expenditures (OOPE) on doctor or nurse fee, medicines, diagnostic tests, medical or surgical procedures, transportation and boarding/lodging which is called as 'cost from patient's perspective'. We measured OOPE incurred by households in seeking health care during pregnancy, delivery and post delivery period from a household survey [14].

Start-up capital cost

We included two cost heads i.e. start-up capital cost and recurrent implementation cost. Start-up costs included all the capital costs incurred during the initial preplanning phase and start-up phase. Technically, any cost whose inputs may last for more than one year was considered as capital cost [25]. This was categorised as costs levied on modules' development and piloting, development and maintenance of software, equipment cost, mobile phones and overhead costs. Apart from these costs; pre-planning meetings, trainings of ASHAs & their supervisors and translation of modules into local dialect were also taken as capital costs because the effect of these inputs were likely to last for the life of the program.

All the capital costs were apportioned in terms of their time value devoted in ReMiND program out of all the programs running simultaneously by the implementing agencies. The program was piloted in two blocks but it was designed such that it could be launched in 821 blocks of Uttar Pradesh. Accordingly, we apportioned the entire start up expenditure for the two blocks of district Kaushambi where intervention was actually piloted. After obtaining the apportioned value, costs in dollars were converted to Indian National Rupee (INR) by applying the dollar conversion rates given by the US Internal Revenue Service for a particular year of purchase of equipment [26]. The converted rates were then inflated from the year of purchase to the current value of product in 2015 by applying Consumer Price Index in India [27]. These inflated values of capital were then annualized as per the average life of utilization of the product at a discount rate of 3% [28]. The annual maintenance rates for capital items as given by the implementing agency were used in calculations.

The average life of software was assumed to be 12 years as the cost incurred on software may last either till strategies of the program remained the same; or if there was a change in technology itself. We chose former based on expert consultation as it is unlikely that any drastic paradigm change may happen in the content of the programme for another 12 years. Further, any change in technology would have had only marginal effect on costs if it requires any revision. The hosting charges were annualized for 3 years as these charges would be revised and added again like recurrent cost if the program extends beyond three years. For mobile phones, laptops, furniture and vehicle, the average life were taken as 3.5 years, 5 years, 6 and 10 years respectively as per the policy of the implementing agencies.

Recurrent implementation cost

The implementation costs included recurrent costs which were required to sustain the intervention. All the recurrent costs were categorized as cost on human resource, travel, ASHA data/internet usage charges for mobile application, utilities like office rent, electricity, telephone bills & internet bills and stationary & printing. Other program support expenses at state and national office like the office rent and salaries were also accounted. Shared costs were apportioned as per the time value devoted by that given resource in performing a particular activity. The office rents were spent at three levels i.e. at district, state and country level. At the district level, entire rent were spent on the activities related to ReMiND program only and hence no apportioning was required. However, at the state and national levels, multiple programs were being handled simultaneously. Therefore, office rent was apportioned in proportion of floor area occupied by the staff involved in ReMiND program to the total office staff. The travel costs in form of vehicle or fuel for carrying out planning and supervisory activities during the start-up and implementation phase were dedicated to ReMiND program only as no other program was being implemented concurrently at the block levels.

For the recurrent costs, we converted the expenses levied by the partner agencies over 37 months i.e. from Aug 2012 to August 2015, into average annual expense. For converting US dollars into Indian rupees, the average dollar rate for these three years was taken as 1 US $ = INR 58.84.

Government health system program cost

Apart from costs spent by implementing agencies, additional costs incurred by district health system were also estimated. It included three components – first, health system cost on monitoring and supervision of ASHA activities under ReMiND program. It includes the time value of the personnel involved either in their supervision through household visits, interactions with ASHA workers or indirectly via review meetings; second, incremental cost of service delivery due to increased utilization of MNCH services as the result of given intervention and third, incremental effect of intervention on ASHAs payment in terms of incentives. The direct supervisory costs were calculated considering that supervisors spend 13% of their total time in monitoring and supervisory activities, as mentioned in another study conducted in developing country [29].

For program implementation, the extra cost of monthly meetings at the block levels, quarterly meetings at district level and bi-annual meetings at the state level were calculated by apportioning the time devoted by government officials in meetings for review of ASHAs' performance under the program. The effect of ReMiND program on overall utilization of MNCH services was evaluated using a quasi-experimental design with a difference in difference analysis [14]. The unit costs for these services were obtained from economic evidence available in the Indian context [30–32].

Economic implications of changes in service utilization in the intervention and control blocks in terms of the performance based incentives for ASHA workers were evaluated using data from health management information system (HMIS) and financial records as obtained from the office of Chief Medical Officer of the district for year 2014–15 [23].

Unit costs

For calculation of unit costs, the population under the intervention area (387,030) was used as denominator for per capita calculation. For cost per pregnant woman, the number of women registered under mHealth was used as denominator. A total of 28,169 women have been registered under ReMiND program since its inception (over three years) as per data provided by Management Information System of the implementing agencies, so the annual number of beneficiaries was taken as 9390.

Scale up costs of ReMiND program for Uttar Pradesh state

The intervention was implemented on pilot basis in two blocks of Uttar Pradesh state. Subsequently the estimates on the cost of implementation of ReMiND program in two blocks were used to estimate the scale up cost of this program, if the government of UP state decided to roll out intervention in the entire 821 blocks in the state. The scale up costs of mHealth intervention in entire state included costs on purchase of mobile phones, internet usage, trainings of ASHAs & their supervisors for use of application and health system costs on review meetings in the entire state. The scale up cost also implicitly included the costs of ASHAs performance based incentives. For scale up, two case scenarios were assumed. First, if current available human resource in the health system could be utilised for monitoring and supervision of this intervention. In UP, Block Community Managers (BCM) and Health Education Officers (HEO) are employed at block and district levels respectively to coordinate and supervise ASHAs' performance. These are regular salaried staff unlike ASHAs whose remunerations were incentive based. In second scenario, a separate supervisory cadre like sector facilitators in ReMiND program were assumed at block level.

At sub-block level also, one ASHA facilitator was employed for monitoring and supervision of 20 ASHAs as guided by the National Health Mission [33], and the same pattern was followed by the implementing agencies. These were promoted ASHAs and did not receive any extra incentives for holding the position. Supervisory training costs of these ASHA facilitators were also included in the scale up cost.

As there was dearth of data on time value spent by different supervisors on various activities in our study and Indian literature [12], we assumed the time apportioned on supervisory and monitoring activities as 13% of total activity time based on findings from a similar study [29]. Though as per directions given by MoHFW, a block ASHA facilitator shall spend 20 days in field in a month [34].

From the perspective of UP state, there would be no requirement to change the content of the software or the built in audio-visual support as the same dialect could be understood in the entire state. Therefore, the start-up capital costs which included the costs on development of software, preplanning meetings, initial translation of modules were not included in scale up cost. Dimagi Inc. developed the software and provided free of cost server support services to first 50 beneficiaries and thereafter charged US$ 1 per year per beneficiary. Therefore, 5 million US$ have to be spent for 5 million (50 lakh) pregnant women in Uttar Pradesh as scale up hosting server charges. Table 1 describes the different types of costs calculated in the study.

Out of pocket expenditures (Patient's perspective)

A patient's perspective is important to consider in costing studies as it includes expenditures borne by households in form of out of pocket expenditures (OOPE) for seeking health care. Aiming patient's perspective helps in adopting policies that intend to provide financial risk protection against OOPE and minimize the losses to households. The data on mean OOP for utilization of

Table 1 Various types of cost with the data sources and methodology

Area	Type of cost	Type of Data collected	Source of data	Method of data collection
At two block levels	Start up/Capital cost	Cost on Module development, translation & piloting. Development of software, Equipment and mobile cost, overheads. Preplanning meetings, ASHA trainings	Official documents of CRS, Vatsalya & Dimagi. Annual budget reports, bills receipts, Personal Interviews	Primary data collection. Time value contributed over the average age of the program
	Implementation cost	Salaries, travel, ASHA internet usage, utilities like office rent, electricity, telephone bills, stationary and printing. Program support cost at state and national office	Official documents like bills, annual budget reports, Personal interview	Primary data collection. Time apportioned as per the time value spent/utilized on the activities related only to ReMiND program
	Health system cost	Health system cost on program implementation. Incremental cost of service delivery due to increased utilization of MNCH services. unit cost for per service utilization) Incremental effect of intervention on ASHA payment.	Financial documents on ASHA incentives from Chief Medical officer's Office, Personal Interviews, Observations during meetings at block, district and state level. Literature review for unit cost per service utilization	Primary data collection. Apportioning of the salaries of the officials as per the time spent on attending meetings at block, district and state level.
	Costs from Patient perspective	Out of pocket expenditure(OOPE) incurred by the households in seeking health care services for various maternal, newborn and child illnesses	OOPE were obtained from the Impact assessment study carried out n two intervention blocks and two control blocks.	Primary data collection
	Annual Program cost	It is sum of startup cost and implementation cost	–	Derived indicator
	Overall annual unit cost per pregnant women	Annual programmatic cost divided by average annual number of women registered under ReMiND	Management information system (MIS) data from CRS on number of registered women	Derived indicator
	Unit health system cost per pregnant women	Annual health system cost divided by average annual number of women registered under ReMiND	MIS data from CRS	Derived indicator
At state level –Uttar Pradesh	Scale up cost	Number of ASHAs in entire state, training cost of ASHA and supervisors, mobile phone cost, hosting service charges, health system cost	NRHM website, Observations, Calculations from available data	Unit costs of pilot at two blocks were expanded to 821 blocks in Uttar Pradesh state.
	Per capita scale up cost	Total scale up cost divided by Total population of state	Census 2011	Derived indicator
	Per pregnant women scale up cost	Total scale up cost in Uttar Pradesh divided by average number of pregnant women in the state in an year	Crude Birth Rate	Derived indictors

ASHA- Accredited Social Health Activist, *CRS*-Catholic Relief Services, *MNCH*- Maternal, Newborn and Child Health, *OOP*- Out of Pocket Expenditure, *ReMiND*- Reducing Maternal and Newborn Deaths

specific MNCH services was obtained from a household survey undertaken to evaluate impact of ReMiND and its cost effectiveness [14]. The detailed information about the household survey and its methodology are described in details in our protocol paper and impact assessment paper [14, 23]. The household questionnaire included questions to assess any cost borne by patients and their families for treatment, consultation from doctors, purchase of drugs and consumables, travel, lodging & boarding, or any money spent elsewhere. Figure 1 illustrates the conceptual framework of costing process of ReMiND program explaining both health system perspective and patient perspective.

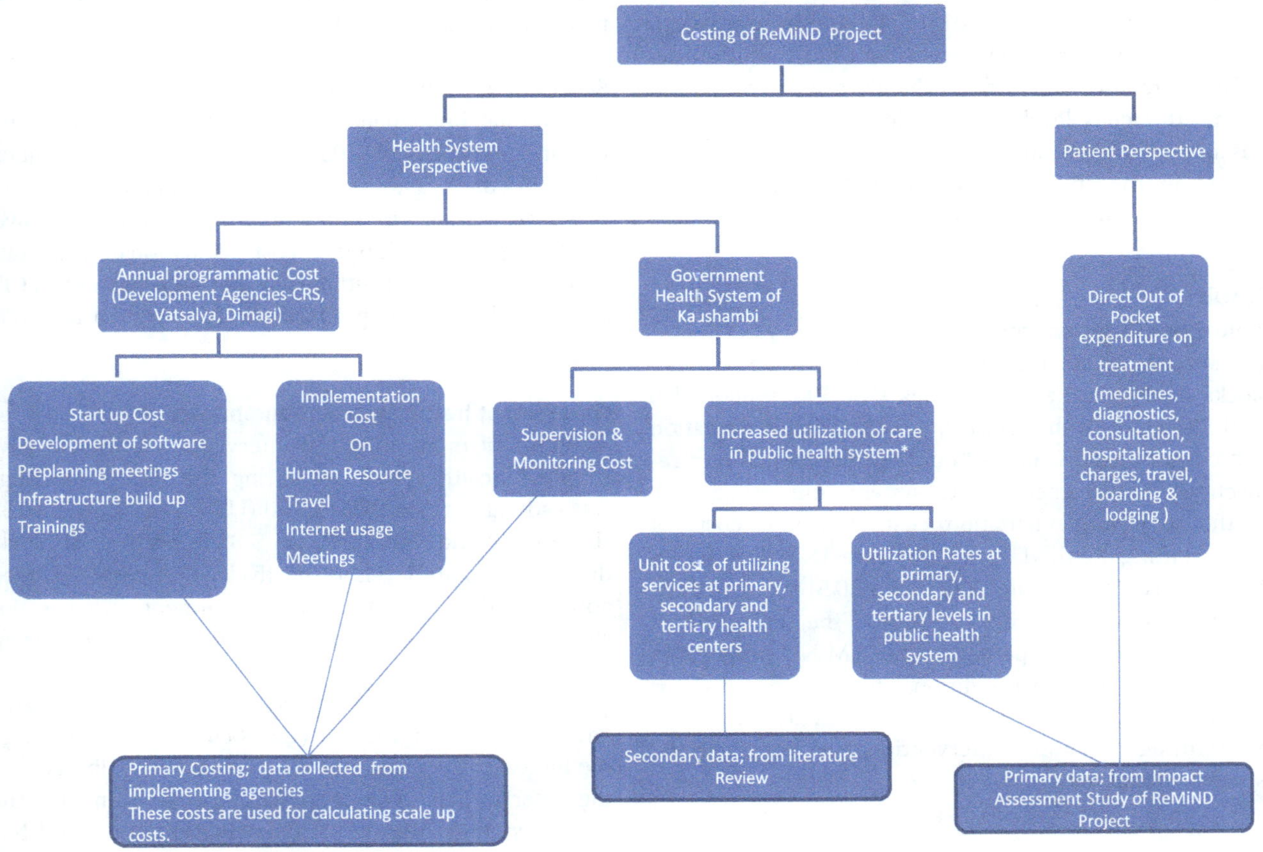

Fig. 1 Conceptual framework for costing process of the ReMiND program. The flow chart describes the procedural detail of costing ReMiND program. The costing was undertaken from both the health system and societal perspectives

Sensitivity analysis

The sensitivity analysis was carried out to understand the effect of variation in input costs on both the base case estimates i.e. annual cost of ReMiND program in two blocks of district Kaushambi and the scale up cost in entire state of Uttar Pradesh. Various case scenarios were considered. The choice of upper and lower bounds for the life of the mHealth application (5 to 15 years) was based on an extensive consultation with the state program managers and development partners. The choice of percentage variation in input prices was based on review of the costing studies done in India [35–37]. It was assumed that the mobile phone and internet data charges may fluctuate to 20%. The cost of training costs of ASHAs and supervisors were fluctuated 10% and 20% respectively; trainings for latter were done in private costlier locations, while a reduction in cost can be achieved if the same were done in Government set-up and monitoring activity was increased to 50% of total time.

A review of economic evaluation studies from India, reported the use of 3%, 3.5%, 8% and 10% as the rates to discount future costs [21]. Further, the WHO-CHOICE and reference case developed by IDSi-BMGF for low and middle income countries recommends use of 3% discount rate [38, 39]. In view of this we used 3% discount rate in the base scenario. Further, since the inflation rate in India is relatively higher than most of the other developing countries [40], a discount rate below 3% was not justifiable. The other most commonly used discount rate for economic costing among developing countries are 5% and 8%. So, we varied the discount rate to 5% and 8%. The company has recently revised its hosting user charges from US$ 1 per beneficiary (pregnant women) per year to US$ 2 per ASHA worker (using mHealth application in phone) per month. In view of this, we undertook a scenario analysis during our scale up cost estimation for UP state to assess the overall and unit cost of ReMiND program in UP with changes in the hosting charges. The results of sensitivity analysis were presented in the form of tornado diagram. Sensit 1.51 software was used for the analysis.

Ethics and consent statement

The Institute Ethics Committee of the Post Graduate Institute of Medical Sciences (PGIMER), Chandigarh provided the ethical clearance for the study vide letter no. 'Program No IEC-01/2015-108'. Administrative approval was obtained from government health authorities of Uttar Pradesh state and Kaushambi district for obtaining health facility level data. In addition, written consent was obtained from all the participants who were interviewed in the study for obtaining the out of pocket expenditures and health system costs.

Results

Annual health system costs

The annual cost for rolling out ReMiND program in two blocks of district Kaushambi was INR 12.1 million (US $191,894). Out of this, start-up cost and implementation cost contributed 9% and 91% of the total annual cost respectively. Government health system contributed 4.8% of the total implementation cost. The unit costs of implementing ReMiND program were INR 31.4 (US $ 0.49) per capita and INR 1294 (US $ 20.5) per registered pregnant women. Figure 2 shows the proportional distribution of total expenditure on ReMiND program in district Kaushambi. An additional file provides detailed description of start-up and implementation costs contributing to annual intervention cost for ReMiND (see Additional file 1).

Start-up capital cost

The start-up cost for the ReMiND program was INR 1.1 million ($17,526). A major portion of this cost was for training of ASHAs and their supervisors (33%) followed by development of software & modules and its piloting (30.3%), mobile phones (29.2%), equipment (5.4%) and programmatic expenses (2.2%). Figure 3 shows the proportional distribution of start-up costs of ReMiND program in district Kaushambi.

Recurrent implementation cost

The annual implementation cost of mHealth intervention in two blocks of Uttar Pradesh was INR 11 million (US $174,368). The costs were predominantly constituted by human resources (62.5%), followed by travel (15.4%), program support cost at national and state office of CRS (8.2%), utilities (5.2%), internet use (3.6%) and health system programme support cost (4.8%) (Fig. 4).

Government health system program cost

The cost of monitoring the intervention from the government health system as during the review meetings was estimated to be INR 94,750 (US $ 1496.8), INR 3133 (US $ 49.5) and INR 2230 (US $ 35.2) per year at block, district and state levels respectively. The costs included apportioned time value of government officials for supervisory activities, with small contribution from travel and overheads.

We estimated that health system in intervention area had to spend INR 430,582 (US $6802) in order to cater the increased coverage of MNCH services attributable to the intervention. The incremental cost borne by the health system during implementation of ReMiND program was INR 39.9 ($ 0.63) per pregnant woman. This cost included the additional cost borne by government on monitoring and supervision of the program; increased utilization of MNCH services by pregnant and lactating mothers and increased performance based incentives to ASHAs as a result of ReMiND program. However, there was no increase in ASHA payments,

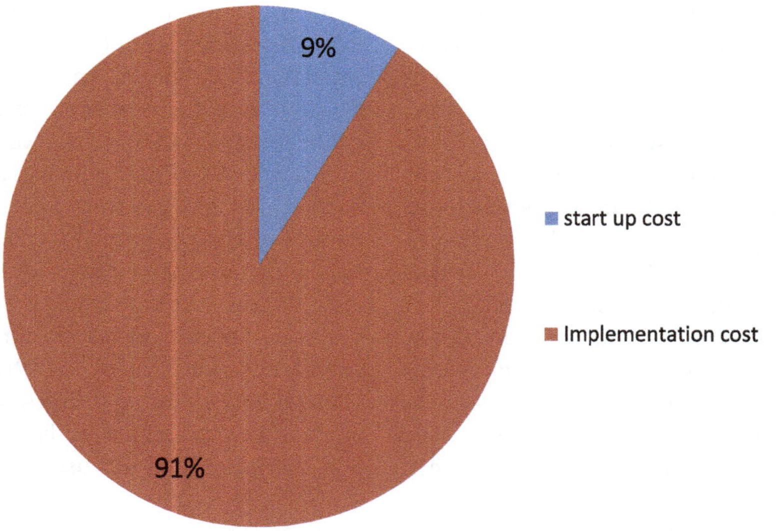

Fig. 2 Proportional distribution of total expenditure on ReMiND program from 2011 to 2015. The figure shows the proportional distribution of start up cost and implementation cost in the total expenditure of ReMiND program

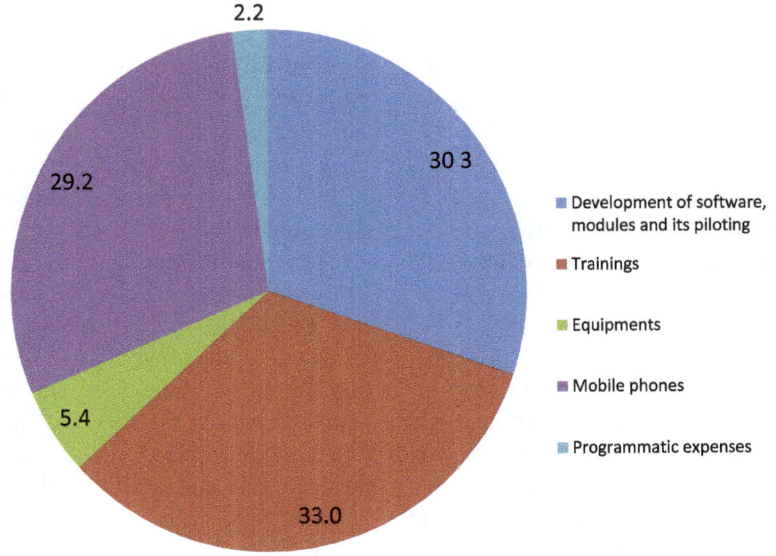

Fig. 3 Proportional distribution of start up costs of ReMiND program in intervent on area of district Kaushambi. The figure shows the proportional contribution of different start up costs in the total start up cost of ReMiND program

hence the incremental health system cost represents the former two, i.e., cost of monitoring & supervision and cost of increase in service utilization. The detailed description of the start-up and implementation costs is given in the Additional file 1.

Out of pocket expenditure (Patient's perspective)

As discussed in methodology, to calculate cost of ReMiND program from patient perspective, the proportion of people bearing OOP expenditure for seeking various MNCH services and the mean OOP expenditure at various levels of health centres in both public and private sector were taken from the Impact Assessment study [14]. It was estimated that the incremental out of pocket expenditure for seeking various health care services in the intervention block was INR 15 million (US $ 240,333). The detailed out of pocket expenditures are shown in Additional file 2.

Scale up costs

In first case scenario where intervention has to be scaled up from two blocks in Kaushambi to 821 blocks in state using the existing human resources for monitoring and supervision, we estimated the scale-up would cost around INR 876 million (US$ 13.8 million). The unit cost of scale up in Uttar Pradesh state would be INR

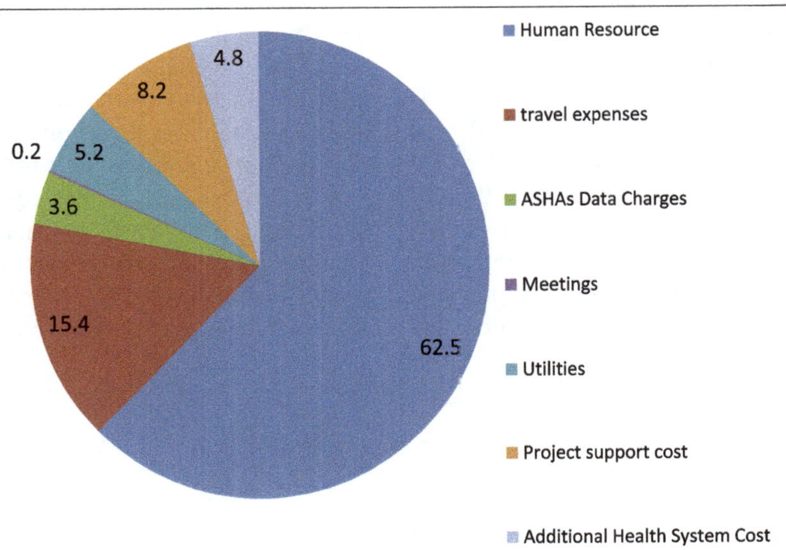

Fig. 4 Proportional distribution of annual cost of implementation of ReMiND program in district Kaushambi. The figure shows the proportional contribution of different recurrent costs in the annual implementation cost of ReMiND program

4.39 (US $0.07) per capita and INR 175.3 (US $2.77) per pregnant women. In second case scenario, additional human resource was assumed to be recruited for monitoring of ASHAs in every block of state. In this case, government has to spend around INR 993 million (US $15.7 million) with INR 4.97 (US $ 0.08) as per capita unit cost and INR 198.8 (US $ 3.14) as unit cost per pregnant woman (Refer Table 2). 'An additional file describes the details of scale up costs (see Additional file 3)'.

Sensitivity analysis

Sensitivity analysis was conducted to estimate costs in various alternate scenarios. Firstly, the total annual cost was estimated assuming that the development of software was done for two blocks of Kaushambi only. In this case, the start-up cost would be INR 4.6 million (USD 73,367) which is 30% of the total annual intervention cost of INR 15 million (USD 247,734). The incremental costs of intervention would be INR 1670 (USD 26.4) per pregnant woman and INR 40.52 (USD 0.64) per capita.

Secondly, the discount rates were varied to 5% and 8%, and the average life of program was taken as 5 and 15 years. On applying the discount rate of 5%, the incremental costs would be INR 1302 (USD 20.6) per pregnant woman and INR 31.60 (USD 0.49) per capita. At 8% discount rate, the incremental cost would be INR 1316 (USD 20.8) per pregnant woman and 31.93 (USD 0.50) per capita.

On assuming the life of programs to be 5 and 15 years, the incremental costs per pregnant woman would change to INR 1338 (USD 21.14) and 1287 (USD 20.34) respectively while per capita costs would be 32.5 (USD 0.51) and 31.23 (USD 0.49) respectively.

The tornado diagrams in Figs. 5 and 6 are the graphical representation of effect of multiple univariate input variables (represented as horizontal bars on y-axis) on the outcome variable (x-axis) i.e. annual cost of ReMiND program in two blocks of Kaushambi district and total cost of scale up of ReMiND project at the level of UP state respectively. The values shown along the both sides of black bars are range (lower and upper side) considered for varying a particular cost input parameter. More is the width of black bar, more sensitive is the outcome variable to change in input parameter. The vertical line between the black horizontal bars shows the base case results. The tornado diagram in Fig. 5 shows that salaries (human resource cost) presents the highest uncertainty and maximum impact on the total annual cost of ReMiND program (90.7% swing) followed by travel cost (5.5% swing) while start up costs like training of ASHAs (0.3% swing), purchase of equipments (0.3% swing) and development of the software (0.0%) had little influence.

Figure 6 showed that the scale up of ReMiND intervention in state of Uttar Pradesh was most sensitive to the variations in the mobile internet data charges followed by hosting charges and purchase of mobile phones. Refer Table S4A and B in 'Additional file 4' which presented the base cost parameter values for different input variables with their upper and lower limits for both case scenarios i.e. program cost in two blocks of Kaushambi district and scale up cost in Uttar Pradesh state.

With the revised hosting charges at the rate of US$ 2 per ASHA worker per month, UP state will have to spend INR 559 million (US $ 8.8 million) per year. The per capita costs of ReMiND program in such a scenario will be INR 2.80 (US $ 0.04) per capita and INR 111.9 (US $ 1.76) per pregnant woman.

Discussion

Use of technology in health and other sectors has been promoted by GOI from the highest level [41]. Several other policy discourses have encouraged the application of mHealth. The High-Level Expert Group on Universal Health Coverage called for harnessing technology for promoting utilization of services [42]. Small to medium scale pilot interventions have been initiated in a variety of geographic settings in India involving a diverse range of health services such as maternal and child health to non-communicable diseases [43]. Various studies from elsewhere have also shown that the application of mHealth results in better delivery of health education, increased awareness & improved uptake of preventive as well as curative services [16, 44–46].

In Indian context, the introduction of ASHA under the National Health Mission holds strong potential for generating demand for health services [34]. However, several evaluations have shown that the knowledge and skills of ASHA workers to counsel pregnant women for

Table 2 Summary of scale up costs of mHealth intervention in Uttar Pradesh in two case scenarios

Cost Description	Scenario1 When currently employed staff is used for supervisory activities INR (US$)	Scenario 2 When additional human resource is employed at the level of blocks INR (US$)
Annual cost of scale up	87,63,69,067 (13,844 693)	99,38,73,262 (15,700,999)
Annual cost per beneficiary	175 (2.77)	198.8 (3.14)
Annual cost per capita	4.39 (0.07)	4.97 (0.08)

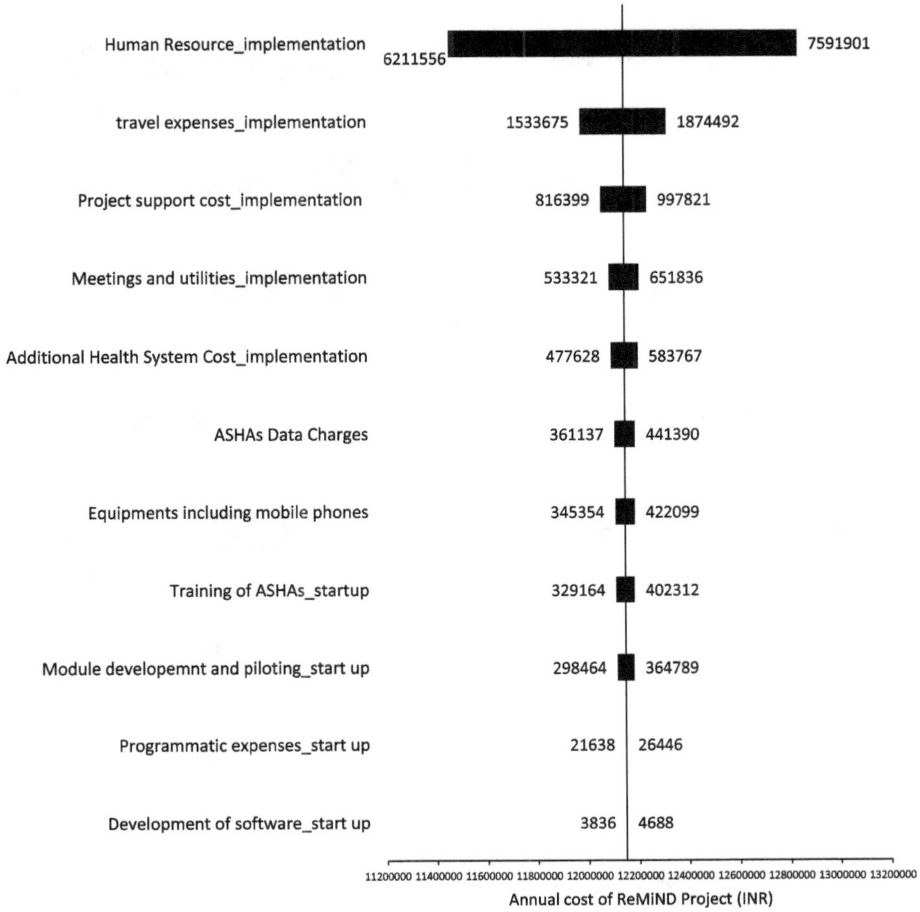

Fig. 5 Tornado diagram illustrates the sensitivity analysis for various input factors on the annual cost (INR) of ReMiND program. The figure shows the sensitivity analysis with the help of tornado diagram to show the effect of variation in different input factors on total annual cost of ReMiND program in two blocks of Kaushambi district

their health care needs during pregnancy and nursing babies requires strengthening [12]. In light of this, use of mobile technology for improving the quality of counselling can serve as a major strategy. This can further improve knowledge and awareness among communities which may directly augment demand for services. However, it is important to understand the feasibility and financial implications of implementating this intervention as part of routine care. Hence our economic analysis holds a significant value for the policy makers in order to estimate the economic implications for implementing and scaling up of such mHealth interventions. The researchers can also use costing studies for carrying out cost effectiveness analysis of such mHealth interventions.

Our study showed that the introduction of mHealth intervention costs INR 31.4 (US $ 0.49) per capita and INR 1294 (US $ 20.5) per pregnant woman registered. The unit costs for scale up within Uttar Pradesh state were INR 4.39 ($0.07) per capita and 175.3($ 2.77) per pregnant women. The overall annual scale up cost for Uttar Pradesh to implement the same intervention in the entire state would be at least INR 876 million (US $ 13.8 million) if no additional human resource were employed for the program monitoring and support. As per our knowledge, this is the first cost outcome analysis targeting MNCH services in India [44].

Fiscal sustainability

From the point of state budget, the total annual money allotted for reproductive & child health (RCH), maternal health (MH) and ASHA incentives for year 2015–16 in Uttar Pradesh were INR 14.6 billion, 6.99 billion and 1.22 billion respectively [47]. The introduction of mHealth intervention and its scale up in the entire state of Uttar Pradesh will represent 6.0%, 12.5% and 71.7% share in the total budget for RCH, MH and ASHA incentive program respectively. It is important to note, this scale up amount does not include introduction of any new cadre of supervisors, and rather considers training the already available cadre for supervision. As per the guidelines of Financial Management Group of National Health Mission-India's flagship health program, it is

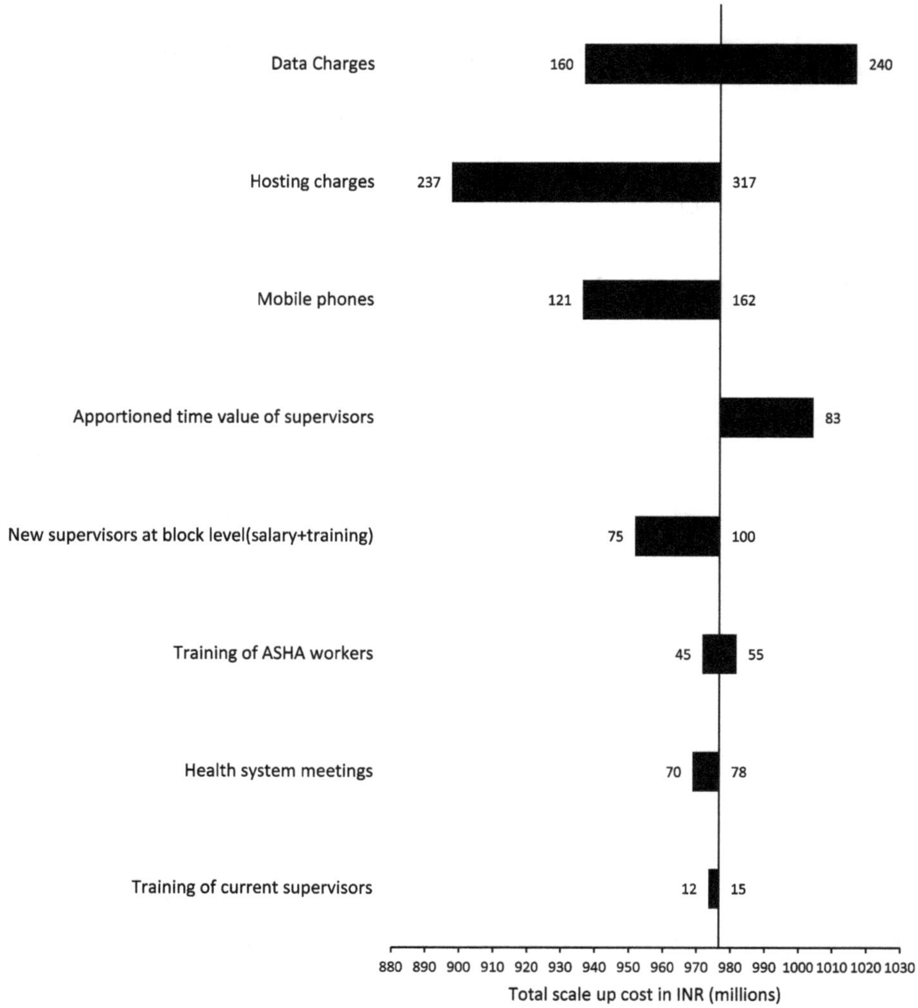

Fig. 6 Tornado diagram illustrates the sensitivity analysis for various input factors on the scale up cost (INR) of ReMiND program in entire Uttar Pradesh. The figure shows the sensitivity analysis with the help of tornado diagram to show the effect of variation in different input factors on the total scale up cost of ReMiND program in entire Uttar Pradesh state

recommended to increase the budget of high priority districts by 10–15% every year [48]. Considering the cost for scale up of ReMiND intervention to be 6% of the total budget allotted to 'Maternal and child health' line item under the NRHM budget of UP state, the intervention appears financially sustainable.

The World Health Report 2005 published a working paper series on scaling up of maternal and newborn interventions to reach universal health coverage by 2015. It estimated that for delivering the whole package of MNCH care (with 95% coverage) for countries in Health System Constraint Category 2 –where India fits – has an incremental cost of USD 1.53 per capita. On inflating this value to the current value of dollar by applying CPI rates in India, the current incremental cost would be USD 2.35 (INR 149.3). The WHO benefit package comprises of universal provision of comprehensive maternal, newborn and child health care services [49]. Our study shows that scale-up of mHealth in UP state will incur an incremental cost of INR 4.77 (USD0.07) per capita, which is 3% of the total incremental value proposed by WHO for achieving universal coverage of MNCH services. This again shows that the scale-up of mHealth is sustainable from fiscal viewpoint.

Policy implications

The need to introduce a service or intervention in the benefit package of care is usually justified based on the burden of health problem which it addresses. However, the amenable burden or the reduction in the health problem which the intervention can potentially bring about is usually not considered. In light of this it is also important to understand that such mHealth application for RMNCH would thus be more useful in weaker states where the reasons for poor coverage are linked more with the demand for service. For example, the Coverage

Evaluation Survey reported that poorer states such as Bihar and Uttar Pradesh have low rates of RMNCH service utilization, a large portion of which is explained by lack of awareness and knowledge about the importance of services [36]. The findings from our impact assessment study suggested an increase in knowledge and thereby utilization of MNCH services after introduction of ReMiND program [14]. Hence, such an intervention which aims at improving counselling of ASHAs, which translates into improved knowledge of community and its demand for health services, is likely to be more beneficial in these states.

Also, ReMiND intervention and its scale up appear feasible from the financial and programmatic perspectives. Currently, a quarter of Indian population who could not access healthcare cited large distances from health facilities as the reason for not being able to access health care. In such situations, mHealth can offer a useful solution. Moreover, the increased penetration of mobile use in the rural areas as well as by community health workers makes it a feasible strategy. Second, mHealth can be used as platform for strengthening programs other than RMNCHA, which are implemented through community health workers. The Government of India's recently announced ambitious scheme of Ayushman Bharat which envisions the transformation of the existing sub-centres as Health and Wellness centres. The proposed health and wellness centres clearly outline a significant role of information technology and digital records for improving service delivery. Further, increased and timely utilization of services at these centres for primary care may decrease out of pocket expenditures on tertiary care. Global evidence suggest that mHealth solutions could lower the total annual per capita healthcare expenditure as it reduced in Brazil and Mexico by 20% and 25% respectively [50].

Also, the scale up cost of ReMiND program in UP would cost INR 993 million (US $15.7 million) if additional supervisors were to be recruited in each block for monitoring as was structured in ReMiND program while the cost would reduce to INR 876 million (US$ 13.8 million) if already employed staff was used for supervision. Dimagi Inc. charged US$ 1 per beneficiary per year as web hosting charges which has now changed to US$ 2 per ASHA worker (using mHealth application in phone) per month. This change in hosting charges would decrease the total scale up cost from INR 876.3 million to 559.8 million. Thus, it is likely that technological advances may further reduce the cost of ReMiND program. Therefore, m health solutions are emerging as useful and sustainable option from a fiscal point of view.

The mHealth program would also impact OOPE which can be understood by the theory of change explained elsewhere in a published study protocol [23]. The introduction of mHealth intervention as a job aid for community health volunteers improved their counselling skills and hence, increased knowledge among pregnant women towards early identification of the complications. This increased the demand for use of preventive and curative healthcare services. The impact assessment analysis showed that mHealth resulted in statistically significant increase in coverage iron and folic acid (IFA) supplementation (12.70%), identification and self-reporting of illnesses/complication during pregnancy (13.20%) and after delivery (19.5%) in the intervention area as compared to the control area. The coverage of > = 3 ANC visits, > = 2 tetanus toxoid, Full ANC, and ambulance usage also increased in the intervention area by 9.7%, 4.5%, 1% and 2.5% respectively, however, the change was statistically insignificant [14]. As far as utilization of public health facilities was concerned, while 50% of women with pregnancy related complications in intervention area sought care in public hospitals, nearly 72% women sought care in private health facilities in the control area [51]. Therefore, the increased uptake of primary and secondary health care services at initial stages of illness may result in reduction in subsequent tertiary care services thus, reducing OOPE on health care. The detailed description of the theory of change and results of impact assessment survey are provided as published literature [14, 23]. The out of pocket expenditures (OOPE) for seeking maternal, newborn and child care services in private and public health facilities in the intervention and control households in reported in the table in Additional file 2. It highlighted that the out of pocket expenditures on utilization of inpatient services for newborn and childhood illnesses were lesser in intervention areas than the control areas, there is limited data available in literature from India to assess the impact of mHealth interventions on out of pocket expenditures. However, assessment reports from other LMICs like Brazil and Mexico highlighted that mHealth could reduce OOPE by US$ 102 per mHealth user thus making healthcare more affordable [50].

Limitations

Our study had few limitations. Firstly, we could not obtain detailed year wise breakup of the expenses during the implementation phase, i.e., August 2012 to August 2015. We assumed that the same amount of expenses happened every year and averaged the cost, which might not be the case in the real situation. Second, in order to know the present worth of the capital involved in the study, we inflated the costs from year 2012 to 2015 considering the CPI Index for calculation of inflation and 3% discount rates. There is a possibility that advancement in technology over time may have actually reduced the price of capital items such as mobile phones, software etc. While this was not considered in the base case, we did undertake a sensitivity analysis to understand the impact of this assumption.

Third, since the retrospective data was collected and many of the officials from implementing agencies had left, there was a possibility of recall bias. However, as most of the data was retrieved from records, possibility of recall bas influencing the validity of our results was relatively less.

Fourth, the scale up cost implicitly included the costs of ASHAs' performance based incentives. However, based on our impact assessment analysis, we found that the ReMiND program increased the coverage of IFA supplementation, identification and self-reporting of illnesses/ complication during pregnancy & after delivery in the intervention area as compared to control area and none of these coverage indicators were linked to any performance based incentives paid to ASHAs [14]. Also, the data obtained from the district health office did not show any substantial difference in incentives received by ASHAs in the intervention and control areas. Therefore, the effect of ASHAs incentives on scale up cost was likely to be minimal on scale up costs.

The scale up cost analysis for Uttar Pradesh state was done from the health system perspective alone. It did not include cost for increased utilization of services because of following reasons. First, the choice of selection of two blocks was not random and specifically blocks were chosen from the worst performing high priority districts. The utilization rates of services in the other districts are likely to be better than the piloted blocks. Therefore, the effectiveness values obtained in these two blocks may not be generalized in the entire Uttar Pradesh state. Moreover, the contribution from the additional cost of increased utilization of services to overall cost is less than 3.5% in the 2 blocks where ReMiND was piloted. Thus, the effect on additional cost of utilization in entire state is expected to be even less than 3.5%. Hence, it is unlikely to make any significant difference in the scale up analysis. Also, scale-up costs were estimated in the ideal conditions without considering any bottlenecks in the implementation of programme which may deviate to some extent in the real life situations. The sudden changes like political & economic instability and introduction of newer programs may affect the program in one way or other. These uncertainties could not be accounted for in our analysis. Also, we acknowledge lack of data on time spent on supervisory and monitoring activities for which the data was taken from another study [29].

Finally, as there is a keen interest globally on the use of mobile health interventions, it is furthermore important to assess the cost- effectiveness of such interventions. Our analysis is a cost-outcome description and an attempt to study the scale-up costs to understand the fiscal challenges of scale-up. However, a full economic evaluation of ReMiND program from a societal perspective was also undertaken, the results of which has been published elsewhere [23, 52]. This economic analysis estimated the incremental cost of implementing ReMiND program per disability adjusted life year averted as a result of program's effectiveness on improving the maternal and child health outcomes. Overall, from a health system perspective, ReMiND incurred an incremental cost of INR 12,993 (USD 205) per DALY averted. From a societal perspective, ReMiND program was a cost saving intervention [52].

Conclusion

This study is the first cost analysis of a mHealth intervention for maternal & child health services in India. Our estimates on cost are useful for policy-makers and program managers in order to plan health programs. Overall the study findings on cost of mHealth are favourable from fiscal sustainability point of view.

Additional files

Additional file 1: Summary table for annualized start up and implementation costs of ReMiND program in district Kaushambi. The table shows the detailed description of annual costs involved during start up and implementation phase of ReMiND program.

Additional file 2: Out of pocket expenditures for seeking maternal, newborn and childhood health care in public and private sector health facilities in Kaushambi, 2015. The out of pocket expenditures were estimated as a part of household survey conducted in the intervention and control areas to assess the impact of the ReMiND program. The Table presents the out of pocket expenditures of households in seeking treatment for maternal, newborn and child illnesses in private and public facilities in two areas.

Additional file 3: Scale up costs for implementation of mobile health in the entire state of Uttar Pradesh in two case scenarios. The table shows the scale up cost of implementing the ReMiND program in state of Uttar Pradesh under two case scenarios. First, if the scale up is undertaken utilizing the existing human resource. Second, if additional staff is recruited for monitoring & supervisory activities at block level.

Additional file 4: Table S4A. showing parameter base values with lower and upper limit (in INR) for implementation of ReMiND program in two blocks of district Kaushambi in Uttar Pradesh, India. **B.** showing scale up parameter base values with lower and upper limit (in INR) for implementation of ReMiND program in entire state of Uttar Pradesh, India. The table shows the base parameter cost of input variables with their lower and upper limits for the sensitivity analysis in two case scenarios.

Abbreviations

AF: Asha Facilitator; AMR: Annual Maintenance Rates; ASHA: Accredited Social Health Activist; BCM: Block Community Manager; CEAHH: Cost Effectiveness Analysis Household Survey; CHW: Community Health Workers; CPI: Consumer Price Index; CRS: Catholic Relief Services; DCPM: District Community Process Manager; HEO: Health Education Officer; IMR: Infant Mortality Rate; INR: Indian National Rupee; M & E: Monitoring and Evaluation; MH: Maternal health; mHealth: Mobile Health; MMR: Maternal Mortality Ratio; MNCH: Maternal, Newborn and Child Health; MoHFW: Ministry of Health and

Family Welfare; NGO: Non- Government Organizations; NRHM: National Rural Health Mission; OOP: Out of Pocket; RCH: Reproductive & Child health; ReMiND: Reducing Maternal and Newborn Deaths; UP: Uttar Pradesh; USD: United States Dollar; WHO: World Health Organization

Acknowledgements

We gratefully acknowledge the implementing agencies of ReMiND program, namely; Catholic Relief Services, Vatsalya and Dimagi Inc., for providing data for undertaking costing of ReMiND program. We also recognize critical inputs from the Study Advisory Committee comprising Rajesh Kumar, Indrani Gupta, Stephen Jan, Krishna Rao, Pavitra Mohan, Meenu Singh, Jitendra Kumar, Rajani Ved, Ashok Jha, Neeta Rao, Suresh Dalpath, Prabhu Dayal, Rajesh Jha and Rajkumar Mishra.

Funding

The present study was funded by the United States' International Aid Agency (USAID), New Delhi, India. The funding agency has no role in the study design, collection of data, analysis or report writing.

Authors' contributions

Conception of study: SP. Study design and preparation of tool: AG, SP, PB. Data collection: AG, RN. Data Analysis: AG, SP. Written first Draft: AG. All authors reviewed the manuscript, provided critical inputs for revision, and approved the final version.

Competing interests

The authors' declare that they have no competing interests.

References

1. Ram U, Jha P, Ram F, Kumar K, Awasthi S, Shet A, Pader J, Nansukusa S, Kumar R. Neonatal, 1–59 month, and under-5 mortality in 597 Indian districts, 2001 to 2012: estimates from national demographic and mortality surveys. Lancet Glob Health. 2013;1(4):e219–26.
2. Press Information Bureau.Government of India. Ministry of Health and Family Welfare. List of High Priority Districts (HPDs) in the country http://pib.nic.in/newsite/PrintRelease.aspx?relid=118620. Accessed 24 May 2018.
3. Ministry of Home Affairs, Annual Health Survey Fact Sheet: Uttar Pradesh 2012–13 http://www.censusindia.gov.in/vital_statistics/AHSBulletins/AHS_Factsheets_2012-13/FACTSHEET-UTTAR_PRADESH.pdf. Accessed 4 Sept 2016.
4. UNICEF: The Situaton of Children in India: A profile. In.; May 2011.
5. Jaggi OP, Chattopadhyaya DP. Medicine in India: modern period. Oxford: Oxford University press; 2000.
6. NHM/MOHFW: InductionTraining Module for ASHAs in Urban Areas. In.
7. MoHFW, ASHA Training Modules, National health mission, Government of India http://nhm.gov.in/communitisation/asha/resources/asha-training-modules.html. Accessed 24 Aug 2016.
8. MoHFW, Training Modules for ASHA on NCD http://www.nhm.gov.in/communitisation/asha/resources/asha-training-modules.html. Accessed 24 Aug 2016.
9. Sundararaman T, Ved R, Gupta G, Samatha M. Determinants of functionality and effectiveness of community health workers: results from evaluation of ASHA program in eight Indian states. In: BMC proceedings: 2012: BioMed Central. 2012:O30.
10. Fathima FN, Raju M, Varadharajan KS, Krishnamurthy A, Ananthkumar S, Mony PK. Assessment of 'accredited social health activists'—a national community health volunteer scheme in Karnataka state, India. J Health Popul Nutr. 2015;33(1):137.
11. Saprii L, Richards E, Kokho P, Theobald S. Community health workers in rural India: analysing the opportunities and challenges accredited social health activists (ASHAs) face in realising their multiple roles. Hum Resour Health. 2015;13(1):95.
12. Bajpai N, Dholakia RH. Improving the performance of accredited social health activists in India. Mumbai: Columbia Global Centres South Asia. 2011.
13. Neogi S, Sharma J, Chauhan M, Khanna R, Chokshi M, Srivastava R, Prabhakar P, Khera A, Kumar R, Zodpey S. Care of newborn in the community and at home. J Perinatol. 2016;36(s3):S13.
14. Prinja S, Nimesh R, Gupta A, Pankaj B, Gupta M, Thakur JS. Impact of m-health application used by community health volunteers for improving utilization of maternal, newborn and child health care (MNCH) services in a rural area of Uttar Pradesh, India. Tropical Med Int Health. 2017. https://doi.org/10.1111/tmi.12895.
15. Little A, Medhanyie A, Yebyo H, Spigt M, Dinant GJ, Blanco R. Meeting community health worker needs for maternal health care service delivery using appropriate mobile technologies in Ethiopia. PLoS One. 2013;8(10):e77563.
16. Meankaew P, Kaewkungwal J, Khamsiriwatchara A, Khunthong P, Singhasivanon P, Satimai W. Application of mobile-technology for disease and treatment monitoring of malaria in the "better border healthcare Programme". Malar J. 2010;9:237.
17. Blanas DA, Ndiaye Y, MacFarlane M, Manga I, Siddiqui A, Velez O, Kanter AS, Nichols K, Hennig N. Health worker perceptions of integrating mobile phones into community case management of malaria in Saraya, Senegal. Int Health. 2015;7(3):176–82.
18. Ajay VS, Prabhakaran D. The scope of cell phones in diabetes management in developing country health care settings. J Diabetes Sci Technol. 2011;5(3):778–83.
19. Surka S, Edirippulige S, Steyn K, Gaziano T, Puoane T, Levitt N. Evaluating the use of mobile phone technology to enhance cardiovascular disease screening by community health workers. Int J Med Inform. 2014;83(9):648–54.
20. Kay M, Santos J, Takane M. mHealth: new horizons for health through mobile technologies. World Health Organ. 2011:66–71.
21. Prinja S, Chauhan AS, Angell B, Gupta I, Jan S. A systematic review of the state of economic evaluation for health care in India. Appl Health Econ Health Policy. 2015;13(6):595–613.
22. Kaushambi District : Census 2011 data http://www.census2011.co.in/census/district/545-kaushambi.html. Accessed 28 Aug 2016.
23. Prinja S, Nimesh R, Gupta A, Bahuguna P, Thakur JS, Gupta M, Singh T. Impact assessment and cost-effectiveness of m-health application used by community health workers for maternal, newborn and child health care services in rural Uttar Pradesh, India: a study protocol. Glob Health Action. 2016;9.
24. CRS. Baseline Study Summary: ReMiND - Reducing Maternal and Newborn Deaths. 2011–12. http://www.crs.org/sites/default/files/tools-research/baseline-study-summary-remind-reducing-maternal-newborn-deaths.pdf. Accessed 30 Aug 2016.
25. Annexure 6b: Module 6. Analysing Health Sector Financing and Expenditure http://www.who.int/hac/techguidance/tools/disrupted_sectors/module_06/en/index10.html. Accessed 10 Feb 2016.
26. Internal Revenue Service US: Yearly Average Currency Exchange Rates Translating foreign currency into U.S. dollars. In., Nov 2, 2015 edn.
27. Muennig P, Bounthavong M: Cost-effectiveness analysis in health: a practical approach: John Wiley & Sons; 2016.
28. Baltussen RM, Adam T, Tan-Torres Edejer T, Hutubessy RC, Acharya A, Evans DB, Murray CJ, World Health Organization. Making choices in health: WHO guide to cost-effectiveness analysis.
29. Larsen-Cooper E, Bancroft E, Rajagopal S, O'Toole M, Levin A. Scale matters: a cost-outcome analysis of an m-health intervention in Malawi. Telemedicine and e-Health. 2016;22(4):317–24.
30. Prinja S, Jeet G, Verma R, Kumar D, Bahuguna P, Kaur M, Kumar R. Economic analysis of delivering primary health care services through community health workers in 3 north Indian states. PLoS One. 2014;9(3):e91781.
31. Prinja S, Gupta A, Verma R, Bahuguna P, Kumar D, Kaur M, Kumar R. Cost of delivering health care services in public sector primary and community health centres in North India. PLoS One. 2016;11(8):e0160986.
32. Prinja S, Balasubramanian D, Jeet G, Verma R, Kumar D, Bahuguna P, Kaur M, Kumar R. Cost of delivering secondary-level health care services through public sector district hospitals in India. Indian J Med Res. 2017;146(3):354.

33. National Planning for Community Health Worker Programs http://www.mchip.net/sites/default/files/mchipfiles/03_CHW_Planning_0.pdf. Accessed 27 May 2018.
34. Policy and Guidelines. Guidelines for Community Processes 2014 http://nhsrcindia.org/index.php?option=com_content&view=article&id=152&Itemid=475. Accessed 2 June 2018.
35. Prinja S, Kaur G, Malhotra P, Jyani G, Ramachandran R, Bahuguna P, Varma S. Cost-effectiveness of autologous stem cell treatment as compared to conventional chemotherapy for treatment of multiple myeloma in India. Indian J Hematol Blood Transfus. 2017;33(1):31–40.
36. Kaur G, Prinja S, Malhotra P, Lad DP, Prakash G, Khadwal A, Ramachandran R, Varma S. Cost of treatment of multiple myeloma in a public sector tertiary Care Hospital of North India. Indian J Hematol Blood Transfus. 2018;34:1–7.
37. Kaur G, Prinja S, Ramachandran R, Malhotra P, Gupta KL, Jha V. Cost of hemodialysis in a public sector tertiary hospital of India, Clinical Kidney Journal, sfx152. https://doi.org/10.1093/ckj/sfx152.
38. Making choices in health: WHO guide to cost-effectiveness analysis http://apps.who.int/iris/bitstream/handle/10665/42699/9241546018.pdf;jsessionid=6AF3430426FB4D38FFD4FCB7393DBDB5?sequence=1. Accessed 2 June 2018.
39. Wilkinson T, Sculpher MJ, Claxton K, Revill P, Briggs A, Cairns JA, Teerawattananon Y, Asfaw E, Lopert R, Culyer AJ. The international decision support initiative reference case for economic evaluation: an aid to thought. Value Health. 2016;19(8):921–8.
40. The World Bank. Inflation, consumer prices (annual %) https://data.worldbank.org/indicator/FP.CPI.TOTL.ZG. Accessed 8 June 2018.
41. Narendra Modi speaks at AAPI Global Healthcare Summit. In.; 2014.
42. High Level Expert Group Report on Universal Health Coverage for India, Planning Commission of India http://planningcommission.nic.in/reports/genrep/rep_uhc0812.pdf. Accessed 24 Aug 2016.
43. Praveen D, Patel A, Raghu A, Clifford GD, Maulik PK, Abdul AM, Mogulluru K, Tarassenko L, MacMahon S, Peiris D. SMART Health India: development and field evaluation of a mobile clinical decision support system for cardiovascular diseases in rural India. JMIR mHealth and uHealth. 2014;2(4):e54.
44. Larsen-Cooper E, Bancroft E, Rajagopal S, O'Toole M, Levin A. Scale matters: a cost-outcome analysis of an m-health intervention in Malawi. Telemedicine and e-Health. 2015.
45. MacLeod BB, Phillips J, Stone A, Walji A, Awoonor-Williams JK. The architecture of a software system for supporting community-based primary health care with mobile technology: the mobile technology for community health (MoTeCH) initiative in Ghana. Online J Public Health Informat. 2012;4(1).
46. Lund S, Hemed M, Nielsen BB, Said A, Said K, Makungu M, Rasch V. Mobile phones as a health communication tool to improve skilled attendance at delivery in Zanzibar: a cluster-randomised controlled trial. BJOG Int J Obstet Gynaecol. 2012;119(10):1256–64.
47. Balasubramanian D, Prinja S, Aggarwal AK. Effect of user charges on secondary level surgical care utilization and out-of-pocket expenditures in Haryana state, India. PLoS One. 2015;10(5).
48. National Rural Health Mission 2005–12. Approval of state program implementation programme: Uttar Pradesh, 2013–14. In.
49. WHO, Estimating the cost of scaling-up maternal and newborn health interventions to reach universal coverage: methodology and assumptions. In.: Technical Working Paper. Prepared by the Department of Making Pregnancy Safer and Health Systems Financing for the World Health Report 2005: World Health Organization; 2005.
50. Socio-economic impact of mHealth. An assessment report for Brazil and Mexico https://www.pwc.in/assets/pdfs/consulting/strategy/socio-economic-impact-of-mhealth-brazil-and-mexico.pdf. Accessed 8 June 2018.
51. Delivery of maternal, neonatal and child health services in district Kaushambi, Uttar Pradesh (2011–2015): A descriptive report.
52. Prinja S, Bahuguna P, Gupta A, Nimesh R, Gupta M, Thakur JS. Cost effectiveness of mHealth intervention by community health workers for reducing maternal and newborn mortality in rural Uttar Pradesh, India. Cost Effectiveness and Resource Allocation : C/E, 16, 25. 2018. http://doi.org/10.1186/s12962-018-0110-2.

15

Effects of oxytocin and anaesthesia on vascular tone in pregnant women: a randomised double-blind placebo-controlled study using non-invasive pulse wave analysis

Sofus Rabow[1,3*], Ull Hjorth[2], Sofia Schönbeck[2] and Per Olofsson[2]

Abstract

Background: Oxytocin is an uterotonic drug with profound cardiovascular effects, which in compromised patients could lead to serious events. The objective was to investigate whether oxytocin affects cardiac function and vascular tone in large and small arteries. We hypothesized that oxytocin decreases arterial vascular tone and elevates cardiac output.

Methods: 51 pregnant women were randomised to treatment with 8.3 μg (5 U) oxytocin or placebo injection during first trimester surgical evacuation of the gravid uterus under general anaesthesia. Oxytocin or placebo was administered once either early or late in the procedure, in a double-blind fashion. Digital photoplethysmography pulse wave analysis variables, heart rate, mean arterial blood pressure and electrocardiographic ST index were recorded before and after anaesthesia and after each injection. Non-parametric statistics were used with a two-sided P value < 0.05 considered significant.

Results: Anaesthesia induced a significant fall in blood pressure, heart rate and vascular tone in small and peripheral arteries. Oxytocin had a vasodilatory effect on small and peripheral arteries and increased the left cardiac ventricular ejection time. The ST index decreased.

Conclusions: Pulse wave analysis indicated peripheral vasodilation and increased cardiac output after oxytocin, implying increased myocardial oxygen demand. These effects might have been enhanced by the vasodilating effects of anaesthesia. Previous studies have demonstrated myocardial ischaemia after oxytocin, as reflected by a decrease in ST index in the present study.

Keywords: Anaesthesia, Arterial stiffness, Oxytocin, Photoplethysmography, Placebo, Pregnancy, Pulse wave analysis, RCT, Vascular tone

* Correspondence: sofus.rabow@med.lu.se
[1]Department of Clinical Sciences Lund, Anaesthesiology and Intensive Care, Skåne University Hospital, Lund University, S-22185 Lund, Sweden
[3]Department. of Intensive and Perioperative Care, Skåne University Hospital, S-22185 Lund, Sweden
Full list of author information is available at the end of the article

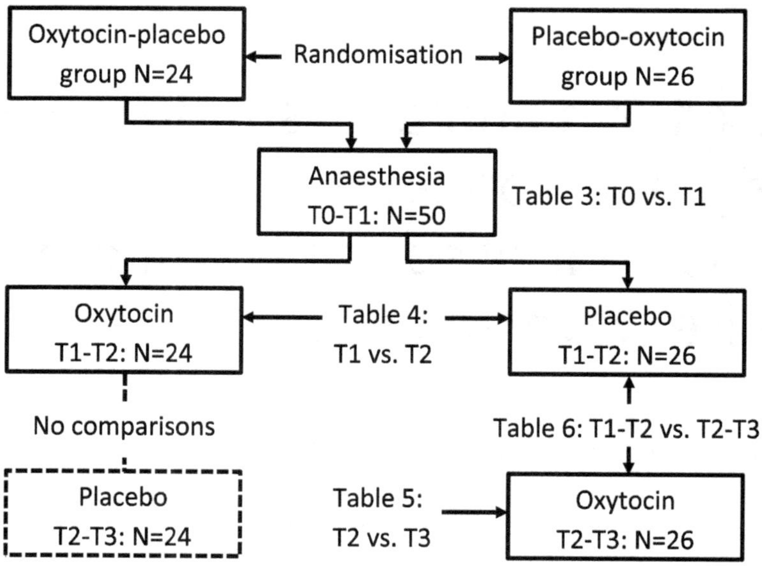

Fig. 1 Flow chart showing the steps of the experiment. The first drugs were administered between the T1 and T2 measurement points, and the second drugs between T2 and T3

Table 1 Description of the digital pulse wave analysis variables used in the study, revised from von Wowern et al. [5]

Variable	Physiological background	Conditions with high values	Conditions with low values	Interpretation of increase	Interpretation of decrease
Pulse height (PH)	Circulation in small finger arteries, perfusion of finger tips	High BP, hyperthyroidism, fever, anemia, excessive blood volume, exercise, well-tuned athlete	Peripheral vaso-constriction, low BP, hypovolemia/ dehydration, hypothyroidism, increased peripheral resistance	Peripheral vasodilatation	Peripheral vasoconstriction
Left ventricular ejection time compensated (ETc)	Represents systole, i.e. time from onset of the systolic upstroke limb to the closure of the aortic valve	Aortic valve stenosis, increased large artery compliance (low vascular tone)[a]	LV failure, decreased preload, hypovolemia, decreased large artery compliance (high vascular tone) [a]	Increase in LV ejection time, Decreased afterload, decreased SVR, increased preload [a]	Decrease in LV ejection time, Increased afterload, increased SVR, decreased preload [a]
Cardiac ejection elasticity index (EEI)	Index for LV ejection capacity and compliance/elasticity of large arteries	Large artery vasodilatation, anemia, increased LV ejection power, hyperthyroidism, congested heart failure	Large artery vasoconstriction, arteriosclerosis, LV ejection insufficiency	Increase in LV ejection power, large artery vasodilatation	Decrease in LV ejection power, large artery vasoconstriction
Dicrotic index (DI)	Represents the peripheral circulation, indicates peripheral resistance	Small artery vasoconstriction	Small artery vasodilatation	Peripheral vasoconstriction	Peripheral vasodilatation
b/a	Early systolic PW peaks identified by second derivatives of the crude PW curve contour; indicates LV ejection capacity and large artery compliance/ elasticity	Low large artery elasticity, increased cardiovascular risk, vasoconstriction, atherosclerosis, increases by age	Young persons, athletes	Large artery vasoconstriction, decreased LV ejection	Large artery vasodilatation, increased LV ejection
d/a	*d* is a late systolic PW peak identified by second derivative of the crude PW curve contour; mainly reflects the intensity of the tidal PW from small peripheral arteries	High small artery elasticity, young persons	A longer negative *d* peak develops by advancing age, indicating arterial stiffness, atherosclerosis	Small artery vasodilatation	Small artery vasoconstriction
Ageing index (AI)	AI = $(b\text{-}c\text{-}d\text{-}e)/a$, representing the global vascular stiffness, i.e. "vascular age"	Atherosclerosis, increases by age	Young persons, athletes	Global arterial vasoconstriction	Global arterial vasodilatation

BP blood pressure, *SVR* systemic vascular resistance, *LV* left heart ventricle, *PW* pulse wave
[a]) See Discussion for interpretation

Background

Oxytocin is used to contract the uterus for prevention and treatment of post-partum haemorrhage after both vaginal delivery and Caesarean section (CS) [1]. It is also used after curettage to prevent post-operative uterine atony and bleeding [2]. Oxytocin has cardiovascular side effects such as tachycardia, vasodilation, hypotension and chest pain. This may lead to serious cardiovascular events in an already compromised patient [3].

We have previously studied the cardiovascular effects of oxytocin using digital photoplethysmographic pulse wave analysis (DPA) during elective CS [4]. We found that oxytocin causes arterial vasodilation of both small and large arteries and has a direct negative chronotropic effect with increased left ventricular (LV) ejection power accompanied by electrocardiographic (ECG) ST changes. However, the combination of CS, spinal anaesthesia, intravenous fluids, vasoactive drugs and delivery of the baby and placenta, made it problematic to study the haemodynamic effects of oxytocin exclusively. Therefore, we wanted to conduct a study in a more stable clinical setting. For this purpose, we chose to study the circulatory effects in first trimester pregnant women undergoing uterine evacuation after miscarriage or for surgical termination of pregnancy.

The DPA method can assess cardiac LV ejection time (LVET) and distinguish between tonus changes in large and small arteries [5]. Using DPA in combination with ECG ST index and mean arterial blood pressure (MAP) measurements adds information whether there are direct cardiac effects of oxytocin [5, 6]. The method has been validated against invasive aortic pressure measurements during vasoconstrictory and vasodilatory manipulations [7][Takazawa 1998], the physiological background to the digital photoplethysmographic volume pulse wave contour characteristics has been thoroughly described [8, 9] and the method correlates well with the gold standard applanation tonometry method [5, 8]. The DPA has the advantage of being rapid, non-invasive, pain-free, and user independent.

Methods

The primary objective of the study was to investigate whether oxytocin affects both large and small arteries, and cardiac LV ejection function, using the DPA method. Based on our own observations [4] and observations by Weis et al. [10], we hypothesised that oxytocin decreases arterial vascular tone and elevates cardiac output (CO). The regional research ethics committee in Lund approved the study (dnr 2012/649) and all enrolled women gave their informed oral and written consent. The study was performed in accordance with The Code of Ethics of the Declaration of Helsinki. The women were recruited consecutively at the Department of Obstetrics and Gynaecology at Skåne University Hospital, Malmö, during the spring 2013, as part of the Master's degree projects by U. H. and S. S. All women scheduled for termination of pregnancy in the first trimester by vacuum aspiration or curettage, who met the inclusion criteria, were asked to participate. Inclusion criteria were healthy women assessed as American Society of Anesthesiologists physical status classes I-II, with a gestational age below 12 weeks, age above 18 years, and understanding oral and written Swedish. In all, 54 women were asked to participate, of whom 3 declined, and the recruitment stopped after 51 included patients. A sample size based on power calculation could not be performed, because in comparison with placebo, the oxytocin effects on DPA variables were unknown.

The women were randomised by P.O. using a web-based random number generator [11] to first treatment with either intravenous (IV) oxytocin or placebo. Before the start of anaesthesia, the nurse anaesthetist opened a sealed opaque envelope containing the treatment allocation. The nature of the injection was blinded to the woman, to the researchers, and to the surgeon. Women given oxytocin as the first injection were given placebo as the second injection (oxytocin-placebo sequence, OP group) and vice versa (placebo-oxytocin sequence, PO group) (Fig. 1). The oxytocin injection comprised 1 mL of Oxytocin Pilum 8.3 μg/mL (5 U) (Orifarm Generics, Stockholm, Sweden) and the placebo injection comprised 1 mL of NaCl 9 mg/mL.

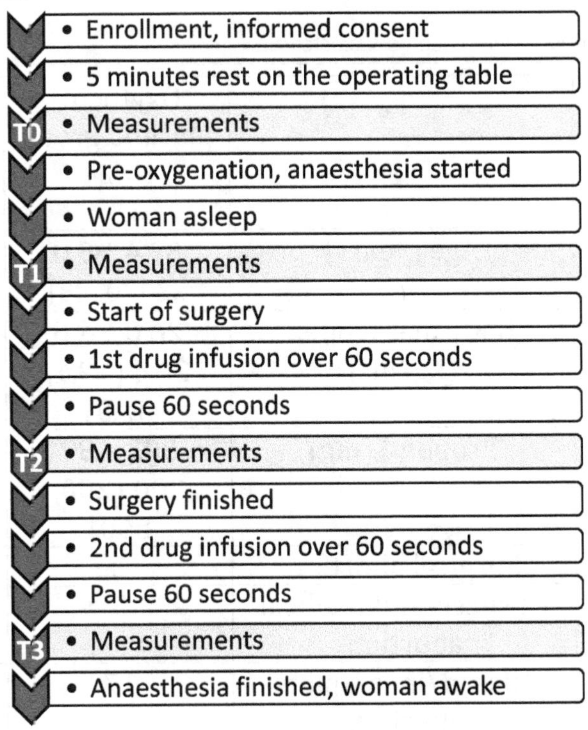

Fig. 2 Study protocol with time sequences of monitoring, anaesthesia and intravenous drug injections

The physiological background to the DPA method has been described previously [6, 8]. The Meridian DPA™ reports 17 different variables, but for this study we selected those variables with the best repeatability and best correlation to gold standard applanation tonometry: pulse height (PH), ageing index (AI), cardiac LV ejection time (LVET) compensated (ETc), cardiac ejection elasticity index (EEI), dicrotic index (DI), and the ratios *b*/*a* and *d*/*a* [5]. The variables are described in Table 1.

The sequences of monitoring and treatments are shown in Fig. 2. Three hours prior to scheduled surgery, the women were pre-medicated with two intravaginal misoprostol 0.2 mg tablets (Cytotec®, Pfizer AB, Sollentuna, Sweden) and two oral paracetamol 500 mg tablets (Alvedon®, GlaxoSmithKline Consumer Healthcare, Bröndby, Denmark). Upon arrival at the operating room, a peripheral IV catheter was introduced. A 5-lead ECG, a blood pressure (BP) cuff and a peripheral oxygen saturation (SaO_2) probe were connected to the surveillance monitor (DASH 4000, GE Medical Systems Information Technologies, Danderyd, Sweden). The ECG ST index was automatically derived from the ECG lead II. Readings of BP, SaO_2, and ST index were manually noted in a case report form.

For the DPA measurements, a customized pulse oximetry probe was placed on the right second or third finger, and then connected to the Meridian DPA™ (Meridian Co. Ltd., Korea, and Salcor AB, Uppsala, Sweden). The Meridian DPA was connected to a laptop (HP 625, Hewlett Packard, Solna, Sweden). Each DPA measurement takes 70 s to perform, during which surgery was halted.

Since the surgery was performed with the woman in the lithotomy position and the DPA measurements are sensitive to body position, the woman was placed in this position on the operating table already before initialising anaesthesia. After 5 min of rest in this position, the baseline measurements (time point T0) were performed (Fig. 2). The woman was then pre-oxygenated with 100% oxygen through a breathing mask. General anaesthesia was commenced with an injection of fentanyl 100 μg (Fentanyl® B. Braun 50 μg/mL) followed by a bolus dose of propofol (Propofol®-Lipuro B. Braun 10 mg/mL), individually titrated to loss of consciousness and eyelid reflex, after which anaesthesia was maintained with propofol only. The women were kept on mask airway during anaesthesia.

At each time point, the measurements were started with a DPA recording (lasting 70 s) paralleled by the ECG ST index reading, followed by a BP measurement. The second measurements were performed after the induction of anaesthesia, but before the start of surgery (time point T1, see Fig. 2). The first drug injection was given when the cervical dilatation was completed and uterine evacuation began. The injection time was one minute. A stopwatch was started and the point T2 DPA recording started 60 s after finishing the injection.

The second drug injection was given at the end of surgery but before end of anaesthesia and the point T3

Table 2 Demographic characteristics

	Oxytocin-placebo group N=24	Placebo-oxytocin group N=26	Total number	Significance of difference (*P*)
Age (years)	32.4 ± 6.0 33 (20, 43)	28.4 ± 6.4 28.5 (18, 41)	50	0.032
Body mass index (kg/m^2)	26.0 ± 4.6 25.4 (19.1, 37,5)	23.0 ± 3.6 22.5 (17.8, 31.2)	50	0.018
Propofol (mg)	303 ± 89 290 (200, 560)	313 ± 65 300 (220, 460)	50	0.36
Surgical abortion	2	6	8/50	
Unsuccessful medical abortion	5	8	13/50	0.19
Missed/incomplete abortion	17	12	29/50	

Figures are mean ± standard deviation and median (range)
Statistics were performed with the Mann-Whitney *U* test or Fisher's exact probability test

Table 3 Haemodynamic effects of general anaesthesia in first trimester pregnant women. For explanation of measurement points T0 and T1, see text and Fig. 2

Variable	Number of cases	Cardiovascular effect of anaesthesia measured T0-T1			
		T0 value Mean ± SD Median (range)	T1 value Mean ± SD Median (range)	Significance of difference (*P*)	Cardiovascular effect
MAP (mmHg)	49	85 ± 12 84 (65, 112)	65 ± 9 64 (49, 89)	0.0001	Blood pressure drop
HR (bpm)	33	73 ± 14 70 (44, 96)	65 ± 9 63 (48, 84)	0.002	Heart rate drop
ECG ST index	48	0.15 ± 0.28 0.20 (− 0.70, 0.90)	0.20 ± 0.22 0.20 (− 0.30, 0.60)	0.13	
PH	33	2.0 ± 1.9 1.3 (0.6, 10.5)	5.3 ± 2.9 4.9 (0.8, 14.9)	0.0001	Peripheral vasodilation
ETc (ms)	33	374 ± 30 372 (313, 442)	361 ± 45 368 (165, 437)	0.56	
EEI	27	0.69 ± 0.28 0.59 (0.27, 1.32)	0.60 ± 0.18 0.58 (0.18, 1.00)	0.19	
EEI@75	27	0.71 ± 0.26 0.74 (0.19, 1.21)	0.68 ± 0.19 0.69 (0.28, 1.14)	0.61	
DI	33	0.66 ± 0.14 0.65 (0.37, 0.93)	0.56 ± 0.14 0.56 (0.36, 0.94)	0.31	
DI@75	33	0.65 ± 0.08 0.65 (0.50, 0.83)	0.56 ± 0.14 0.58 (0.25, 0.80)	0.0009	Small-artery vasodilation
b/a	33	−0.63 ± 0.14 − 0.64 (−1.05, − 0.39)	− 0.60 ± 0.15 − 0.56 (− 1.02, − 0.26)	0.46	
d/a	33	− 0.20 ± 0.10 − 0.17 (− 0.49, − 0.07)	− 0.18 ± 0.14 − 0.15 (− 0.54, − 0.01)	0.24	
AI	33	− 0.48 ± 0.30 − 0.53 (− 1.03, 0.24)	−0.32 ± 0.28 − 0.38 (− 0.77, 0.42)	0.010	Global vasoconstriction

MAP, mean arterial blood pressure, *HR* heart rate *ECG*, electrocardiogram. *PH* pulse height, *ETc* cardiac left ventricular ejection time compensated, *EEI*, cardiac ejection elasticity index, *EEI@75*, EEI adjusted to a HR of 75 bpm, *DI* dicrotic index; DI@75, DI adjusted to a HR of 75 bpm; *b/a*, ratio between second derivatives of crude pulse wave contour; *d/a*, ratio between second derivatives of crude pulse wave contour; AI, ageing index
Statistics performed with Wilcoxon matched-pairs signed-rank test

measurements were performed in the same way as for the T2 measurements (Fig. 2).

Since the plasma half-time elimination of oxytocin is 3–20 min [12], the comparison of oxytocin vs. placebo could not be performed in the OP group after the second injection due to a too short wash-out time of oxytocin after the first injection. Thus, the oxytocin effect was in comparison with placebo studied cross-sectionally in the OP group at T1-T2 and longitudinally in the PO group for T1-T2 vs. T2-T3 (Fig. 1). For each studied variable, the difference from before until after administration was calculated, denoted Δ value. A positive Δ value denotes an increase and a negative value a decrease.

The DPA data were automatically exported to an Excel file in the laptop and later converted to a statistics software document (StatView version 5.0.1, SAS Institute, Cary, NC, USA). The Meridian manufacturer recommends that at least 80% of the pulse waves should be recorded to ensure good quality of the mathematical analyses of the pulse wave contour, so recordings with < 80% recognition were excluded from statistical analyses.

The Mann-Whitney U test was used to compare continuous variables between groups. For longitudinal comparisons within groups the Wilcoxon signed-ranks matched-pairs test was used. Categorical data were compared with Chi-2 test or Fisher's exact probability test. Fisher's exact test in 2 × 3 tables was performed with software available on the web [13]. Two-sided *P* values < 0.05 were considered statistically significant.

Some of the DPA variables are heart rate (HR) dependent [5] and the statistical analyses were accordingly performed with both crude and HR-adjusted DPA values. If simple linear regression analyses yielded a statistically significant correlation ($P < 0.05$) between HR and a DPA variables at T0, and the intervention (anaesthesia, oxytocin or placebo administration) also resulted in a significant change in HR, the DPA variables in question was adjusted to a HR of 75 bpm, denoted DPA@75, with the equation DPA@75 = DPA ± *C*(75-HR). *C* denotes the slope constant. The DPA

Table 4 Haemodynamic effects of 5 U (8.3 μg) oxytocin and placebo (NaCl) given intravenously to first trimester pregnant women undergoing surgical evacuation of the uterus. For explanation of time points T1 and T2, see text and Figs. 1 and 2

Variable	Effect of drug injection measured T1-T2								
	Oxytocin (OP group) N = 24				Placebo (PO group) *N* = 26				Δ value[a] *P*
	T1 value Mean ± SD Median (range)	T2 value Mean ± SD Median (range)	P^b	Effect	T1 value Mean ± SD Median (range)	T2 value Mean ± SD Median (range)	P^b	Effect	
MAP (mmHg)	67 ± 10 65 (49, 89)	76 ± 12 76 (57, 97)	0.001	BP increase	64 ± 9 62 (52, 88)	73 ± 8 74 (57, 87)	0.0001	BP increase	0.61
HR (bpm)	64 ± 8 63 (48, 82)	68 ± 9 71 (53, 84)	0.011	HR increase	66 ± 9 65 (51, 84)	66 ± 8 65 (53, 82)	0.90	No change	0.020
ECG ST index	0.21 ± 0.24 0.30 (−0.20, 0.60)	0.15 ± 0.19 0.10 (− 0.40, 0.60)	0.30	No change	0.19 ± 0.21 0.10 (− 0.30, 0.60)	0.33 ± 0.21 0.30 (0.00, 0.80)	0.0005	ST increase	0.0008
PH	5.3 ± 2.9 4.8 (0.8, 13.3)	9.6 ± 2.5 8.8 (6.1, 15.0)	< 0.0001	Peripheral vasodilation	5.3 ± 3.0 4.9 (1.8, 14.9)	9.9 ± 3.3 9.5 (4.9, 16,0)	< 0.0001	Peripheral vasodilation	0.45
ETc (ms)	360 ± 39 366 (245, 418)	381 ± 41 383 (267, 444)	0.021	Decreased afterload, decreased SVR, increased preload	362 ± 51 369 (165, 437)	356 ± 55 371 (156, 404)	0.70	No change	0.069
EEI	0.58 ± 0.19 0.58 (0.18, 0.93)	0.59 ± 0.16 0.60 (0.26, 0.77)	0.65	No change	0.61 ± 0.18 0.60 (0.31, 1.00)	0.53 ± 0.13 0.51 (0.36, 0.83)	0.12	No change	0.17
EEI@75	0.67 ± 0.18 0.66 (0.28, 0.98)	0.65 ± 0.16 0.67 (0.32, 0.95)	0.95	No change	0.69 ± 0.20 0.72 (0.32, 1.14)	0.61 ± 0.15 0.57 (0.41, 0.96)	0.23	No change	0.43
DI	0.65 ± 0.15 0.67 (0.36, 0.94)	0.55 ± 0.11 0.55 (0.33, 0.77)	0.001	Small-artery vasodilation	0.66 ± 0.13 0.66 (0.41, 0.92)	0.67 ± 0.14 0.66 (0.41, 0.99)	0.84	No change	0.015
DI@75	0.55 ± 0.14 0.57 (0.25, 0.77)	0.49 ± 0.11 0.50 (0.32, 0.65)	0.023	Small-artery vasodilation	0.58 ± 0.14 0.58 (0.28, 0.80)	0.59 ± 0.15 0.61 (0.22, 0.88)	0.97	No change	0.10
b/a	− 0.59 ± 0.16 − 0.54 (− 0.95, − 0.26)	−0.57 ± 0.13 − 0.57 (− 0.85, − 0.25)	0.74	No change	−0.62 ± 0.14 − 0.61 (− 1.02, − 0.40)	−0.56 ± 0.08 − 0.55 (− 0.78, − 0.39)	0.094	No change	0.19
d/a	−0.17 ± 0.14 − 0.14 (− 0.54, − 0.01)	− 0.20 ± 0.09 − 0.20 (− 0.39, − 0.08)	0.38	No change	−0.18 ± 0.14 − 0.18 (− 0.50, − 0.01)	− 0.23 ± 0.13 − 0.20 (− 0.76, − 0.08)	0.084	No change	0.84
AI	− 0.31 ± 0.29 − 0.38 (− 0.77, 0.21)	−0.27 ± 0.24 − 0.27 (− 0.63, 0.24)	0.99	No change	−0.32 ± 0.29 − 0.37 (− 0.70, 0.42)	−0.25 ± 0.20 − 0.30 (− 0.50, 0.25)	0.086	No change	0.27

OP group, women given oxytocin at first injection and placebo at second injection; PO group, women given placebo at first injection and oxytocin at second injection

[a)] The Δ values are not shown, but represent the T2 value minus T1 value. *P* denotes significance of difference in Δ value between oxytocin and placebo injections, performed with the Mann-Whitney *U* test

[b)] *P* denotes significance of difference between T1 and T2 values, performed with the Wilcoxon matched-pairs signed-ranks test

variable ETc and the ECG variable ST index are automatically adjusted for HR when reported by the respective apparatus.

Results

One patient in the OP group did not receive the allocated intervention due to a surgical complication with perforation of the uterus. Thus, 24 women allocated to the OP group and 26 to the PO group were included in the study. Their demographic characteristics are shown in Table 2.

At time point T0, in 17/50 (34%) women the PH was below the 80% threshold for receiving adequate signals for pulse wave contour analysis, thus disabling reliable calculations of DPA variables. This excluded the longitudinal comparisons T0-T1 (effects of anaesthesia) in 34–46% of cases. For recordings T1-T3, the recording error rate was 4–8%.

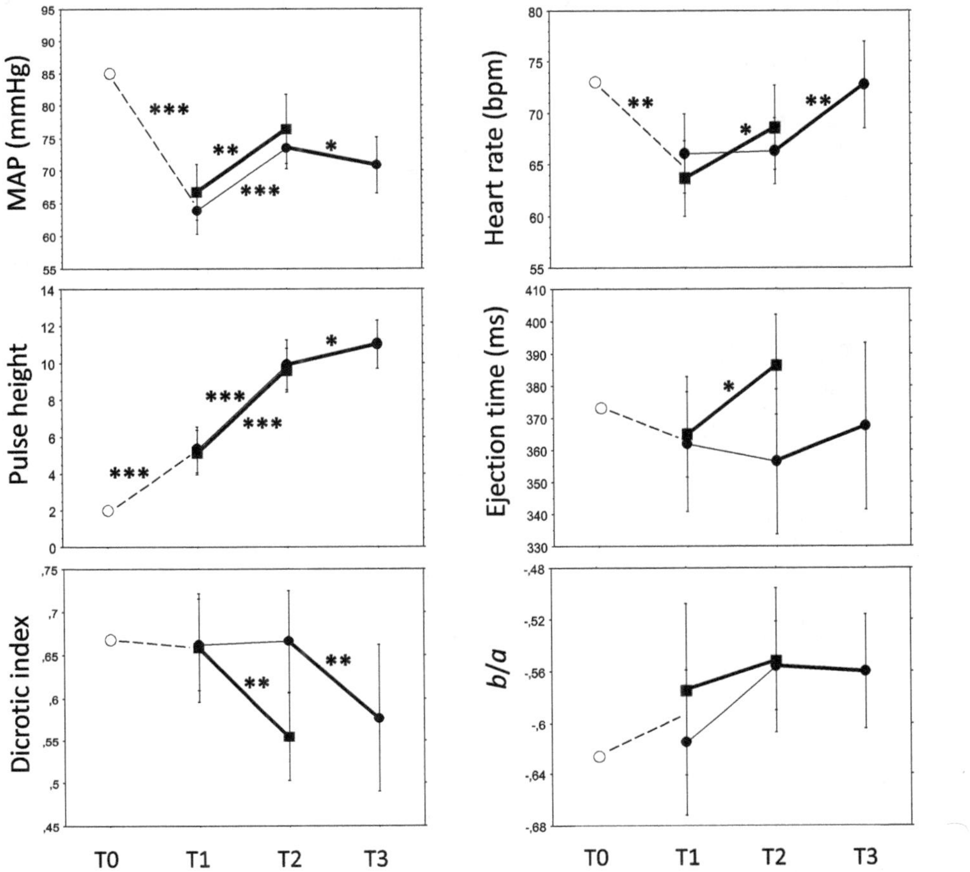

Fig. 3 Sequential changes of mean arterial blood pressure (MAP), heart rate, pulse height, left ventricular ejection time, dicrotic index and *b/a* from time point T0 through T3 (for details, see text). Dashed lines represent the effect of general anaesthesia. Oxytocin/placebo were administered between T1 and T2 and vice versa between T2 and T3, where filled squares represent the oxytocin-placebo group and filled circles the placebo-oxytocin group. The oxytocin-placebo group were not analysed at T2-T3, as explained in the text. Bold lines represent oxytocin effects and thin lines placebo effects. Values are mean with 95% confidence interval. The asterisk * denotes a *P* value < 0.05, ** denotes $P < 0.01$ and *** $P < 0.001$, calculated with the Wilcoxon signed-ranks matched-pairs test.

At point T0, a significant relationship was found between HR and DI ($P < 0.0001$, r^2 0.67) and EEI ($P = 0.017$, r^2 0.17) and these variables were accordingly adjusted in the statistical analyses (called DI@75 and EEI@75). AI, *b*/*a* and *d*/*a* were not significantly related to HR ($P \geq 0.50$).

Anaesthesia caused a decrease in MAP and HR and a small-artery and peripheral vasodilation, as indicated by PH and DI@75, and a global vasoconstriction was indicated by AI (Table 3).

The surgery started after point T1 (Fig. 2), and oxytocin and placebo showed from T1 to T2 the following effects (Table 4, Fig. 3):

- MAP increased by equal magnitudes in the OP and PO groups, i.e. no matter the sort of injection.
- An increase in HR was seen only after oxytocin, and the difference to placebo was confirmed by comparison of ΔHR values.
- The ECG ST index changed only after placebo, confirmed by a difference in Δ values.
- PH increased (peripheral vasodilation) by equal magnitudes after oxytocin and placebo, confirmed by the absence of difference in ΔPH values.
- ETc increased (increase in LVET, increased preload, and/or decreased afterload) only after oxytocin, but the difference in ΔETc values did not reach significance ($P = 0.069$).
- EEI and EEI@75 were not affected by oxytocin or placebo.
- Changes of DI and DI@75 after oxytocin indicated small-artery vasodilation, and the difference was confirmed by a difference in ΔDI values.
- *b*/*a*, *d*/*a* and AI did not change significantly in any group.

Due to a probable insufficient wash-out effect of oxytocin given as the first injection in the OP group,

Table 5 Haemodynamic effects of 5 U (8.3 μg) oxytocin given as the second injection at T2-T3 in women given placebo as the first injection

Variable	Oxytocin (PO group) $N = 26$			
	T2 value Mean ± SD Median (range)	T3 value Mean ± SD Median (range)	P^a	Effect
MAP (mmHg)	73 ± 8 74 (57, 87)	71 ± 11 71 (51, 90)	0.046	BP decrease
HR (bpm)	66 ± 8 65 (53, 82)	73 ± 10 72 (53, 88)	0.001	HR increase
ECG ST index	0.33 ± 0.21 0.30 (0.00, 0.80)	0.18 ± 0.29 0.20 (− 0.40, 0.70)	0.014	ST decrease
PH	9.9 ± 3.3 9.5 (4.9, 16,0)	11.0 ± 3.0 11.5 (5.5, 16.0)	0.019	Peripheral vasodilation
ETc (ms)	356 ± 55 371 (156, 404)	367 ± 60 381 (179, 430)	0.39	No change
EEI	0.53 ± 0.13 0.51 (0.36, 0.83)	0.50 ± 0.13 0.48 (0.33, 0.80)	0.33	No change
EEI@75	0.61 ± 0.15 0.57 (0.41, 0.96)	0.52 ± 0.15 0.52 (0.31, 0.84)	0.33	No change
DI	0.67 ± 0.14 0.66 (0.41, 0.99)	0.58 ± 0.20 0.53 (0.26, 0.99)	0.006	Small-artery vasodilation
DI@75	0.59 ± 0.15 0.61 (0.22, 0.88)	0.56 ± 0.20 0.55 (0.12, 1.06)	0.013	Small-artery vasodilation
b/a	−0.56 ± 0.08 − 0.55 (− 0.78, − 0.39)	− 0.56 ± 0.10 − 0.57 (− 0.74, − 0.35)	0.056	No change
d/a	−0.23 ± 0.13 − 0.20 (− 0.76, − 0.08)	− 0.22 ± 0.09 − 0.21 (− 0.40, − 0.04)	0.42	No change
AI	−0.25 ± 0.20 − 0.30 (− 0.50, 0.25)	−0.20 ± 0.19 − 0.20 (− 0.68, 0.05)	0.15	No change

[a] *P* denotes significance of difference between T2 and T3, performed with the Wilcoxon matched-pairs signed-ranks test

the effects of placebo given as the second injection T2-T3 were not analysed (Fig. 1). Table 5 shows the effects of oxytocin when comparing T2 and T3 values. Effects were found on MAP, HR, ST index, PH, DI and DI@75, whereas no effects were found on ETc, EEI, EEI@75, *d/a* and AI. A decrease in *b/a* did not reach statistical significance ($P = 0.056$, which would indicate large-artery vasodilation and increase in LV ejection if significant).

At point T3 surgery had finished, but the women were still under anaesthesia (Fig. 2). In longitudinal comparisons in the PO group, the effects of oxytocin measured T2-T3 were compared with the effects of placebo measured T1-T2 (Table 6, Fig. 1). EEI and EEI@75 statistics could not be performed due to too few cases in comparisons ($N = 10$). The results in Table 6 are interpreted in Table 7, together with an overall interpretation of oxytocin effects displayed in Tables 4-6.

Figure 3 shows the sequential variable changes throughout the experiment from T0 to T3, and Table 7 shows a comprehensive interpretation of oxytocin effects, where some interpretations need further explanations. The MAP increased at T1-T2 in both the oxytocin and placebo groups with no significant difference in magnitude (Table 4), whereas the difference to placebo in the comparison T1-T2 vs. T2-T3 was significant (Table 6); as oxytocin at T2-T3 caused a decrease (Tables 5 and 6) and placebo at T1-T2 an increase (Table 4), the comprehensive interpretation is that MAP decreased after oxytocin (Table 7).

The ECG ST index was unchanged after oxytocin, whereas it increased after placebo at T1-T2 comparisons (Table 4). The difference to placebo in the comparison T1-T2 vs. T2-T3 was significant, where oxytocin showed a decrease and placebo an increase (Tables 4-6). The interpretation is that ECG ST index decreased after oxytocin (Table 7).

The ETc increased at T1-T2 after oxytocin whereas placebo had no effect (Table 4). In the longitudinal comparison with placebo at T1-T2 vs. T2-T3 (Table 6) there was no difference to placebo, and at T2-T3 oxytocin had no effect on ETc (Table 5). The findings were then not unanimous.

Table 6 Haemodynamic effects of oxytocin (administered during sequence T2-T3) relative to placebo (sequence T1-T2) in first trimester pregnant women in the placebo-oxytocin group ($N = 26$). For interpretation and comparisons of oxytocin effects, see Table 7

Variable	Placebo Δ value T1-T2[a] Mean ± SD Median (range)	Oxytocin Δ value T2-T3[b] Mean ± SD Median (range)	Significance of difference[c] (*P*)
MAP (mmHg)	10 ± 9 10 (− 13, 23)	− 3 ± 7 − 2 (− 16, 12)	0.0002
HR (bpm)	0 ± 5 0 (− 13, 9)	6 ± 7 4 (− 4, 22)	0.020
ECG ST index	0.14 ± 0.16 0.10 (− 0.10, 0.50)	− 0.15 ± 0.28 − 0.10 (− 0.90, 0.30)	0.001
PH	4.7 ± 2.9 4.1 (− 0.8, 10.1)	1.0 ± 1.8 0.9 (− 2.8, 3.4)	0.005
ETc (ms)	−3 ± 48 5 (− 200, 55)	2 ± 48 6 (− 160, 107)	0.70
DI	0.00 ± 0.18 − 0.02 (− 0.41, 0.46)	− 0.11 ± 0.16 − 0.14 (− 0.34, 0.30)	0.016
DI@75	0.00 ± 0.18 0.00 (− 0.39, 0.49)	−0.06 ± 0.17 − 0.01 (− 0.25, 0.50)	0.11
b/a	0.06 ± 0.15 0.02 (− 0.19, 0.53)	−0.02 ± 0.08 − 0.05 (− 0.14, 0.21)	0.024
d/a	−0.04 ± 0.13 − 0.03 (− 0.39, 0.27)	−0.02 ± 0.09 − 0.00 (− 0.18, 0.16)	0.78
AI	0.07 ± 0.23 0.08 (− 0.55, 0.62)	0.06 ± 0.20 0.04 (− 0.26. 0.47)	0.94

[a] Δ value calculations *T2* value minus T1 value
[b] Δ value calculations: T3 value minus T2 value
[c] Statistics performed with Wilcoxon matched-pairs signed-ranks test, comparing the changes (Δ value) obtained by oxytocin and placebo

No harmful side effects were noted during the study and no woman complained of chest discomfort.

Discussion

This study supports the hypothesis that oxytocin decreases vascular tone. The changes in DPA variables after an oxytocin bolus suggest vasodilation and decreased vascular tone of small and peripheral arteries. This was established at both cross-sectional and longitudinal comparisons with placebo. The PH, an indicator of the peripheral circulation, increased after anaesthesia and then further after the first drug injection, of equal magnitude after oxytocin and placebo. PH has previously been found to increase with increasing depth of anaesthesia due to reduced sympathetic activity [14]. Then, a continuously increasing PH with increasing depth of anaesthesia might explain the placebo effect of the first injection.

The second injection was given when surgery was finished and the depth of anaesthesia was at steady state or ceasing. Then, oxytocin caused small-artery and peripheral vasodilation, fall of MAP and increase in HR, which further supports the conclusion that oxytocin causes a small-artery and peripheral vasodilation.

The increase in MAP in both groups at the start of surgery might be the result of an increase in sympathetic activity due to painful stimuli. It is, however, possible that a fall in MAP of a very short duration failed to be captured in our study protocol, as MAP was measured after the one-minute DPA recording was completed. The BP measurement takes up to 30 s, meaning that MAP was measured 2–3 min after the end of the oxytocin injection. It has been demonstrated in previous studies that the MAP reduction reaches its nadir already within 1–2 min, and returns to normal after another minute [15, 16]. The ECG changes also occur within 1–2 min [17]. Furthermore, oxytocin has a biphasic effect, with a rapid initial HR increase and decrease in systolic BP followed by a fall in HR and increase in BP [3, 18]. We might then not have captured the rapid initial effect of oxytocin in our study. Also the duration of the bolus injection has been attributed to the nadir lag time. Some researchers used *statim* bolus and others, like us, used a 60 s injection time. A short injection time might maximise the initial effects. Since the BP measurements could interfere with the DPA measurements, we had no choice but to await finishing the DPA measurement before we could record the BP.

The ETc increased after oxytocin at T1-T2 whereas placebo had no effect. Considering the whole experiment, the effect of oxytocin on ETc was not unanimous, but as the T1-T2 comparison was the only one performed during equal conditions in the OP and PO groups, our overall interpretation is that oxytocin caused an increase in ETc. According to our previous communications with the South Korean manufacturer of the Meridian DPA, an increase in ETc could mean aortic valve stenosis or LV failure, as previously described [4, 5]. It might be true concerning aortic valve disease, but is more complex concerning LV failure [19]. Both ETc and the similar measure Flow Time Corrected, derived from oesophageal Doppler velocimetry of aortic blood flow, correlate strongly with the LVET [5, 20]. Lewis et al. pointed out already in 1977 that LV muscle failure and diminished preload is associated with a shortened LVET, and that a marked increase in SV would lengthen the LVET [19].

Later on, Singer et al. [21, 22] using oesophageal Doppler velocimetry, demonstrated that the LVET was increased when preload was increased from a hypovolemic state, but also when preload was decreased from an overload state. Thus, LVET is reaching its maximum at optimal filling pressures. As preload diminishes, compensatory peripheral vasoconstriction causing increased systemic vascular resistance (SVR) usually occur. In effect, vasodilating agents alone also produce an increase in LVET, leaving preload unaffected. Taken together, in

Table 7 Summary of observations based on haemodynamic effects of oxytocin administered at first injection T1-T2 (Table 4) and second injection T2-T3 (Tables 5 and 6). For further explanation of comparisons, see Fig. 1, and for explanation of interpretations, see text

Variable	Table 4 T1-T2 in OP group *N* = 24	Table 5 T2-T3 in PO group *N* = 26	Table 6 T1-T2 vs. T2-T3 in PO group *N* = 26	Summary of observations
MAP (mmHg)	No change[a]	Decrease	Decrease	Decrease
HR (bpm)	Increase	Increase	Increase	Increase
ECG ST index	No change	Decrease	Decrease	Decrease
PH	No change[b]	Increase ➔ peripheral vasodilation	Increase ➔peripheral vasodilation	Increase ➔ peripheral vasodilation
ETc (ms)	Increase ➔ large-artery vasodilation, decreased afterload, decreased SVR, increased preload	No change	No change	Increase ➔ large-artery vasodilation, decreased afterload, decreased SVR, increased preload
EEI	No change	No change	N/A[c]	No change
EEI@75	No change	No change	N/A[c]	No change
DI	Decrease ➔ small-artery vasodilation	Decrease ➔ small-artery vasodilation	Decrease ➔ small-artery vasodilation	Decrease ➔ small artery vasodilation
DI@75	Decrease ➔ small-artery vasodilation	Decrease ➔ small-artery vasodilation	No change	Decrease ➔ small artery vasodilation
b/a	No change	No change	No change/decrease ➔ large-artery vasodilation, increase in LV ejection	No change
d/a	No change	No change	No change	No change
AI	No change	No change	No change	No change

[a] *MAP* increased after both oxytocin and placebo
[b] *PH* increased after both oxytocin and placebo, indicating peripheral vasodilation
[c] *EEI* and *EEI@75* statistics could not be performed due to too few cases in comparisons (N = 10)

healthy patients without fluid overload, LVET increases not only by increased preload but also by decreased afterload, i.e. from decreased SVR [23].

From this argumentation, we believe that the rise in ETc after the first oxytocin injection indicates a reduction in SVR, since preload is assumed unaffected. As HR increased without a fall in MAP, an increase in CO is assumed. An increase in CO leads to an increase in myocardial oxygen demand. Signs of myocardial ischemia have previously been noted after oxytocin injection [17], and that observation could explain the different responses in ECG ST index after oxytocin and placebo.

Thirty-four percent of DPA values were missing at T0 due to cold fingers, probably caused by pre-operative stress-induced peripheral vasoconstriction [14]. Among confounding factors, sympathetic activity induced by noxious stimuli from the surgical procedure might explain changes seen in the placebo group between T1 and T2. Although there were no differences between the groups in the total doses of propofol given, variations in anaesthetic depth is another possible confounding factor.

The cardiovascular effects of anaesthesia included decreases in BP and HR and dilatation of small and peripheral arteries. However, the global index AI indicated vasoconstriction. AI is a composite index of four indices reflecting different phases of the pulse wave from early systole to early diastole, i.e. *b/a*, *c/a*, *d/a* and *e/a* [5]. The two indices reported separately in the present study, i.e. *b/a* and *d/a*, did not change significantly, and the variable reflecting large arteries, EEI, did not change either. Then, the significant change of AI can be interpreted as the amalgamated result of non-significant changes of the subset of indices, or it was a result of a type 1 error. Oxytocin has both vasodilatory and vasoconstrictory properties via the same receptor, V1aR [24], and various vascular beds and organs display different distributions and receptor sensitivity [25]. Although not possible to demonstrate in the present study, vasoconstriction in medium-sized arteries could be a physiological response to peripheral vasodilation and falls in BP and HR.

DPA with digital photoplethysmography is a non-invasive, operator-friendly and rapid method to study vascular tone and pharmacological hemodynamic effects in a clinical setting where the effects come swift. As illustrated by the DPA measurements before initializing anaesthesia, cold fingers must be avoided as they distort the results. That applies to finger movements as well.

A strength of the study is the randomised double-blinded placebo-controlled design in a normal clinical setting. In comparison with our previous study on oxytocin during CS, where the procedures with spinal anaesthesia, IV fluids, vasoactive drugs and delivery of the baby made it problematic to interpret the hemodynamic effects of oxytocin [4], the present study was less compromised by confounding factors. Another strength is the DPA method's ability to investigate effects on large and small arteries separately, by using derivative mathematics to analyse the systolic and diastolic segments of the pulse wave contour. It is a limitation that the study protocol could not be adapted to capture short biphasic courses of events. As surgery needed to be stopped during DPA and BP measurements, for the safety of the women we could not perform double measurements, as would have been experimentally preferred. Variations in anaesthetic depth and sympathetic activity are possible confounders that could not be controlled for.

Misoprostol 0.4 mg was administered vaginally 3 h prior to scheduled surgery. The drug has a plasma half-time of about 30 min, but due to slow absorption by the vaginal route the bioactivity could remain for a few hours [26]. It is therefore possible that remainders of misoprostol persisted at the time of the experiments. However, the lasting bioactivity has been shown on the myometrium [26], whereas no cardiovascular effects of misoprostol have been demonstrated [27, 28]. We therefore believe possible remainders of misoprostol did not confound the results. The placebo-controlled design of the study could ensure it was not misoprostol effects that we measured, and the longitudinal measurements were performed during a short time-span when steady-state concentrations of misoprostol would not bias the results.

Conclusions

This study confirmed the hypothesis that oxytocin decreases vascular tone in small and peripheral arteries, resulting in a lower BP and a compensatory increase in HR. These effects might have been enhanced by the vasodilating effects of anaesthesia. We could not confirm any effect on vascular tone in large arteries. The net oxytocin effect on the heart is likely to be an increased CO, implying increased myocardial oxygen demand. The demonstrated multiple effects of oxytocin on the cardiovascular system suggest a cautious use of oxytocin in pregnant women.

Abbreviations

AI: Ageing index; b/a: Second derivative quotient of the acceleration phase the percussion pulse wave; BP: Blood pressure; CO: Cardiac output; CS: Caesarean section; d/a: Second derivative quotient of percussion wave clashing the reflected tidal wave; DI: Dicrotic index; DI@75: DI adjusted to a heart rate of 75 bpm; DPA: Digital pulse wave analysis; ECG: Electrocardiogram; EEI: Ejection elasticity index; EEI@75: EEI adjusted to a heart rate of 75 bpm; ETc: Left ventricular ejection time compensated (for heart rate); Ftc: Flow time corrected; HR: Heart rate; IV: Intravenous; LV: Left ventricle of the heart; LVET: Left ventricular ejection time; MAP: Mean arterial blood pressure; OP: Oxytocin-placebo sequence; PH: Pulse height; PO: Placebo-oxytocin sequence; ST index: Difference in ECG ST segment from the isoelectric baseline; SVR: Systemic vascular resistance; Δ value: Difference between measurement at time point T_n minus measurement at point T_{n-1}

Funding

The study was funded by grants from the Medical Faculty at Lund University (ALF) and from Region Skåne. The funders had no role in study design, data collection and analysis, decision to publish, or preparation of the manuscript.

Authors' contributions

PO conception and design of the study, PO and SR planning and carrying out the study, analysing data and writing the article, UH and SS carrying out the study, analysing data, reviewing the manuscript. All authors have read and approved the manuscript.

Competing interests

The authors declare that they have no competing interests.

Author details

[1]Department of Clinical Sciences Lund, Anaesthesiology and Intensive Care, Skåne University Hospital, Lund University, S-22185 Lund, Sweden. [2]Department of Clinical Sciences Malmö, Obstetrics and Gynaecology, Skåne University Hospital, Lund University, Malmö, Sweden. [3]Department. of Intensive and Perioperative Care, Skåne University Hospital, S-22185 Lund, Sweden.

References

1. Royal College of Obstetrician and Gynaecologists. Prevention and management of postpartum haemorrhage. London: RCOG Greentop Guidel; 2009. p. 1–24. Available from: https://doi.org/10.1111/1471-0528.14178.
2. Nygaard IHH, Valbø A, Heide HC, Kresovic M. Is oxytocin given during surgical termination of first trimester pregnancy useful? A randomized controlled trial. Acta Obstet Gynecol Scand [Internet], vol. 90. Blackwell Publishing Ltd; 2011. p. 174–8. Available from: https://doi.org/10.1111/j. 600-0412.2010.01025.x
3. Thomas JS, Koh SH, Cooper GM. Haemodynamic effects of oxytocin given as i.v. bolus or infusion on women undergoing caesarean section. Br J Anaesth. 2007;98:116–9.
4. Rabow S, Olofsson P. Pulse wave analysis by digital photoplethysmography to record maternal hemodynamic effects of spinal anesthesia, delivery of the baby, and intravenous oxytocin during cesarean section. J Matern Neonatal Med. 2016;7058:1–26.
5. von Wowern E, Östling G, Nilsson PM, Olofsson P. Digital Photoplethysmography for assessment of arterial stiffness: repeatability and comparison with Applanation tonometry. West J, editor. PLoS One [Internet]. 2015;10:e0135659. Available from: http://dx.plos.org/10.1371/journal.pone.0135659
6. Elgendi M. On the analysis of fingertip photoplethysmogram signals. Curr Cardiol Rev. 2012;8:14–25.
7. Takazawa K, Tanaka N, Fujita M, Matsuoka O, Saiki T, Aikawa M, et al. Assessment of vasoactive agents and vascular aging by the second derivative of Photoplethysmogram waveform. Hypertension [Internet]. 1998; 32:365–70. Available from: https://www.ahajournals.org/lookup/doi/10.1161/01.HYP.32.2.365. [cited 2013 May 24].
8. Millasseau SC, Ritter JM, Takazawa K, Chowienczyk PJ. Contour analysis of the photoplethysmographic pulse measured at the finger. J Hypertens. 2006;24:1449–56.
9. Millasseau SC, Guigui FG, Kelly RP, Prasad K, Cockcroft JR, Ritter JM, et al.

Noninvasive assessment of the digital volume pulse. Comparison with the peripheral pressure pulse. Hypertens. (Dallas, Tex 1979) [Internet]. 2000;36: 952–6.
10. Weis FR, Markello R, Mo B, Bochiechio P. Cardiovascular effects of oxytocin. Obstet Gynecol. 1975;46:211–4.
11. Stat Trek Random Number Generator [Internet]. [cited 2013 Oct 2]. Available from: http://stattrek.com/statistics/random-number-generator.aspx
12. FASS, Farmaceutiska specialiteter i Sverige [Internet] www.fass.se. Available from: http://www.fass.se/LIF/product?userType=0&nplId=20091203000014 . [cited 2017 Nov 30].
13. VassarStats: website for statistical computation. Fisher exact probability test: 2x3 [Internet]. [cited 2017 Apr 6]. Available from: http://vassarstats.net/fisher2x3.html
14. Enekvist B, Johansson A. Pulse perfusion value predicts eye opening after sevoflurane anaesthesia: an explorative study. J Clin Monit Comput. 2015;29:461–5.
15. Johnstone M, Anaesth BJ. The cardiovascular effects of oxytocic drugs. Brit J Anaesth. 1972;44:826–34.
16. Langesaeter E, Rosseland LA, Stubhaug A. Hemodynamic effects of oxytocin during cesarean delivery. Int J Gynaecol Obstet. 2006;95:46–7.
17. Svanström MC, Biber B, Hanes M, Johansson G, Näslund U, Bålfors EM. Signs of myocardial ischaemia after injection of oxytocin: a randomized double-blind comparison of oxytocin and methylergometrine during caesarean section. Br J Anaesth. 2008;100:683–9.
18. Moertl M, Friedrich S, Kraschl J, Wadsack C, Lang U, Schlembach D. Haemodynamic effects of carbetocin and oxytocin given as intravenous bolus on women undergoing caesarean delivery: a randomised trial. BJOG. 2011;118:1349–56.
19. Lewis RP, Rittgers SE, Forester WF, Boudoulas H. Reviews of Contemporary Laboratory Methods Arnold M. Weissler M D, A critical review of the systolic time intervals Circulation. 1977;56:146–158.
20. GSH C, Middleton PM, Celler BG, Wang L, Lovell NH, Asada HH, Shaltis P, RS RA, HRC, et al. Automatic detection of left ventricular ejection time from a finger photoplethysmographic pulse oximetry waveform: comparison with Doppler aortic measurement. Physiol Meas IOP Publishing. 2007;28:439–52.
21. Singer M, Bennett ED. Noninvasive optimization of left ventricular filling using esophageal Doppler. Crit Care Med. 1991;19:1132–7.
22. Singer M, Allen MJ, Webb AR, Bennett ED. Effects of alterations in left ventricular filling, contractility, and systemic vascular resistance on the ascending aortic blood velocity waveform of normal subjects. Crit Care Med. 1991;19:1138–45.
23. Deltex Medical CardioQ-ODM Manual [Internet]. [cited 2016 Dec 8]. Available from: http://www.deltexmedical.com/cardioq-odm/flow-parameters/
24. Japundžić-Žigon N. Vasopressin and oxytocin in control of the cardiovascular system. Curr Neuropharmacol. 2013;11:218–30.
25. Thibonnier M, Conarty DM, Preston JA, Plesnicher CL, Dweik RA, Erzurum SC. Human Vascular Endothelial Cells Express Oxytocin Receptors. Endocrinology. 1999;140:1301–9.
26. Gemzell-Danielsson K, Bygdeman M, Aronsson A. Studies on uterine contractility following mifepristone and various routes of misoprostol. Contraception. 2006;74:31–5.
27. Brecht T. Effect of misoprostol on human circulation. Prostaglandins. 1987; 33:51–60.
28. Ramsey PS, Hogg BB, Savage KG, Winkler DD, Owen J. Cardiovascular effects of intravaginal misoprostol in the mid trimester of pregnancy. Am J Obstet Gynecol. [Internet] Elsevier; 2017;183:1100–2. Available from: https://doi.org/10.1067/mob.2000.108886.

16

Maternal mortality ratio in selected rural communities in Kebbi State, Northwest Nigeria

Usman Gulumbe[1], Olatunji Alabi[2*], Olusola A. Omisakin[2] and Semeeh Omoleke[3]

Abstract

Background: Maternal mortality remains a topical issue in Nigeria. Dearth of data on vital events posed a huge challenge to policy formulation and design of interventions to address the scourge. This study estimated the lifetime risk (LTR) of maternal death and maternal mortality ratio (MMR) in rural areas of Kebbi State, northwest Nigeria, using the sisterhood method.

Methods: Using the sisterhood method, data was collected from 2917 women aged 15–49 years from randomly selected rural communities in 6 randomly selected local government area of Kebbi State. Retrospective cohort of their female siblings who had reached the childbearing age of 15 years was constructed. Using the most recent total fertility rate for Kebbi State, the lifetime risk and associated MMR were estimated.

Result: A total of 2917 women reported 8233 female siblings of whom 409 had died and of whom 204 (49.8%) were maternal deaths. This corresponds to an LTR of 6% (referring to 11 years before the study) and an estimated MMR of 890 deaths/100,000 live births (95% CI, 504–1281).

Conclusion: The findings provide baseline information on the MMR in rural areas of the State. It underscores the need to urgently address the bane of high maternity mortality, if Kebbi State and Nigeria in general, will achieve the health for all by year 2030 as stated in the Sustainable Development Goals (SDGs).

Keywords: Maternal mortality, Sisterhood method, Kebbi state, Northwest Nigeria

Introduction

Maternal mortality remains a topical issue, and it is often used as one of the indicators for assessing the health status of a population as well as classifying countries into "developed" and "developing" countries. According to the tenth revision of International Classification of Diseases (ICD-10), pregnancy-related death is death of a woman during pregnancy or within 42 days of the termination of such pregnancy without considering the cause of death [1]. The occurrence of maternal death has huge consequences not only for the family but also the society in general. As pointed out by Ogunjimi et al. [2], survival of infants and under-five children closely depends on the survival of the mother. They opined that maternal mortality could reduce the life span and life chances of young children because children whose mothers are dead would lack daily care and often become delinquent.

It is clearly evident from literature that Nigeria has persistently ranked as one of the countries with most appalling maternal mortality ratio (MMR), accounting for an estimated 14% of global maternal deaths [3]. Reducing the high level of maternal mortality to an acceptable level agreed upon by the global community is a collective as well as individual national government's efforts. This quest to achieve an acceptable maternal mortality level is often hampered by lack of accurate and reliable data to monitor progress. In most developing countries, vital registration is non-existent. Therefore, many rely on population census and survey — which oftentimes are not conducted at regular interval.

In Nigeria, Northern regions —north central, north east and north west — have the highest MMR with

* Correspondence: alabi.olatunji@fubk.edu.ng
[2]Department of Demography and Social Statistics, Federal University, Birnin-Kebi, Kebbi State, Nigeria
Full list of author information is available at the end of the article

estimated maternal mortality of more than 1000/100,000 live births in some of the states [4–6]. For example, Kebbi State, one of the north western states, has one of the worst reproductive health indices in Nigeria. More than two-third (71%) of pregnant women in the state never attended antenatal care; 91% of the women delivered at home; less than 10% had skilled birth attendance during the most recent birth, among others [1].

In recognition of this appalling statistics, the Nigeria Minister of Health recently inaugurated the "Task Force on Accelerated Reduction of Maternal Mortality in Nigeria" and stated that six northern States including Kebbi were among States with the highest burden in Nigeria [7]. Prior to this, the State Government of Kebbi and Adamawa in 2013 accessed a grant of 30 million Euros (six billion naira) from The European Union Commission to help reduce MMR in the two states [8]. Despite these, achieving a drastic reduction in MMR in Kebbi State remains a challenge. The effort is further hampered by the low utilization of health facilities for any kind of health services including child birth, low literacy level and strong socio-cultural dictates which prevent documentation of mortality events [9]. In a bid to overcome these challenges associated with evidence for policy formulation, an indirect method of estimating MMR is often resorted to in most developing countries.

The use of indirect technique of estimation of MMR, such as the sisterhood methods, is best suited for settings like Nigeria where vital statistics are deficient or non-existent [10]. Sisterhood method requires a smaller number of respondents, data collection is retrospective, simple, quick and based on information about maternal deaths among sisters of the respondents [5]. However, the method does not measure current level of MMR estimate for the current year of the survey but provides retrospective estimate for 10–12 years preceding the survey. The method has been widely used in some States in Nigeria. For instance, Doctor et al. [4] estimated MMR in four states of Jigawa, Katsina, Yobe and Zamfara in Northern Nigeria as 1271 deaths per 100,000 live births. In Plateau State, MMR of 905 per 100,000 live births was estimated using sisterhood method [11]. Also in Kaduna State, a MMR of 1400 deaths per 100,000 live births was estimated using sisterhood method [12]. However, there has not been any such study in Kebbi State.

In addition, the recent assertion by the Honourable Minister of Health underscores the need for a baseline study in Kebbi State to estimate MMR in a bid to measuring her progress towards the achievement of Sustainable Development Goal number three. Furthermore, the recent influx of non-governmental organisations (NGOs) working to improving maternal and child health in Kebbi State also necessitates the generation of baseline data on MMR situation in the State to monitor and evaluate the contributions of the NGOs towards the reduction.

This study sets out to estimate the lifetime risk (LTR) of maternal death and the associated MMR in selected rural villages in Kebbi State. Thus, the study will provide policy makers, government and stakeholders with baseline information on the MMR situation in the State and bring to fore the need to urgently address the scourge of high MMR in Kebbi State and in general, if Nigeria will achieve the health for all by year 2030 as stated in the Sustainable Development Goals (SDGs).

Methods and materials

Study area

Kebbi State, northwest Nigeria is a unique state due to its geographical location bordering two countries of Niger and Benin, and three other northern Nigerian States of Sokoto, Niger and Zamfara- with similar poor maternal and child health indicators. The study was carried out in randomly selected villages across the three senatorial zones of Kebbi State, northwest Nigeria. A total of six Local Government Areas (LGA) were randomly selected from the twenty-one LGAs in Kebbi State (i.e two LGAs were selected from each Senatorial Zone). Within the LGAs, rural communities were randomly selected.

Kebbi State is unique for this kind of study due to its position as one of the six states in the country with the highest number of maternal deaths due to inefficient and inadequate social amenities and health infrastructures- characteristic of a typical rural northern setting. There is also low rate of out-of-wedlock births despite sexually active population, which may suggest a high rate of abortion— a factor that may influence the estimate— in the study area [13].

Data collection

The study adopted a retrospective cross-sectional design which utilizes quantitative data collection methods. The quantitative data was a cross-sectional household survey conducted in August, 2017. Six LGAs were randomly selected from the twenty-one LGAs from the three Senatorial zones in the State. Within the selected LGAs, a number of communities were randomly selected with a target sample size of an average of 500 (translating to 3000 women aged 15–49 in all the six LGAs) women of reproductive age from each LGA as proposed by Graham et al. [10].

Ethical clearance for the study was obtained from the research and ethics committee of the Federal University, Birnin kebbi. The ethics committee approved the use of verbal consent obtained from respondents before the commencement of the survey. The need to obtain parental consent for respondents under age of 16 was further waived by the committee. In each of the community sampled, approval was first sought from the district heads and village heads (*mai-anguwar)* before commencement of field work. During the field work, verbal consent was obtained from each respondent before administering questionnaires. There was a response rate of 97.2% during the survey as few of the respondents did not give their consent. Thus, 2917 sisters of childbearing age were interviewed.

Field team was trained on the use of electronic data collection methods and interview skills. During the training, the team was trained using questionnaire translated to Hausa and, back to English for ease of comprehension and administration in Hausa language on the field. Role plays were conducted in Hausa language during the training. An electronic-based sisterhood questionnaire (see Additional file 1) was administered on randomly selected women aged 15–49 years. Respondents were asked of the total number of sisters they had (born to the same mother). Out of these female siblings, the number exposed to the risk of childbearing i.e., married, was recorded (since child bearing is only accepted within the confines of marital union and there is high rate of early marriage in the study area). Specifically, the following questions were asked: "of the maternal sisters exposed to the risk of childbearing, how many of them were alive and how many were dead? Of the dead sisters, how many died while they were pregnant, or during childbirth, or during the six weeks after the end of pregnancy?" Age at death and place of death of sisters who died as a result of maternal death was also collected for each of the sisters.

The use of electronic-based data collection and recording of geo-coordinates of all household sampled afforded real time data analysis as well as minimising data entry error and data falsification. Data was checked for consistency and quality assurance. The data verified was downloaded from the dedicated surveyCto server into the computer using Excel spreadsheet. The data was exported to MMR calculation template developed for the purpose to generate the LTR and the associated MMR. Migration, which is an important factor in completeness of data was very minimal in the selected communities as most migration of women of reproductive age are due to marriage and intra-state. Thus, respondents accounted for all the female siblings with the help of consistency checks built into the e-based questionnaire.

Analysis

Sibling history data was analysed and disaggregated into five-year age group. Number of maternal sisters exposed to the risk of maternal death and duration of exposure to the risk for each age group was computed by multiplying the number of reported sisters by an adjustment factor for the age groups. The lifetime risk (LTR) of maternal death was calculated using the total number of maternal deaths divided by the estimated total number of sisters exposed. Estimate of total fertility rate (TFR) of 6.7 for Kebbi State was obtained from the 2013 Nigeria Demographic and Health Survey (NDHS). MMR was computed using the formula: $MMR = 1 - [(1\text{-}LTR)^*(1/TFR)]$ and 95% Confidence Interval (CI) was obtained using formula for calculating CI outlined in Hanley et al., (1996).

Result

Table 1 shows the socio-demographic characteristics of respondents interviewed. Of the 3000 women of child bearing age interviewed, 83 (2.8%) did not consent to be interviewed yielding a response rate of 97.2%. Highest number of respondents that consented were in 25–29 age group. As observed, more than half of the respondents had Islamic education (57.9%) while 3 in 10 of them had no formal education. Majority (96.3%) of the respondents were however married as at the time of the study.

Table 2 shows the sisters' vital status by five-year age group and the computation of LTR and MMR for the study area. In all, a total of 2917 women of child bearing age reported 8233 maternal sisters. Of the 8233 female siblings, 409 were reported dead and 204 of the dead sisters died a pregnancy and childbearing related death (maternal death). Lifetime risk of maternal death was 6% or 1:16 and TFR of Kebbi State was 6.7, thus a MMR of 890 deaths/100,000 livebirths (95% CI, 504–1281) was estimated for the State. The approximate time reference for the MMR estimate was the year 2006 corresponding to 11 years before the interviews.

Estimating MMR for more recent periods, we replicated the analysis for women under age 30. A total of 1871 women aged below 30 years reported 4668 maternal sisters. Of the 4668 sisters reported, 155 are dead and 93 (60%) died of pregnancy and childbearing related deaths. The MMR computed for this age group was 1286 deaths/ 100,000 live births (95% CI, 1026–1545) referring to a period of 7 years before the survey.

Discussion

The estimated MMR of 890 deaths/100,000 live births (and the estimate for respondents below 30 years of 1286 deaths/100,000 live births) in Kebbi State are higher than the national average of 576 deaths/ 100,000 live births and is equally one of the highest in the world [1]. The estimates again underscore the assertion that highest burden of maternal mortality in Nigeria are from rural northern Nigeria communities [14]. This remains consistently high due to poor and weak health system in the region, in terms of facilities and human resource

Table 1 Respondents socio-demographic characteristics

Respondents characteristics	Frequency N = 3000	Percentage
Local Government		
Birnin kebbi	582	19.4
Maiyama	429	14.3
Fakai	310	10.3
Shanga	500	16.7
Augie	720	24.0
Bunza	459	15.3
Consent granted?		
Yes	2917	97.2
No	83	2.8
Age group		
15–19	494	16.9
20–24	666	22.8
25–29	711	24.4
30–34	412	14.1
35–39	314	10.8
40–44	202	6.9
45–49	118	4.1
Level of Education		
No formal education	907	31.1
Islamic education	1691	57.9
Primary education	162	5.6
Secondary education	139	4.8
Post secondary education	18	0.6
Marital Status		
Single	42	1.4
Married	2809	96.3
Divorced	34	1.2
Separated	5	0.2
Widowed	27	0.9

among other factors. The situation in Kebbi State is more worrisome where utilisation of maternal health services remains very low. Indicators of maternal health services in Kebbi State shows that 71 % of pregnant women did not attend antenatal care; 1135 of the 1247 births were delivered at home and 261 were assisted by traditional birth attendants (TBA) during delivery while another 318 delivered with "no one present" (NOP) [1].

This study provides the first evidence-based baseline data on MMR in Kebbi State as there has never been such study in the State to the best of our knowledge. Our finding is also consistent with similar studies in neighbouring states in northwest Nigeria estimating MMR for the region to be higher than the national average- usually above 1000 deaths/ 100,000 live births [4, 6, 14]. This finding pointed to the fact that if much is to be achieved in the quest for reduction of MMR in Kebbi State, stakeholders need to urgently review the strategies with a renewed tenacity to institute evidence-based interventions to achieve the goal of reduction of MMR in Kebbi State, and Nigeria in general.

Evidence-based interventions geared towards addressing the 3-delays in accessing obstetrics care services such as improving health infrastructures, provision of skilled manpower at the Primary Heath Care (PHC) facilities, community engagement activities. Community engagement activities should include training of TBA on identification of pregnancy and delivery danger signs, sensitization of community and religious leader e,t,c. Further, Emergency Transport Scheme (ETS) should be piloted within communities with highest maternal mortality burden and later scaled-up to cover the entire State.

Furthermore, the MMR of 890/100,000 live births in the study area as computed from the formula was mainly due to high TFR in the study area. Studies have documented several socio-cultural practices sustaining high fertility levels in northern Nigeria [15, 16]. Practices

Table 2 Responses of 2917 respondents about their sister's vital status and the lifetime risk of maternal death in Kebbi State

Age group of respondent (years)	No. of respondents (%)	No. of maternal sisters ever married	No. of sisters who died (%)	No. of maternal deaths (%)	Adjustment factor	Sisters exposed (Col3×Col6)	Lifetime risk (Col 5/Col 7)
15–19	494 (16.9)	1120	26 (6.4)	16 (7.8)	0.107	120	
20–24	666 (22.8)	1586	40 (9.8)	30 (14.7)	0.206	327	
25–29	711 (24.4)	1962	89 (21.8)	47 (23.1)	0.343	673	
30–34	412 (14.1)	1214	63 (15.4)	29 (14.2)	0.503	611	
35–39	314 (10.8)	1125	65 (15.8)	32 (15.7)	0.664	747	
40–44	202 (6.9)	743	74 (18.1)	31 (15.2)	0.802	596	
45–49	118 (4.1)	483	52 (12.7)	19 (9.3)	0.900	435	
Total	2917 (100.0)	8233	409 (100.0)	204 (100.0)		3508	0.06

MMR, 890/100,000 live births; CI, 504–1281

such as early girl marriage (less than 18 years) should be addressed with the right policies and interventions in the State, if the State is to reduce the scourge of high TFR and maternal mortality. Kebbi State is one of the states with the lowest age at first marriage among women (as low as 12 years) [1]. Thus, community engagement activities to address the age at first marriage among women should be prioritised by the government. Interventions that encourages girl child education beyond secondary school like the Bill and Melinda Gates-funded Girls-for-Health (G4H) project in the State should be adequately monitored as it has potentials of further helping to reduce maternal deaths by raising the age at marriage and thus reduce fertility.

Issues around effects of migration and abortion on MMR estimate are very minimal within the study area. Most women migration are intra-state and are usually due to marriages. Pregnancy is also usually within union due to strict adherence to cultural norms and religious tenets in the study area.

However, limitations of this study are those that are generally associated with similar studies using the sisterhood method of estimating MMR. One of such limitation is that the estimates refers to a period of about 11 years from the period of data collection. Secondly, information on place of residence of dead sisters is not available, therefore the location of respondent is used as a proxy for dead sisters' location. Thirdly, the estimate was from six LGAs (about one-third) out of the twenty-one LGAs in Kebbi State. However, the randomisation in sampling technique addressed the issue of potential sampling bias. Moreover, the health service utilisation level in the sampled communities is similar to that of other areas in the state.

Conclusion

Our study provided an estimated lifetime risk (LTR) of maternal death which indicates that 1:16 women will have a pregnancy or childbearing related death. Also, the study found MMR of 890 deaths/100,000 live births in selected rural villages in Kebbi State. The findings provide the policy- makers, government and stakeholders with the baseline information on the MMR situation in the State. Our study results underscore the need to urgently address the scourge of high MMR, if Kebbi State and Nigeria in general will achieve the health for all by year 2030 as stated in the Sustainable Development Goals (SDGs).

Abbreviations

CI: Confidence Interval; ETS: Emergency Transport Scheme; G4H: Girls for health; LGA: Local Government Area; LTR: Lifetime risk; MMR: Maternal mortality ratio; NOP: No one present; PHC: Primary health care; SDG: Sustainable Development Goal; SMoH: State ministry of health; TBA: Traditional birth attendants; TFR: Total fertility rate

Acknowledgements

We acknowledged the management of Federal University, Birnin Kebbi for the support in accessing and releasing the fund. The village heads and the community members of the study area, the research assistants and the IT personnel are duly acknowledged.

Funding

This study was conducted with funding from the Tertiary Education Trust Fund Institution Based Research 2016 (TETFund IBR, 2016).

Authors' contributions

UG and OA wrote the initial proposal to access the TETFund grant and wrote the draft manuscript, supervised the whole process from data collection to analysis. OAO was involved in the data management and analysis. SO was involved in the drafting and critical review of the manuscript. All authors read and approved the final manuscript.

Authors' information

The authors UG, OA, and OAO are academic staff at the Federal University, Birnin Kebbi.SO is a medical doctor and National Professional Officer-Surveillance/State Coordinator at World Health Orgnization, Kebbi State Office, Nigeria.

Competing interests

The authors declare that they have no competing interests.

Author details

[1]Department of Mathematics and Statistics, Federal University, Birnin-Kebbi, Kebbi State, Nigeria. [2]Department of Demography and Social Statistics, Federal University, Birnin-Kebi, Kebbi State, Nigeria. [3]Immunisation, Vaccines and Emergencies Unit, World Health Organisation, Abuja, Nigeria.

References

1. NPC [Nigeria] and ICF International. Nigeria Demographic and Health Survey 2013. In: National Population Commission. Rockville, MD: Abuja and ICF International. p. 2014.
2. Ogunjimi, L. O., Ibe, R. T.,and Ikorok, MM. Curbing maternal and child mortality: the Nigerian experience. Int J Nurs Midwifery (2012)Vol. 4(3), pp. 33–39. https://doi.org/10.5897/IJNM11.030. Available online at http://www.academicjournals.org/IJNM (Assessed 6/7/2016).
3. World Health Organisation (2014). Trends in maternal mortality: 1990 to 2013. Estimates by WHO, UNICEF, UNFPA, the World Bank and the United Nations population division. Available at: apps.who.int/iris/bitstream/10665/112682/2/9789241507226_eng.Pdf (assessed 5/9/2017).
4. Doctor HV, Findley SE, Afenyadu GY. Estimating maternal mortality level in rural northern Nigeria by the sisterhood method. Int J Popul Res. 2012;2012. ISSN 2090-4029.
5. Doctor HV, Alabi O, Findley SE, Afenyadu GY, Abdulwahab A, Jumare A. Maternal mortality in northern Nigeria: findings of a health and demographic surveillance system in Zamfara state, Nigeria. Trop Dr. 2012;42: 140–3. https://doi.org/10.1258/td.2012.120062.
6. Guerrier G, Oluyide B, Keramarou M, Grais R. High maternal and neonatal mortality rates in northern Nigeria: an 8-month observational study. Int J Women's Health. 2013;5:495–9. https://doi.org/10.2147/IJWH.S48179.
7. THISDAY NEWSPAPER (July 27, 2017). Adewole: Nigeria to Achieve Below 100 Maternal Mortality Ratio by 2030. Available at: https://www.thisdaylive.com/index.php/2017/07/27/adewole-nigeria-to-achieve-below-100-maternal-mortality-ratio-by-2030/ (Assessed 5/9/2017).
8. Abdul'Aziz, I. (2013). Maternal Mortality: Adamawa, Kebbi Get 30 Million Euro Grant. Available at: https://newsdiaryonline.com/maternal-mortality-adamawa-kebbi-get-30-million-euro-grant/. Accessed 5 Sept 2017.

9. Alabi O, Doctor HV. The potential role of a health and demographic surveillance system in rural northern Nigeria to reduce maternal and child deaths. Health. 2015;7:1741–6. https://doi.org/10.4236/health.2015.712189.
10. Graham W, Brass W, Snow RW. Estimating maternal mortality: the sisterhood method. Stud Fam Plann. 1989;20(3):125–35.
11. Abubakar, IS, Zoakah, AI, Daru, HS and Pam, IC. Estimating maternal mortality rate using sisterhood methods in plateau state Nigeria. Highland Med Res J, (2003) Vol1 (4), 28–34. Available at: https://doi.org/10.4314/hmrj.v1i4.33820 (Assessed 6/7/2016).
12. Idris H, Tyoden C, Ejembi C, Taylor K. Estimation of Maternal Mortality using the Indirect Sisterhood Method in Three Communities in Kaduna State, Northern Nigeria. Afr. J. Reprod Health. 2010;14(3):77–81.
13. Bankole A, Adewole IF, Hussain R, Awolude O, Singh S, Akinyemi JO. The incidence of abortion in Nigeria. Int Perspect Sex Reprod Health. 2015;41(4): 170–81. https://doi.org/10.1363/4117015.
14. Sharma V, Brown W, Kanuwa MA, Leight J, Nyqvist MB. High maternal mortality in Jigawa state, northern Nigeria estimated using the sisterhood method. BMC Pregnancy Childbirth. 2017;17:163. https://doi.org/10.1186/s12884-017-1341-5.
15. Mberu BU, Reed HE. Understanding subgroup fertility differentials in Nigeria. Popul Rev. 2014;53(2):23–46. https://doi.org/10.1353/prv.2014.0006.
16. Solanke BL. Marriage age, fertility behaviour, and women empowerment in Nigeria. SAGE Open. 5(4) 2158244015617989.

17

Unpredictability dictates quality of maternal and newborn care provision in rural Tanzania - A qualitative study of health workers' perspectives

Ulrika Baker[1,2*], Farida Hassan[3], Claudia Hanson[1,4], Fatuma Manzi[3], Tanya Marchant[4], Stefan Swartling Peterson[1,5,6] and Ingrid Hylander[2]

Abstract

Background: Health workers are the key to realising the potential of improved quality of care for mothers and newborns in the weak health systems of Sub Saharan Africa. Their perspectives are fundamental to understand the effectiveness of existing improvement programs and to identify ways to strengthen future initiatives. The objective of this study was therefore to examine health worker perspectives of the conditions for maternal and newborn care provision and their perceptions of what constitutes good quality of care in rural Tanzanian health facilities.

Methods: In February 2014, we conducted 17 in-depth interviews with different cadres of health workers providing maternal and newborn care in 14 rural health facilities in Tandahimba district, south-eastern Tanzania. These facilities included one district hospital, three health centres and ten dispensaries. Interviews were conducted in Swahili, transcribed verbatim and translated into English. A grounded theory approach was used to guide the analysis, the output of which was one core category, four main categories and several sub-categories.

Results: 'It is like rain' was identified as the core category, delineating unpredictability as the common denominator for all aspects of maternal and newborn care provision. It implies that conditions such as mothers' access to and utilisation of health care are unreliable; that availability of resources is uncertain and that health workers have to help and try to balance the situation. Quality of care was perceived to vary as a consequence of these conditions. Health workers stressed the importance of predictability, of 'things going as intended', as a sign of good quality care.

Conclusions: Unpredictability emerged as a fundamental condition for maternal and newborn care provision, an important determinant and characteristic of quality in this study. We believe that this finding is also relevant for other areas of care in the same setting and may be an important defining factor of a weak health system. Increasing predictability within health services, and focusing on the experience of health workers within these, should be prioritised in order to achieve better quality of care for mothers and newborns.

Keywords: Maternal and newborn health, Health workers, District health services, Quality of care, Sub Saharan Africa, Grounded theory

* Correspondence: ulrika.baker@ki.se
[1]Department of Public Health sciences, Global health - Health Systems and Policy Research, Widerströmska huset, Karolinska Institutet, Tomtebodavägen 18 A, 171 77 Stockholm, Sweden
[2]Department of Neurobiology, Care Sciences and Society, Division of Family Medicine, Karolinska Institutet, Nobels allé 12, 141 83 Huddinge, Sweden
Full list of author information is available at the end of the article

Background

In rural Tanzania, mothers' utilisation of health care during pregnancy and childbirth is increasing [1–4]. This implies a huge potential to reduce maternal and newborn deaths, but there is a significant 'quality gap' in the services provided [5, 6]. While contact coverage of health services is high, effective coverage of the same is low with a small proportion of mothers and newborns receiving those key medical interventions that can prevent or treat complications [1, 7]. This is mirrored in estimates that as many as 83% of all maternal deaths globally could be averted by 2020 through improving quality of care in health facilities alone, without any further increases in institutional delivery [8].

Health workers are the key to realising this potential to increased survival. Without them, mothers and newborns will not receive the care they need [9, 10]. Poor readiness of health facilities in terms of lack of drugs and equipment [11] together with a critical shortage of health workers [12], especially in rural areas, is repeatedly mentioned as causing bottlenecks in health service delivery [13]. Many health workers are also inadequately trained, subject to erratic supervision and work in isolated settings [12]; insufficiently supported for the tasks at hand.

In the face of these challenges, several programs have focused on enhancing the performance of health workers in order to improve quality of care in Tanzania and other low-income settings. These include e.g. Pay-for-Performance (P4P) schemes [14], Standards-Based Management and Recognition (SBM-R) [15], Computer-based Decision Support Systems (CDSSs) [16], the 5-S-approach [17] and collaborative quality improvement using Plan-Do-Study-Act (PDSA) cycles [18]. The theory underpinning these programs is that notwithstanding the challenges of providing care in the context of an under-resourced health system, quality can be improved.

Health workers constitute the core of these programs; both as targets for and implementers of program activities. To understand why and how these programs work, it is therefore vital to investigate the conditions for care provision from a health worker perspective and also, how health workers themselves perceive good quality of care. A few studies have explored health worker motivation and perceptions of working conditions in rural Tanzania [19–22]. Assessments of quality have largely however been analysed from a user perspective, e.g. through exit-interviews on satisfaction [23, 24], or from assessments of health service readiness, e.g. through measuring signal functions for obstetric and newborn care [25, 26].

Our objective was therefore to examine health worker perspectives of the conditions for maternal and newborn care provision and their perceptions of what constitutes good quality of care in rural Tanzanian health facilities.

Methods

Study design

This was a qualitative study using a grounded theory approach to guide the analysis [27], based on 17 in-depth interviews with health workers in Tandahimba district, Mtwara region, south-eastern Tanzania. It was nested within a district-wide quality improvement project, called EQUIP (Expanded Quality Management Using Information Power) [28].

Setting

Tandahimba district is located on the Makonde plateau in rural southern Tanzania, close to the border of Mozambique. The population of about 200,000 people is predominantly subsistence farmers but also engage in cashew nut farming. The road network within the district becomes muddy during the rainy season, making emergency transport difficult.

The district has 32 health facilities providing maternal and child care, all government apart from one faith-based. The district hospital provides comprehensive Emergency Obstetric and Neonatal Care (EmONC) [25] as well as regular childbirth care. The three health centres are supposed to manage basic EmONC and efforts are underway to upgrade their services to include caesarean sections [29]. In reality however, the functions required to provide even basic EmONC are rarely fulfilled, especially in terms of assisted delivery and provision of Magnesium sulphate for eclampsia. The 28 dispensaries provide childbirth care according to their abilities including the administration of Oxytocin when available, both to prevent and manage postpartum haemorrhage. Capacity to provide neonatal resuscitation has recently increased in all facilities through provision of equipment and targeted training [28].

There is a severe shortage of health workers with 52% of clinical posts vacant in the district [29]. Lower cadre health workers, such as medical attendants, often have to take on the responsibilities of higher cadre health workers such as nurses and midwives; an example being to assist women during childbirth (Additional file 1) [29].

Utilisation of health care during pregnancy is high with all mothers attending Antenatal care (ANC) at least once during pregnancy, although only 47% attend at least four times [1, 2]. The proportion of mothers giving birth in health facilities has increased substantially in recent years and was estimated as high as 87% (CI 95%: 77–93) in 2014 [28]. The maternal mortality ratio however remains high at 579 deaths/100,000 live births in the Mtwara region, which is higher than the national MMR average of 432 [30]. Neonatal mortality in was estimated at around 31 per 1000 in 2013 [2].

Data collection

Interviews with an open sample of 17 health workers providing maternal and newborn care were conducted in 14 health facilities between the 4th and 14th of February, 2014 (Table 1). Respondents were selected purposively, to represent different cadres of health workers and levels of health facilities, with the aim to achieve variation in the data (Table 1).

Permission to conduct the interviews was obtained from the District Medical Officer in Tandahimba district. Respondents were contacted in advance, by telephone where possible, else by going to see them in the health facility. They were asked if they would be willing to participate and when a suitable time for the interview would be. At the time of the interview, informed written consent was then sought from all respondents. An information sheet about the study was provided and read out by one of the interviewers. Respondents were informed that they could refuse to participate, withdraw or stop the interview without having to state any reason and without any consequences. All respondents chose to participate. Interviews were held in a private area of the health facility. Only the respondent and interviewers were present. Interruptions to allow respondents to attend to their patients were made and for this reason, some interviews took place over the course of a few hours. The median effective interview time was 1 h 12 min (range 1 h 3 min to max 2 h 7 min).

Interviews were co-conducted in Swahili by the first (UB) and second (FH) authors. UB is a Swedish medical doctor with 2 years' experience of working as a clinician and program manager in rural Tanzania. FH is a Tanzanian social scientist with experience from several qualitative studies in southern Tanzania. Both are fluent Swahili-speakers and minimal translation into English by FH to UB was done during the interviews. Neither UB nor FH were known to the respondents beforehand. The interview guide was semi-structured and developed in collaboration between all authors of the study. It was adapted after the first interviews as some questions did not yield sufficient response and to reflect new ideas emerging during the data collection (see Additional file 2). While the number of interviews was pre-determined, it was felt that saturation in the interview material was reached before the last few interviews were conducted as no or little new information emerged. No repeat interviews with respondents were done.

Interviews were audio recorded and transcribed verbatim. Subsequent translation into English was conducted with careful attention to quality to ensure preservation of the original meaning. Extensive field-notes were taken during and at the end of each interview. Transcripts were not shared with respondents.

Table 1 Characteristics of health workers interviewed

Cadre of health worker	Interviewed total	Hospital	Health centre	Dispensary
Medical attendant	3		1	2
Nurse/midwife	9	2	3	4
Clinical Officer	4			4
Assistant Medical Officer	1	1		
TOTAL	17	3	4	10

Data analysis

Data analysis was conducted using Microsoft Word 2010. It was led by the first author, UB, with frequent and substantial input by the senior author, IH. A grounded theory approach was used for the analysis, the end result of which was a core category [27]. Transcripts and field-notes were initially read and re-read to capture the whole. Transcripts were initially coded inductively, using so called open coding close to the text to capture 'what was going on' [31]. Similar codes were categorised into higher order categories. After analysing half of the transcripts, a code list was prepared to harmonise emergent codes and categories, agreed upon through discussions between UB and IH. Subsequent transcripts were coded applying these new codes and categories where possible, using focused coding. Theoretical coding was applied early on using the conditional matrix by Corbin and Strauss [31], focusing on the conditions in which health workers provide care and the consequences these have for care provision. As the analysis progressed, theoretical coding continued using the concepts of mothers' utilisation of care, the availability of resources in health facilities and the actions taken by health workers, i.e. clinical practice, as it became apparent that the data fitted well into these categories. Main categories contained health worker perceptions of the conditions for care provision and their perspectives of what constitutes good quality care. All main categories were linked to the core category. As the core category emerged, interviews were also reread to find more examples of the core category and to saturate the description of the links between the core category and the main categories. Results were not checked by the respondents.

Results

The result of our analysis is a model (Fig. 1) illustrating the core category 'It is like rain' with its four main categories: 'Uncertain availability of resources', 'Unreliable utilisation of care (mothers)', 'Health workers have to help' and 'Unpredictable outcomes of care'. Each main category contains two sub-categories, one of which contains conditions that challenge care provision or perceptions of poor quality care. The other sub-category contains enabling conditions for care provision or

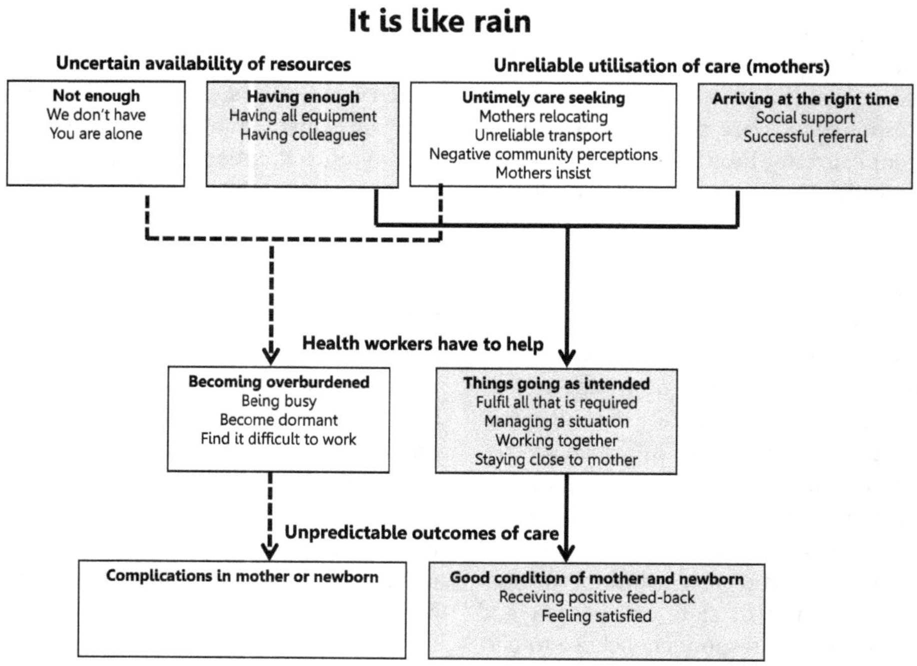

Fig. 1 Results framework. 'It is like rain' is the core category. The four main categories are outlined in bold with sub-categories contained within the boxes below. Sub-categories in *white* boxes are the ones perceived to challenge quality of care while those in *grey* boxes are perceived to represent conditions for or signs of good quality care. Codes within sub-categories, where applicable, are listed within the boxes. Arrows between boxes illustrate relationships between categories: dashed lines emanate from *white* boxes and full lines from grey

perceptions of good quality of care. The results follow the flow in Fig. 1 and are outlined in detail below.

It is like rain

The notion of uncertainty, represented by the expression 'it is like rain', was identified as the core category. Its essence is the inherent unpredictability of the conditions underlying maternal and newborn care provision, as experienced by health workers. One cannot be certain that mothers will come at the right time or that transport will be available. One cannot depend on a regular supply of sufficient drugs or functioning equipment. Colleagues may or may not be available to help manage an unforeseeable work load or a difficult case.

'It is like rain' also represents a sense of being out of control; that circumstances are dictated from higher levels of the system while as a health worker, one is left with no choice but to handle the situation on the ground. It is closely linked to how health workers identify good quality of care. When things go as intended, when circumstances are predictable and the system reliable, care provision is more likely perceived to be successful.

Unreliable utilisation of care (mothers)

Mothers' utilisation of health services is determined by their access to those services, and is a prerequisite for the provision of timely and appropriate care. Health workers perceived mothers' utilisation of care as unreliable and determined by factors largely outside their control. Untimely care seeking practices were perceived to affect care provision negatively, while mothers 'arriving at the right time' was experienced as an important factor for good quality care provision.

Untimely care seeking

Mothers relocating

Around the time of delivery, some mothers would move to stay close to their parents. Many families would also relocate during the farming season, causing mothers not to be able to visit their usual health facility. This was perceived to disrupt continuity of care and result in an unpredictable work load.

> *[...] sometimes people are many because there are people coming here for farming activities, so you may get even ten people for Mtwara [...]* (Health worker I5)

Unreliable transport

Unreliable transport for referral was indicated as the biggest problem for care provision by several health workers. While there was one district ambulance and a few tricycles with side-cars for transporting mothers, these could not be used consistently due to other engagements, unreliable fuel supply, punctures or absence of a driver. Moreover, drivers would sometimes be reluctant to transport a mother who was in a critical condition.

> *I was in the health facility where the driver came and he was shocked with the blood all over the place [...] We asked him to take the patient to the hospital but he refused [...] he was afraid to take her.* (Health worker I5)

Negative community perceptions

Community perceptions were perceived to influence mothers' utilisation of care. Commonly held beliefs about when to seek health care, reliance on traditional healers, and negative attitudes towards health workers and health facilities were mentioned as negative influences.

> *They see us as people who are there to provide bad service to them [...]. They don't perceive the hospital to be a friendly place.* (Health worker I16)

Mothers insist

Mothers at high risk of developing complications would be advised to go straight to hospital at the time of delivery. Those who had given birth many times before would however often insist on delivering in the dispensary anyway.

> *You can find that many don't follow what we say.* (Health worker I11)

Health workers similarly perceived that it was difficult to motivate mothers who felt healthy to attend all scheduled postpartum and postnatal care visits.

> *We normally advise mothers to come to postnatal care for examination. That's where we get problems: if a woman thinks she is ok, she doesn't come.* (Health worker I15)

Although many mothers would attend antenatal care and arrive in time to deliver in the health facility, some would leave before they had received appropriate care such as being tested in ANC. It was common that mothers asked to leave before having been observed for the required 48 h postpartum.

> *They [mothers] often stay for 24 h only [...]. They are the ones who are asking to leave; they say that they don't have money.* (Health worker I8)

Arriving at the right time

Health workers described mothers' timely arrival at a health facility as key for adequate management of labour and delivery. When mothers arrived in time, health workers were satisfied.

> *Most of them come when the labour pain starts, [...], so it is just a reasonable time* (Health worker I13)

Social support

Mothers would usually arrive with one or more members of their family which health workers viewed positively and essential in case of an emergency. Increasingly, mothers were accompanied by their husbands. This was experienced as a positive development and in contrast with traditional values, where men didn't see it as their role to be involved during pregnancy and childbirth.

> *[...] The fathers [before] had the mentality that once they have impregnated a woman then it is the woman's responsibility to care for the pregnancy, [...] his job is done.* (Health worker I4)

Successful referral

Successful referral of mothers and newborns to the district hospital mirrored the concern for transport availability and was perceived as an important aspect of good quality care. Several health workers described situations when they had phoned for help and the district vehicle had been able to come or alternative transport had been organised.

> *Good luck, we managed to refer the baby [with asphyxia]. [...] we succeeded to do that.* (Health worker I13)

Uncertain availability of resources

Health facilities' availability of material and human resources determines their capacity to provide care. This was experienced as uncertain by health workers; of frequently not having essential drugs and equipment available and of often being alone. The perceptions of quality mirrored this uncertainty.

Not enough

We don't have

In many health facilities, essential equipment and infrastructure was either not available, not in working order or not enough for the needs of the facility. This was often mentioned as the biggest challenge in providing maternal and newborn care.

> *[...] you were eager to provide a good service as it is supposed to be, but you failed because of tools. [...] so we are working in a very difficult environment.* (Health worker I17)

Like now, we have patients who just delivered. If another patient comes, she will not have a place to sleep [because we only have one bed]. (Health worker I2)

Health workers expressed placing orders of drugs and equipment according to their needs but often receiving an insufficient amount. While lower level health facilities relied on the hospital to have drugs in stock, this wasn't always the case.

They [at the lower level health facility] don't have Oxytocin and therefore decided to send her [to the hospital] but when she arrived there, there was also no Oxytocin – you can imagine how it is confused! (Health worker I7)

You are alone

Being alone was expressed as a critical determinant of health workers' capacity to provide care. This included a lack of colleagues, not having adequate knowledge and not being able to influence one's working conditions.

Some health workers described working alone as a punishment and expressed the lack of colleagues as influencing their clinical practice negatively. Insufficient knowledge to provide specific aspects of care was experienced by some health workers, e.g. how to monitor labour using a Partograph, deciding what pain relief to administer postpartum or how to administer magnesium sulphate for pre-eclampsia.

I am always alone here [in the health facility] and they [the district health management] are aware of this situation. I went to ask the nursing officer that did you locate me here as a punishment or what? Eeh it is just like a punishment. (Heath worker I5)

Health workers experienced inaction from higher levels of the health system when voicing deficiencies in infrastructure, requesting equipment or claiming allowances for working out of hours. This created a sense of not being seen, of being on your own.

For the problem of supplies, truly we have been requesting Tandahimba [the district health management]. [...] we only see that they don't respond. (Health worker I5)

Having enough

Having all equipment

Having all drugs and equipment was perceived as fundamental to be able to provide good quality care. This was also consistently mentioned as key to improve health services for mothers and newborns.

Sometimes you have all equipment and necessary things, so you provide good services. (Health worker I16)

Having colleagues

Having colleagues to consult or to assist in difficult situations was perceived as important. Sharing tasks was perceived to improve services and to promote provision of good quality care.

Health workers have to help

Mothers' unpredictable utilisation of health services along with the uncertain availability of resources affects care provision. Health workers expressed having to help regardless of whether these essential elements were fulfilled and trying to balance resources to continue to provide care.

I am medical attendant, but because of the problem [shortage of staff], I am also doing deliveries. I can't tell a patient that the midwife is not around so it is impossible. I must receive the patient. (Health worker I14)

[...] we were trying to balance the situation [of lack of Oxytocin] that you can provide [Oxytocin] to one [mother] whom you think is in need and monitor others. (Health worker I4)

Having to help and balance would sometimes lead to health workers becoming overburdened, but sometimes, of things going as intended.

Becoming overburdened

Health workers frequently felt overburdened and found it hard to manage due to the lack of resources and colleagues. This was experienced as affecting their performance negatively.

Being busy

Being the sole provider of maternal and newborn care in a health facility sometimes resulted in competing demands. This was perceived to result in untimely delivery of care.

You cannot serve [mothers] in time if you are just alone [...] (Health worker I9)

Become dormant

Health workers who bore the sole responsibility for maternal and newborn care in a facility described never being able to rest; having to be prepared to work whenever a mother needed assistance, to remain in the facility at night and not being able to fulfil family commitments.

I was alone in the facility [...] for a year and a half. [...] I didn't have Saturdays, Sundays, even holidays. Except for the week-ends if there was no patient, I would rest. (Health worker I6)

Being alone in a work place was also perceived to influence clinical practice negatively in terms of not having somebody to discuss with.

[In a previous workplace] we were able to share ideas and discuss how to do things, but if you are here alone, you become dormant. (Health worker I5)

Finding it difficult to work

Trying to balance care provision by compromising certain aspects of care was often done, e.g. in terms of maintaining adequate hygiene in the health facility. This was sometimes experienced as a threat to one's own health and while compromises in care provision would be found, these were sometimes experienced as upsetting.

To sterilise [when chlorine is not available], after delivery you just wash with normal water then you boil them [equipment]. I'm not accepting this method, but it is our circumstance. What will we do? I don't accept it at all. (Health worker I13)

Things going as intended

When care provision was predictable, when things were going as intended, health workers felt that good quality care could be provided.

If you attend a woman according to your estimation, you feel happy and proud. (Health worker I7)

Fulfilling all that is required

To be able to provide all the services that a mother is supposed to receive was expressed as a sign of good quality.

The things I was supposed to provide to the mother who was delivered, I provided [...]. That is why I feel that I have performed well. (Health worker I10)

Managing a situation

Even when complications occurred, health workers expressed satisfaction when they had managed to solve the problem and provide care despite the difficult situation.

[...] So we had to stitch that tear. She was also bleeding a bit; we had to give her normal saline. Now she is a bit better, she says she is fine. [...] So I am very happy my patient has improved. (Health worker I3)

Working together

Working together was mentioned as a sign of good clinical practice and health workers described critical situations where they would leave other duties to help each other.

All together when an expectant mother emerges, nobody isolates herself. All together we stop other duties to concentrate on that case until we make sure that the case has been properly attended. (Health worker I11)

Staying close to mother

Health workers expressed staying close to a mother as a sign of quality; physically, to be able to monitor and follow-up, but also emotionally in terms of being kind and respectful. Health workers sometimes accompanied a referred mother to the hospital, or went there afterwards for information about her outcome.

I mean after delivery, she was bleeding excessively and she was getting weaker. Therefore I took her with me, because her spouse had a car so we left together to Tandahimba. I dealt with her until blood transfusion started; that is when I left. (Health worker I4)

Unpredictable outcomes of care

Health workers described varying outcomes of care. Some had experienced situations when a mother or newborn had developed serious complications and even died. More frequent were the examples of normal deliveries, free of complications.

Complications in mother or newborn

Complications such as severe illness or death of a mother or newborn were experienced as deeply upsetting.

I tried to wipe the baby but the baby didn't cry at all and then the baby died. Although the baby was abnormal I felt bad, because she [the mother] carried the baby for 9 months and she got nothing - I felt bad. (Health worker I6)

Health workers also described situations where a mother or newborn had suddenly deteriorated although at first everything had seemed fine. Assisting a mother or baby in such circumstances was experienced as stressful.

> *I was alone here when I attended her on delivery. The placenta came out well but suddenly she started bleeding severely. After providing the medicine to control bleeding, I struggled to call them [the district ambulance].* (Health worker I14)

> *After severe bleeding, she became unconscious and I decided to put a drip. [...] To be honest, I trembled. I was worried, but through experience I put a drip and it was successful.* (Health worker I6)

Good condition of mother and newborn

Observing a mother and baby to be in a good condition was mentioned as an important sign of having provided good quality care. An active and crying baby who managed to breastfeed was especially appreciated.

> *What made me think I had provided good service is the safety of both the baby and its mother; they left this place in a good condition.* (Health worker I11)

Receiving positive feed-back

Positive feed-back, from mothers, the community or colleagues, was also described as a way of knowing that the services provided had been of good quality. Mothers expressing gratitude was commonly expressed as a sign of quality.

> *It is quite certain that when somebody appreciates my service by saying thank you, she only says so when she is satisfied or by asking me when she has to return or when she comes back again whenever she gets problems.* (Health worker I9)

Another sign perceived to indicate that quality of care was provided in a facility was that mothers would come to deliver from villages outside the immediate catchment area.

Feeling satisfied

A feeling of having done one's best, of personal satisfaction, was repeatedly expressed as an indicator of having provided good quality care.

> *I am satisfied with the service I provided because I had all equipment. [...] The good thing was that gloves, Oxytocin and syringes were available so I used them.* (Health worker I5)

Discussion

Unpredictability was found to be the common denominator for all aspects of maternal and newborn care provision as experienced by health workers. 'It is like rain' implies irregular conditions, outside of health workers' control, including mothers' access to and utilisation of care, the availability of drugs and equipment and the presence of colleagues in the health facility. This unpredictability does not however imply that care provision is perceived to be of consistently poor quality. Rather, quality of care fluctuates as health workers try to balance available resources with their feelings of being overburdened and their desire for things to go as intended with the outcome being a good condition of mother and newborn, perceived as a sign of good quality care.

The main categories of our findings reflect different aspects of unpredictability. Mothers' relocating around the time of birth was perceived as one reason for their unreliable access to care. It has previously been associated with low levels of institutional delivery in nomadic pastoralist populations in northern Tanzania [32] but not been explored in other settings. Interestingly, it was perceived to affect both mothers' ability to seek care and cause an unpredictable work load for health workers.

The uncertain availability of transport, especially in the case of referral, was frequently described as limiting access to care. A recent study from southern Tanzania found that maternal mortality from direct obstetric causes, such as haemorrhage and eclampsia, was nearly four times higher in women living far away from a hospital [33], reinforcing the importance of a reliable referral transport service. Successful referral was equally described as an important aspect of quality care by many health workers.

Tensions between mothers' and health workers' assessment of risk were perceived to result in unpredictable care utilisation. This was true especially for multiparous women who were more likely to insist to deliver at home or to deliver in a dispensary rather than the hospital. Similar findings were reported from the same area of Tanzania in a study from the year 2000 [34] and also from western Tanzania, where multiparous women were 30% less likely to deliver in a health facility than nulliparous women [35]. The opposite has been shown for women in their first pregnancy or for women with previous Caesarean sections [36].

Health workers put much emphasis on the uncertain availability of resources and its consequences for care delivery, mirroring findings from a recent study of health service bottlenecks in Tandahimba district [1]. The unreliability of drugs and medical supplies for maternal care has also been observed in other studies from Tanzania as well as Uganda [13, 20].

Health workers expressed feeling alone in the midst of these unpredictable conditions; of not being able to affect much of what determines their ability to provide care. Previous studies from Tanzania have shown similar results, of health workers feeling abandoned and unsupported by the system [21, 37]. Being forced to balance the uncertain availability of resources and mothers' unpredictable utilisation of health services; often having to help with the knowledge that they weren't equipped to do so, was expressed by many health workers. This was perceived as demotivating; also corroborating other study findings from the same area of Tanzania [22, 37]. At the same time, managing a difficult situation was experienced as satisfying and expressed as a sign of quality.

These results resonate with research on the "demand-control" model, originally developed by Karasek and Theorell [38]. This model pose that high demands in combination with feeling a lack of control are the most important stressors in the work environment, but that these can be compensated through support from supervisors and co-workers [38, 39]. Similarly, a recent study showed that high job strain and few days off was related to depressive symptoms and burnout but that support from co-workers had a buffering effect [40]. In our study, the core category 'it is like rain' clearly describes the out of control aspect and health workers expressed having to help regardless of their capacity to do so. Similarly, the importance of colleagues was emphasised.

Overall, health workers' perceptions of quality spanned the three dimensions of good quality care as being effective, safe and a good experience for the patient [41]. To 'fulfil all that is required', to observe a 'good condition of mother and newborn' and 'feeling satisfied' can all be seen as health worker perceptions of effective care. Safe care was expressed as 'managing a situation' and 'working together'. 'Staying close to mother' can be interpreted as an expression of safety, to monitor closely; and also of health workers understanding the importance of the mother's experience. 'Receiving positive feed-back' was expressed as important and reliable indication that a mother was satisfied with the health services.

Policy implications

Our findings are a reminder that without appropriate support for health workers; such as a reliable supply of drugs, functioning equipment, colleagues to share the work with and regular supportive supervision from the district or higher level health facilities; little can be achieved in terms of improving quality of care for mothers and newborns. This goes back to the quality ethos for family planning services: "clients' rights and providers' needs" [42].

Our findings also point to a need to consider the influences that programs aimed at improving care may have on unpredictability within health services, whether positive or negative. Adding predictability to the dimensions of quality of care and to include this in processes of planning, improving and evaluating health programs could be a way forward. Acknowledging predictability as an important outcome in its own right could help to refocus improvement initiatives around those changes that can be supported reliably and sustained over time. Centralisation of obstetric care, although controversial in terms of its negative impact on access, is likely to have a positive impact on predictability and has been suggested as one way to improve quality of maternal and newborn care in low-income settings [5]. Another example would be to draw fewer conclusions from cross-sectional assessments of health facility readiness and more from fluctuations in the availability of resources over time; recognising that this approach would demand concurrent strengthening of HMIS data and increased funding or redesign of standard approaches to enable repeat surveys. Incorporating alternative options and contingency plans for when conditions for care provision change could be important when creating strategies and guidelines for the implementation of health programs.

Methodological considerations

This study included health workers of different cadres from a large proportion of facilities within Tandahimba district and as such achieved good variation in the data. Interviews were co-conducted by a social scientist and a physician, both with experience of working in rural Tanzania, allowing for complementary perspectives.

One limitation of our study was that theoretical sampling according to grounded theory methodology wasn't conducted. However, the first open sample yielded answers to several of the questions that were raised during the analyses. Also, interview questions were revised based on preliminary analyses of the first interviews and the coding followed grounded theory praxis.

Another consideration is the extent to which health workers felt able to share their full experiences with the interviewers. Health workers rarely expressed that they had ever provided sub-optimal care, despite their detailed descriptions of the unpredictable and often challenging conditions for care provision. This finding may be due to social desirability bias, of health workers wanting to make a good impression.

Conclusions

In the context of weak health systems, improving quality of care is challenging and cannot be done without the engagement of health workers. For health programs to be effective, they need to tackle the inherent unpredictability dictating both conditions for and quality of care provision. We argue that unpredictability may indeed be an important definer of a weak health system and that this finding can be extended beyond maternal and newborn care. Increasing predictability within health services, and focusing on the experience of health workers within these, should be prioritised in order to achieve better quality of care for mothers and newborns.

Abbreviations

ANC: Antenatal care; CDSS: Computer based decision support system; EmONC: Emergency obstetric and newborn care; EQUIP: Expanded Quality management using information power; PDSA: Plan-Do-Study-Act; QI: Quality improvement; SBM-R: Standard based management and recognition

Acknowledgements

We would like to thank all the health workers who shared their time with us during this study. We also extend our gratitude to the District Medical Officer in Tandahimba District who gave the study his support and who facilitated communication with the health facilities.

Funding

The study was funded by the European Union Seventh Framework Programme (FP7/2007–2013) under grant agreement no. 265827. Ulrika Baker also received funding for her salary from Karolinska Institutet and Stockholm County Council, Sweden. The funders had no role in the development or implementation of the study.

Authors' contributions

UB led the study including development of the interview guide, analysis of transcripts and writing of the manuscript. She also acted as a co-interviewer. FH contributed to the development of the interview guide, acted as a lead interviewer, transcribed interviews, participated in translation and contributed to analysis. CH contributed to the development of the interview guide, interpretation of results and writing of the discussion. FM facilitated the data collection and helped to interpret results. TM helped to revise the results frame work, interpret results and contributed to the writing of the manuscript. SP contributed to the development of the study and interpretation of results. IH led the development of the interview guide and analysis of transcripts and development of the results framework together with UB. She also made substantial contributions to all parts of the manuscripts. All authors reviewed and approved the final version of the manuscript before submission.

Competing interests

The authors declare that they have no competing interests.

Author details

[1]Department of Public Health sciences, Global health - Health Systems and Policy Research, Widerströmska huset, Karolinska Institutet, Tomtebodavägen 18 A, 171 77 Stockholm, Sweden. [2]Department of Neurobiology, Care Sciences and Society, Division of Family Medicine, Karolinska Institutet, Nobels allé 12, 141 83 Huddinge, Sweden. [3]Ifakara Health Institute, Plot 463 Kiko Avenue, Mikocheni, Dar es Salaam, P.O. Box 78 373, Tanzania. [4]Department for Disease Control, London School of Hygiene and Tropical Medicine (LSHTM), Keppel Street, London WC1E 7HT, UK. [5]International Maternal and Child Health, Uppsala University, Drottninggatan 4, 751 85 Uppsala, Sweden. [6]Makerere School of Public Health, Kampala, Uganda.

References

1. Baker U, Peterson S, Marchant T, Mbaruku G, Temu S, Manzi F, Hanson C. Identifying implementation bottlenecks for maternal and newborn health interventions in rural districts of the United Republic of Tanzania. Bull World Health Organ. 2015;93(6):380–9.
2. Hanson C, Manzi F, Mkumbo E, Shirima K, Penfold S, Hill Z, Shamba D, Jaribu J, Hamisi Y, Soremekun S, et al. Effectiveness of a Home-Based Counselling Strategy on Neonatal Care and Survival: A Cluster-Randomised Trial in Six Districts of Rural Southern Tanzania. PLoS Med. 2015;12(9), e1001881.
3. Ministry of Health CD, Gender, Elderly and Children (MoHCDGEC), [Tanzania Mainland], Ministry of Health (MoH) [Zanzibar], National Bureau of Statistics (NBS), Office of the Chief Government Statistician (OCGS), and ICF International: Tanzania Demographic and Health Survey and Malaria Indicator Survey (TDHS-MIS) 2015–16. Key Indicators. In. Dar es Salaam, Tanzania, and Rockville, Maryland, USA; 2016.
4. Afnan-Holmes H, Magoma M, John T, Levira F, Msemo G, Armstrong CE, Martinez-Alvarez M, Kerber K, Kihinga C, Makuwani A, et al. Tanzania's countdown to 2015: an analysis of two decades of progress and gaps for reproductive, maternal, newborn, and child health, to inform priorities for post-2015. Lancet Global Health. 2015;3(7):e396–409.
5. Campbell OM, Calvert C, Testa A, Strehlow M, Benova L, Keyes E, Donnay F, Macleod D, Gabrysch S, Rong L, et al. The scale, scope, coverage, and capability of childbirth care. Lancet. 2016;388:2193–208.
6. Campbell OMR, Graham WJ. Maternal survival 2 - Strategies for reducing maternal mortality: getting on with what works. Lancet. 2006;368(9543): 1284–99.
7. World Health Organization, The Aga Khan University, and Partnership for Maternal, Newborn & Child Health. In: A Global Review of the Key Interventions Related to Reproductive, Maternal, Newborn and Child Health (RMNCH). 2011.
8. Bhutta ZA, Das JK, Bahl R, Lawn JE, Salam RA, Paul VK, Sankar MJ, Sankar JM, Blencowe H, Rizvi A, et al. Can available interventions end preventable deaths in mothers, newborn babies, and stillbirths, and at what cost? Lancet. 2014;384(9940):347–70.
9. Campbell J. The route to effective coverage is through the health worker: there are no shortcuts. Lancet. 2013;381:725.
10. World Health Organisation. Working together for health. Geneva: World Health Organisation; 2006.
11. Hanson C, Ronsmans C, Penfold S, Maokola W, Manzi F, Jaribu J, Mbaruku G, Mshinda H, Tanner M, Schellenberg J. Health system support for childbirth care in Southern Tanzania: results from a health facility census. BMC Res Notes. 2013;6(1):435.
12. Manzi F, Schellenberg JA, Hutton G, Wyss K, Mbuya C, Shirima K, Mshinda H, Tanner M, Schellenberg D. Human resources for health care delivery in Tanzania: a multifaceted problem. Hum Resour Health. 2012;10:3.
13. Baker U, Okuga M, Waiswa P, Manzi F, Peterson S, Hanson C. Bottlenecks in the implementation of essential screening tests in antenatal care: Syphilis, HIV, and anemia testing in rural Tanzania and Uganda. Int J Gynaecol Obstet. 2015;130(1):S43–50.
14. Binyaruka P, Patouillard E, Powell-Jackson T, Greco G, Maestad O, Borghi J. Effect of Paying for Performance on Utilisation, Quality, and User Costs of Health Services in Tanzania: A Controlled Before and After Study. PLoS ONE. 2015;10(8), e0135013.
15. Necochea E, Tripathi V, Kim YM, Akram N, Hyjazi Y, Da Luz VM, Otolorin E, Pleah T, Rashidi T, Bishanga D. Implementation of the Standards-Based Management and Recognition approach to quality improvement in maternal, newborn, and child health programs in low-resource countries. Int J Gynaecol Obstet. 2015;130 Suppl 2:S17–24.
16. Blank A, Prytherch H, Kaltschmidt J, Krings A, Sukums F, Mensah N, Zakane A, Loukanova S, Gustafsson LL, Sauerborn R, et al. "Quality of prenatal and maternal care: bridging the know-do gap" (QUALMAT study): an electronic clinical decision support system for rural Sub-Saharan Africa. BMC Med Inform Decis Mak. 2013;13:44.
17. Kanamori S, Sow S, Castro MC, Matsuno R, Tsuru A, Jimba M. Implementation of 5S management method for lean healthcare at a health center in Senegal: a qualitative study of staff perception. Glob Health Action. 2015;8:27256.
18. Hanson C, Waiswa P, Marchant T, Marx M, Manzi F, Mbaruku G, Rowe A, Tomson G, Schellenberg J, Peterson S, et al. Expanded Quality Management Using Information Power (EQUIP): protocol for a quasi-experimental study to improve maternal and newborn health in Tanzania and Uganda. Implement Sci. 2014;9(1):41.
19. Mbaruku GM, Larson E, Kimweri A, Kruk ME. What elements of the work environment are most responsible for health worker dissatisfaction in rural primary care clinics in Tanzania? Hum Resour Health. 2014;12:38.
20. Mkoka DA, Goicolea I, Kiwara A, Mwangu M, Hurtig AK. Availability of drugs and medical supplies for emergency obstetric care: experience of health facility managers in a rural District of Tanzania. BMC Pregnancy Childbirth. 2014;14:108.
21. Mkoka DA, Mahiti GR, Kiwara A, Mwangu M, Goicolea I, Hurtig AK. "Once the government employs you, it forgets you": Health workers' and managers' perspectives on factors influencing working conditions for provision of maternal health care services in a rural district of Tanzania. Hum Resour Health. 2015;13:77.

22. Penfold S, Shamba D, Hanson C, Jaribu J, Manzi F, Marchant T, Tanner M, Ramsey K, Schellenberg D, Schellenberg JA. Staff experiences of providing maternity services in rural southern Tanzania - a focus on equipment, drug and supply issues. BMC Health Serv Res. 2013;13:61.
23. Kujawski S, Mbaruku G, Freedman LP, Ramsey K, Moyo W, Kruk ME. Association Between Disrespect and Abuse During Childbirth and Women's Confidence in Health Facilities in Tanzania. Matern Child Health J. 2015; 19(10):2243–50.
24. Larson E, Hermosilla S, Kimweri A, Mbaruku GM, Kruk ME. Determinants of perceived quality of obstetric care in rural Tanzania: a cross-sectional study. BMC Health Serv Res. 2014;14:483.
25. Family Health I, Joseph LMSoPH, Unicef, United Nations Population F, World Health O. Monitoring emergency obstetric care: a handbook. Geneva: World Health Organization; 2009.
26. Gabrysch S, Civitelli G, Edmond KM, Mathai M, Ali M, Bhutta ZA, Campbell OMR. New Signal Functions to Measure the Ability of Health Facilities to Provide Routine and Emergency Newborn Care. PLoS Med. 2012;9(11), e1001340.
27. Charmaz K. Constructing grounded theory. 2nd ed. Thousand Oaks: Sage Publications; 2013.
28. Waiswa P, Manzi F, Mbaruku G, Rowe A, Marx M, Tomson G, Marchant T, Willey B, Schellenberg J, Peterson S, et al. A quasi-experimental study of the Expanded Quality Management Using Information Power (EQUIP) strategy to improve maternal and newborn health in Tanzania and Uganda. 2015.
29. Tandahimba-District-Council. Revised Comprehensive Council Health Plan For the Year 2011–2012. In: United Republic of Tanzania-Prime Minister's Office-Regional Administration and Local Government. Mtwara Region; 2011–2012. 2012.
30. National Bureau of Statistics MoF. Mortality and Health. Dar es Salaam: United Republic of Tanzania; 2015.
31. Corbin JM. Basics of qualitative research: techniques and procedures for developing grounded theory. 3rd ed. Los Angeles: Sage Publications, Inc; 2008.
32. Kruger C, Olsen OE, Mighay E, Ali M. Where do women give birth in rural Tanzania? Rural Remote Health. 2011;11(3):1791.
33. Hanson C, Cox J, Mbaruku G, Manzi F, Gabrysch S, Schellenberg D, Tanner M, Ronsmans C, Schellenberg J. Maternal mortality and distance to facility-based obstetric care in rural southern Tanzania: a secondary analysis of cross-sectional census data in 226 000 households. Lancet Global Health. 2015;3(7):e387–95.
34. Kowalewski M, Jahn A, Kimatta SS. Why do at-risk mothers fail to reach referral level? Barriers beyond distance and cost. Afr J Reprod Health. 2000; 4(1):100–9.
35. Ndao-Brumblay SK, Mbaruku G, Kruk ME. Parity and institutional delivery in rural Tanzania: a multilevel analysis and policy implications. Health Policy Plan. 2013;28(6):647–57.
36. Hanson C. The Epidemiology of Maternal Mortality inSouthern Tanzania. London: London School of Hygiene and Tropical Medicine; 2013.
37. Prytherch H, Kakoko DC, Leshabari MT, Sauerborn R, Marx M. Maternal and newborn healthcare providers in rural Tanzania: in-depth interviews exploring influences on motivation, performance and job satisfaction. Rural Remote Health. 2012;12:2072.
38. Muntaner C, Schoenbach C. Psychosocial work environment and health in U.S. metropolitan areas: a test of the demand-control and demand-control-support models. Int J Health Serv. 1994;24(2):337–53.
39. Saijo Y, Yoshioka E, Kawanishi Y, Nakagi Y, Itoh T, Yoshida T. Relationships of job demand, job control, and social support on intention to leave and depressive symptoms in Japanese nurses. Ind Health. 2015;54:32–41.
40. Saijo Y, Chiba S, Yoshioka E, Kawanishi Y, Nakagi Y, Itoh T, Sugioka Y, Kitaoka-Higashiguchi K, Yoshinda T. Effects of work burden, job strain and support on depressive symptoms and burnout among Japanese physicians. Int J Occup Med Environ Health. 2014;27(6):980–92.
41. Godlee F. Effective, safe, and a good patient experience. BMJ. 2009;339:4346.
42. Huezo C, Diaz S. Quality of care in family planning: clients' rights and providers' needs. Adv Contracept. 1993;9(2):129–39.

18

The influence of physical activity during pregnancy on maternal, fetal or infant heart rate variability

Pavel Dietz[1*], Estelle D. Watson[2], Matteo C. Sattler[1], Wolfgang Ruf[1], Sylvia Titze[1] and Mireille van Poppel[1,3]

Abstract

Background: Physical activity (PA) during pregnancy has been shown to be associated with several positive effects for mother, fetus, and offspring. Heart rate variability (HRV) is a noninvasive and surrogate marker to determine fetal overall health and the development of fetal autonomic nervous system. In addition, it has been shown to be significantly influenced by maternal behavior. However, the influence of maternal PA on HRV has not yet been systematically reviewed. Therefore, the aim of this systematic review was to assess the influence of regular maternal PA on maternal, fetal or infant HRV.

Methods: A systematic literature search following a priori formulated criteria of studies that examined the influence of regular maternal PA (assessed for a minimum period of 6 weeks) on maternal, fetal or infant HRV was performed in the databases Pubmed and SPORTDiscus. Quality of each study was assessed using the standardized Quality Assessment Tool for Quantitative Studies (QATQS).

Results: Nine articles were included into the present systematic review: two intervention studies, one prospective longitudinal study, and six post-hoc analysis of subsets of the longitudinal study. Of these articles four referred to maternal HRV, five to fetal HRV, and one to infant HRV. The overall global rating for the standardized quality assessment of the articles was moderate to weak. The articles regarding the influence of maternal PA on maternal HRV indicated contrary results. Five of five articles regarding the influence of maternal PA on fetal HRV showed increases of fetal HRV on most parameters depending on maternal PA. The article referring to infant HRV (measured one month postnatal) showed an increased HRV.

Conclusions: Based on the current evidence available, our overall conclusion is that the hypothesis that maternal PA influences maternal HRV cannot be supported, but there is a trend that maternal PA might increase fetal and infant HRV (clinical conclusion). Therefore, we recommend that further, high quality studies addressing the influence of maternal PA on HRV should be performed (methodological conclusion).

Keywords: Pregnancy, Public health, Heart rate variability, Childbirth, Stress, Offspring

Background

During pregnancy, maternal physiological systems progressively adapt to accommodate the increasing demands of fetal growth and development [1]. This includes an increase in cardiovascular and respiratory output, an increase in renal function as well as endocrine and metabolic changes [2–4]. Due to these changes, pregnancy is a 'stress test' for the metabolic and physiologic system of women, and can lead to pregnancy-induced complications and adverse health effects. Pregnancy associated conditions such as gestational diabetes, hypertension, mental disorders and maternal obesity have been shown to alter fetal development and increase the risk of diseases in the offspring and the infant's later life [5–8]. Furthermore, the risk for some of these maternal adverse health effects has been shown to be associated with increased sympathetic activity during gestation [9].

* Correspondence: pavel.dietz@uni-graz.at
[1]Department of Physical Activity and Public Health, Institute of Sports Science, University of Graz, Mozartgasse 14, Graz 8010, Austria
Full list of author information is available at the end of the article

One method to monitor sympathetic and parasympathetic control of the autonomic nervous system (ANS) is heart rate variability (HRV). It describes beat-to-beat variation in cardiac R-R interval. Analyzing these R-R intervals in different frequency and time domains provides information on whether changes in heart rate (HR) are mediated primarily by the sympathetic or parasympathetic arm of the ANS [10, 11]. In adults, increased HRV has been associated with higher aerobic fitness and may therefore lead to possible maternal health benefits [12]. Furthermore, several studies indicated that exercise has positive effects on HRV in both healthy adults and children [13, 14]. With regard to the influence of overweight and obesity (OaO) on HRV, increased BMI has been associated with reduced HRV and increased sympathetic and decreased parasympathetic activity [15–18]. Part of this might be due to reduced physical activity (PA) levels in people with higher BMI, since in OaO adults who were regularly physically active HRV was higher compared to sedentary peers [19].

In healthy pregnant women, sympathetic control also increases with progressing gestation as consequence of physiological adaptations of the maternal body, resulting in an altered HRV compared to healthy non-pregnant women [20]. In the growing fetus, HRV is used as a surrogate marker to determine the development of fetal ANS and overall fetal health [11, 21, 22]. However, fetal HRV is strongly influenced by maternal behavior (e.g. cigarette smoking and alcohol consumption) [23, 24].

Throughout pregnancy, regular PA, which is defined as 'any bodily movement produced by skeletal muscles that results in energy expenditure' [25], has been shown to improve maternal cardiovascular and respiratory output, improve insulin resistance and metabolic control, reduce the risk of gestational diabetes mellitus as well as depressive symptoms [26–31]. In non-pregnant women, adult men as well as in children, PA has further been shown to affect cardiovascular autonomic control and HRV [32–35].

Although HRV is a noninvasive method to monitor control of ANS of the mother as well as overall fetal development, the influence of maternal PA on HRV has not yet been systematically reviewed. Therefore, within the present article we systematically reviewed studies that assessed the influence of PA during pregnancy on maternal, fetal or infant HRV. Based on the review, a more definitive conclusion on the influence of maternal PA on maternal, fetal and infant HRV can be obtained. In addition, recommendations for future studies in this field will be formulated.

Methods

Literature search

A systematic literature search of studies that examined the influence of regular maternal PA on maternal, fetal or infant HRV was performed in the databases Pubmed and SPORTDiscus. Therefore, a search term was created that combines 'physical activity', 'pregnancy', and 'cardiovascular outcomes'. The final search term for Pubmed can be found in Appendix 1. For the search on SPORTDiscus, this search term was adapted following the SPORTDiscus search guidelines. Since the search term was very specific, no further limits were used to specify search. The search was completed on February 2nd 2016.

Inclusion criteria and selection process

In this systematic review, all studies had to fulfil the following inclusion criteria: (1) assessing the influence of PA during pregnancy on HRV in (a) mother, (b) fetus or (c) infant; (2) dealing with human subjects; (3) dealing with any kind of PA (e.g. aerobic exercise, resistance exercise, yoga, gymnastics, etc.); from a public health point of view, the effects of regular PA and not the effects of acute PA are of interest, consequently (4) PA levels should be assessed for a minimum period of 6 weeks; (5) abstracts had to be available in English, German or Dutch language; (6) only full papers published in peer-reviewed journals were considered. Since the aim of this systematic review is providing an overview of all studies assessing HRV dependent on PA in pregnancy, (7) all study designs were included (e.g. prospective studies, retrospective studies, intervention studies, observational studies etc.) in order to draw an overall conclusion.

Altogether, 124 articles were identified (Fig. 1). After removing three duplicates, 121 articles were screened by abstract and title for possible inclusion. Of these, 108 articles were excluded due to not passing all of the a priori formulated criteria. Finally, full texts of 13 articles were screened [34, 36–47]. Of these, 4 were excluded for specific reasons (Fig. 1) so that nine articles were included into the final systematic review.

Quality assessment and strength of evidence

For assessing the quality of the included articles, the standardized Quality Assessment Tool for Quantitative Studies (QATQS) [48], a well-established and validated tool for assessing the quality of studies in the field of public health research [49, 50], was used. It consists of six components: (1) the extent to which the participants are representative of the target population (selection bias), (2) study design, (3) control of confounding factors, (4) blinding of outcome assessors and participants, (5) reliability and validity of the data-collection tools, and (6) the number of and reasons for withdrawals and drop-outs. The component 'blinding of outcome assessors and participants' was considered not applicable for observational and intervention studies in this review. The reason for considering 'blinding' not applicable for intervention studies in this case is that in studies with

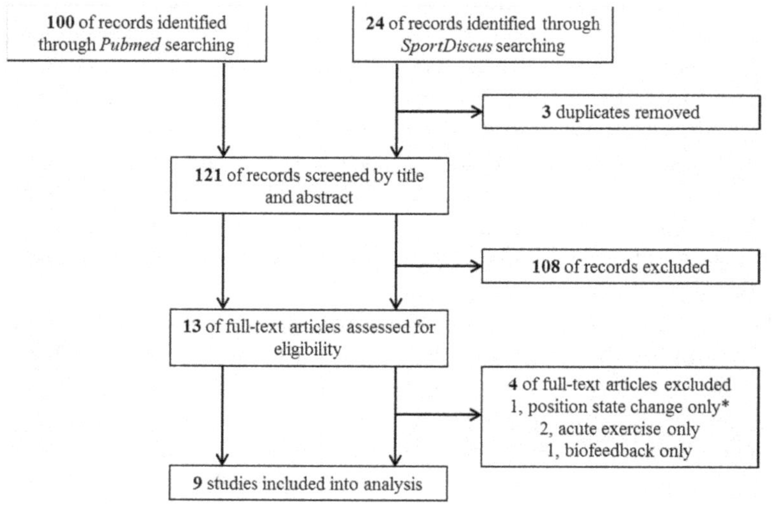

Fig. 1 Flow chart of the literature search. *'Position state change only' means that the only measured activity was the change from sitting to standing position

PA intervention the assessors (i.e. researchers) and the participants are very likely to know the outcome of the randomization [51]. According to standardized criteria, each component (1-6) of each article was rated as 'strong', 'moderate' or 'weak'. Finally, an overall rating was calculated on the basis of the individual ratings also following standardized criteria: the overall rating was 'strong', when there was no 'weak' component rating, 'moderate' when there was only one 'weak component rating, and 'weak' when there were two or more 'weak' component ratings. A detailed description of, as well as the criteria for, the six component ratings can be found online [48].

Data extraction

The systematic literature search using the above described search terms as well as the a priori formulated inclusion criteria has been performed by PD and was checked by a second researcher (ST). Of the nine included articles, all relevant data were extracted by PD following a commonly used table format including study design, sample and subjects, methods, outcomes, statistics. Extracted data were checked by two researchers (EW, MvP). Quality assessment for each study using the QATQS has been performed by two researchers independently (PD, MS). When researches came to different results, these points were discussed within the research team to come to a consensus.

Results

Study descriptions

Nine articles were included into the present systematic review of which three refer to maternal HRV, four to fetal HRV, one to both maternal and fetal HRV, and one to infant HRV. In summary, four articles provide results on maternal HRV, five on fetal HRV, and one on infant HRV. Of these, two articles were intervention studies [36, 43]. The intervention study performed by Stutzman et al. [43] assessed the effects of low intensity exercise in normal weight (NW) and overweight and obese (OaO) pregnant women on maternal HRV. The intervention study performed by Satyapriya et al. [36] assessed the effect of yoga specifically designed for the second and third trimester of pregnancy, compared to standard prenatal exercise (intensity not specified) on maternal HRV. One article was a prospective longitudinal study which was designed to determine the influence of self-reported maternal exercise on fetal cardiac ANS development [40]. To assess self-reported maternal exercise, the authors used the 'Modifiable Physical Activity Questionnaire' (MPAQ). Finally, the remaining six articles [37–39, 41, 42, 47] were post-hoc analyses of subsets of the before mentioned longitudinal study of May et al. [40]. Four of these post-hoc analyses referred to maternal or fetal HRV measurements performed in gestational week 36, one to maternal HRV measurements performed at 28, 32, and 36 weeks of gestation, and one to infant HRV measurements at one month of age. The different HRV parameters assessed in the nine studies as well as their physiological association are summarized and described in Table 1. The cohort and study characteristics are summarized in Table 2.

The HRV outcomes depending on PA of the two intervention studies from pre to post, the longitudinal study, as well as of the six post-hoc analyses are presented in Tables 3, 4, and 5. It has to be stressed that for the longitudinal study as well as for the six post-hoc analyses the MPAQ had been used to assess leisure-time PA (LTPA)

Table 1 HRV parameters and their physiological association

Parameter	Abbreviation	Physiological association
Time domain		
Standard deviation of NN intervals	SDNN	Overall HRV, sympathetic and parasympathetic innervation
Root mean square of successive difference between NN intervals	RMSSD	Short-term HRV, primarily parasympathetic innervation
Frequency domain		
Total power	TP	Total HRV (as the band encompasses all frequencies)
High frequency	HF	Parasympathetic control
Ratio high frequency and total power	HF/TP	Parasympathetic control
Intermediate frequency	IntF	Sympathetic and parasympathetic arm of the ANS
Low frequency	LF	Sympathetic and parasympathetic arm of the ANS
Very low frequency	VLF	Sympathetic control
Ratio very low frequency and high frequency	VLF/HF	Sympatho-vagal balance
Ratio very low frequency and low frequency	VLF/LF	Sympatho-vagal balance
Ratio low frequency and high frequency	LF/HF	Sympatho-vagal balance

(*ANS* autonomic nervous system, *NN* normal-to-normal)

performed during the 9 months of pregnancy plus 3 months before pregnancy. On the basis of these self-reports, the sample(s) of pregnant women were characterized into exercise or control group (more or less maternal PA) or continuous or non-continuous LTPA group. LTPA had not been objectively measured using, for example, accelerometers in any of the included articles.

Study outcomes on HRV

Maternal outcomes

Four articles presented results concerning the influence of regular maternal PA on *maternal* HRV [36, 41, 43, 47]. May et al. [47] showed that the standard deviation of normal-to-normal intervals (SDNN), the root mean square of successive difference (RMSSD), very low frequency (VLF) HRV parameter, low frequency (LF) HRV parameter as well as high frequency (HF) HRV parameter were significantly increased in women who consistently exercised for a minimum of 30 min on three or more days (exercise group) at least at one time point of measurement in pregnancy compared to women of the control group who exercised less (detailed information see Tables 3, 4, and 5). Van Leeuwen et al. [41] showed no significant differences in maternal HRV parameters but showed a trend of increased maternal RMSSD ($p =$ 0.07) in women who exercised for a minimum of 30 min on three or more days a week (exercise group) compared to women of the control group who exercised less during pregnancy.

Stutzman et al. [43] showed that total power frequency (TP) HRV parameter was significantly decreased from pre-to-post intervention only in the OaO control group. LF was also significantly decreased over time in both control groups (NW and OaO) but not in the two exercise groups (NW and OaO). HF and the ratio of LF and HF (LF/HF), as well as the ratio of HF and TP (HF/TP) showed no significant changes from pre-to-post intervention in any of the four groups.

Satyapriya et al. [36] tested maternal HRV of an exercise group which performed yoga and a control group which performed standard prenatal exercise. They assessed changes pre and post the exercise session (acute effects of PA) at gestational week 20 and gestational week 36 (intervention effect over time). At gestational week 20, no significant changes from pre-to-post exercise session were found for any HRV parameter (LF, HF, LF/HF) neither in the yoga nor in the prenatal exercise group. At gestational week 36, LF was significantly decreased from pre-to-post exercise session in the yoga group but not in the prenatal exercise group. Both groups showed a significant increase of HF from pre-to-post exercise session at gestational week 36 and a significant decrease of LF/HF from pre-to-post exercise session at gestational week 36. In summary, significant acute effects of yoga and standard prenatal exercise on HRV were only measured at gestational week 36 and not at gestational week 20 (Tables 3, 4, and 5).

Fetal outcomes

Five articles presented results concerning the influence of regular maternal PA on *fetal* HRV [37, 38, 40–42].

Van Leeuwen et al. [41] showed that the SDNN and the RMSSD were significantly increased in fetuses of women who exercised for a minimum of 30 min on three or more days a week (exercise group) compared fetuses of women in the control group. May, Suminski et al. [37] assessed whether fetal HRV was correlated with continuous or non-continuous maternal LTPA. The SDNN significantly correlated with both continuous and

Table 2 Cohort and study characteristics

First author, year	Study design	Sample (pregnant women)	Intervention, exercise mode, PA determination	HRV outcomes (maternal/fetal/infant)	HRV measure technique	Time(s) of measurement	Data analysis
May, [47]	Post-hoc analysis of maternal magnetocardiograms (May et al. [40]) to assess maternal heart measures depending on maternal exercise behavior (exercise vs. control group) at different weeks of gestation	$N = 56$ (gw36 $N = 51$); 20–39 years singleton, low-risk pregnancies	MPAQ to retrospectively categorize women into exercise (≥30 min. aerobic exercise/ 3 times a week) and control group[a]	maternal M: SDNN, RMSSD, VLF, LF, HF, LF/HF	3 continuous, 18 min simultaneous fetal-maternal MCG were recorded for each subject using an investigational 83-channel dedicated fetal biomagnetometer	Gw28, gw32, and gw36	Students t-test and Wilcoxon rank sum test to contrast variables between exercise and control groups
Van Leeuwen, [41]	Post-hoc analysis of fetal-maternal magnetocardiograms (May et al. [40]) to assess maternal and fetal heart measures depending on maternal exercise behavior (exercise vs. control group)	$N = 40$; 20–35 years singleton, low-risk pregnancies	MPAQ to retrospectively categorize women into exercise (≥ 30 min. of moderate to vigorous aerobic exercise/ 3 times a week; $n = 21$) and control group ($n = 19$)[a]	maternal, fetal M: SDNN, RMSSD F: SDNN, RMSSD	A continuous, 18 min simultaneous fetal-maternal MCG was recorded for each subject using an investigational 83-channel dedicated fetal biomagnetometer	Gw36	Comparison between control and exercise groups using Mann-Whitney-U test
May, Suminski, [37]	Post-hoc analysis of fetal magnetocardiograms (May et al. [40]) to assess fetal heart measures depending on the duration of maternal continuous and non-continuous leisure-time physical activity	$N = 40$; 23–39 years singleton, low-risk pregnancies	MPAQ to retrospectively classify whether the women perform continuous (e.g., walking, jogging) or non-continuous (e.g. weight lifting, yoga)[a] leisure-time physical activity	fetal F: SDNN, RMSSD, VLF, LF, HF	A continuous, 18 min simultaneous fetal-maternal MCG was recorded for each subject using an investigational 83-channel dedicated fetal biomagnetometer	Gw36	Pearson Product Monument correlation to assess relationships between duration (min) of maternal continuous and non-continuous LTPA and fetal heart measures; Multiple regression analyses to predict fetal heart measures
May, Scholtz, [39]	Post-hoc analysis of a subset of infants from a prospective longitudinal pregnancy study (May et al. [40]) to assess infant heart measures depending on maternal exercise behavior (exercise vs. control)	$N = 43$; 20–35 years, singleton, low-risk pregnancies	MPAQ to retrospectively categorize infants of women who were in the exercise (≥ 30 min. of moderate to vigorous aerobic exercise/ 3 times a week; $n = 16$) and control group ($n = 27$)[a]	infant I: SDNN, RMSSD, LF, HF	A continuous, 18 min simultaneous fetal-maternal MCG was recorded for each subject using an investigational 83-channel dedicated fetal biomagnetometer	One month of age	Student´s t-tests to compare infant HRV measures between exercise and control group
Gustafson, [42]	Post-hoc analysis of fetal magnetocardiograms (May et al. [40]) to assess fetal heart measures depending on maternal exercise (exercise vs. control)	$N = 30$; 20–35 years, singleton, low-risk pregnancies	MPAQ to retrospectively categorize women into exercise (≥ 30 min. of moderate to vigorous aerobic exercise/ 3 times a week; $n = 15$) and control group ($n = 15$)[a]	fetal F: RMSSD, VLF, LF, LF/HF, VLF/LF, VLF/HF, INT	A continuous, 18 min simultaneous fetal-maternal MCG was recorded for each subject using an investigational 83-channel dedicated fetal biomagnetometer	Gw36	Mixed-effects models with post-hoc comparisons. Comparisons for exercise vs. control were adjusted for breathing patterns (breathing vs. apnea)
May, [38]	Post-hoc analysis of fetal magnetocardiograms (May et al. [40]) to assess effects of maternal exercise dose on fetal heart measures	$N = 50$; 23–39 years, singleton, low-risk pregnancies	MPAQ to retrospectively assess maternal physical activity behavior, specifically duration and intensity[a]	fetal F: SDNN, RMSSD, VLF, LF, HF, VLF/LF, VLF/HF, LF/HF	A continuous, 18 min simultaneous fetal-maternal MCG was recorded for each subject using an investigational 83-channel dedicated fetal biomagnetometer	Gw36	Spearman correlations were used to assess relationships between maternal LTPA (intensity, duration) during third trimester and fetal heart measures

Table 2 Cohort and study characteristics *(Continued)*

							Multiple regression were additionally performed to assess how well LTPA intensity and duration predict fetal heart measures
Stutzman [43]	Prospective controlled interventional study to assess pre-to-post changes of exercise conditioning on HRV in normal and overweight women. HRV was measured in supine position and during low-intensity exercise	$N = 22$; healthy, singleton pregnancy; $n = 10$ NW (BMI < 25.0 kg/m^2), $n = 12$ OaO[b] (BMI > 25.0 kg/m^2)	Measurements: laboratory testing at gw20 ± 2 and gw36 Intervention: E: Instructed on a16 week progressive low-intensity walking exercise[c], 5 days/ week; $n = 6$ OaO, $n = 5$ NW C: Activity log only; $n = 6$ OaO, $n = 5$ NW →4 group design: a) walking/NW, b) non-walking/NW, c) walking/OaO, d) non-walking/OaO	maternal M: LF, HF, TP, HF/TP, LP/HP	Beat-by-beat R-R intervals were obtained and recorded continuously during testing using three latex-free standard surface ECG electrodes and a Spacelab 514 cardiac monitor	Gw20 and gw36	ANOVAs were used to obtain within and between group changes from gw20 to gw36
May, [40]	Prospective, longitudinal, non-blinded study to assess fetal heart measures depending on self-reported maternal exercise and fetal state	$N = 61$; 20–35 years singleton, low-risk pregnancies	MPAQ to retrospectively categorize women into exercise (≥ 30 min. of moderate to vigorous aerobic exercise/ 3 times a week; $n = 26$) and control group ($n = 35$)[a]	fetal F: SDNN, RMSSD, VLF, LF, IntF, HF	3 continuous, 18 min simultaneous fetal-maternal MCG were recorded for each subject using an investigational 83-channel dedicated fetal biomagnetometer	Gw28, gw32, and gw36	Post-hoc comparisons to obtain changes in fetal heart outcomes between exercise and control groups depending on fetal state (active vs. passive) at gw28, gw32, and gw36
Satyapriya [36]	Prospective, RCT to assess the influence of yoga on maternal HRV (two-group, pre-post-design). Measurements were changes in HRV pre and during exercise session as well as pre and post exercise session (acute effects) at gw20 and gw36 (effects over intervention time; not tested for significance)	$N = 90$; 20–35 years; mean BMI: 25.1 (E) and 25.6 (C)	Intervention: E: two modules of integrated yoga, specifically designed for the second and third trimester of pregnancy ($n = 45$) C: standard prenatal exercise ($n = 45$)	Maternal M: LF, HF, LF/HF	Electrocardiogram was recorded continuously for 5 min before, 10 min during and 5 min after intervention	Gw20 and gw36 Measuring pre, during, and post each session	ANOVAs to obtain within and between group differences in maternal HRV between exercise and control group

(*C* control group, *E* exercise group, *ECG* electrocardiograph, *F* fetal, *gw* gestational week, *HF* high frequency, *HRV* heart rate variability, *I* infant, *IntF* intermediate frequency, *LF* low frequency, *M* maternal, *MCG* magnetocardiogram, *MPAQ* Modifiable Physical Activity Questionnaire, *NW* normal weight, *OaO* overweight and obese, *RMSSD* root mean square of successive difference, *SDNN* standard deviation of normal-to-normal intervals, *TP* total power, *VLF* very low frequency)

[a]The MPAQ was used to retrospectively assess all leisure-time physical activities (LTPA) performed during the last 9 months of pregnancy, plus 3 months before pregnancy (self-reported). Note that no exercise intervention was performed within the highlighted studies

[b]pre-pregnancy BMI; pre-pregnancy weights of the participants were obtained by self-report from the women and confirmed from medical records

[c]the steady-state testing protocol involved a 3-min warm-up at 20 W, followed by a ramp increase in work rate with 30 s to a level corresponding to 40 % of the maximal heart rate reserve

Table 3 Outcome measurements of each study

First author, year	Type of analyses	SDNN (ms)	RMSSD (ms)	TP (ms^2)
May, [47]	Difference in maternal HRV between exercise and control group at gw28, gw32, and gw36	maternal gw28: exercise: 53.9 ± 27.4 control: 38.7 ± 12.9 ($p = 0.01$) gw32: exercise: 53.0 ± 19.8 control: 38.1 ± 13.7 ($p = 0.002$) gw36: exercise: 55.8 ± 20.6 control: 44.6 ± 14.0 ($p = 0.03$)	maternal gw28: exercise: 40.2 ± 34.1 control 25.9 ± 13.5 ($p = 0.05$)[d] gw32: exercise: 32.7 ± 24.9 control: 22.9 ± 11.7 (n.s.) gw36: exercise: 32.4 ± 24.9 control: 21.3 ± 11.2 ($p = 0.05$)[d]	—
Van Leeuwen, [41]	Examining the occurrence of fetal-maternal heart rate synchronization in which the mothers were either exercising regularly or were sedentary	maternal exercise: 57.6 ± 22.2 control: 44.9 ± 12.5 (n.s.) fetal exercise: 29.3 ± 9.6 control: 21.4 ± 6.2 ($p = 0.01$)	maternal exercise: 35.2 ± 26.9 control: 20.8 ± 9.1 (n.s.) fetal exercise: 8.6 ± 3.8 control: 6.2 ± 2.1 ($p = 0.02$)	—
May, Suminski, [37]	Correlation between continuous and non-continuous maternal LTPA and fetal HRV	fetal continuous LTPA $R = 0.38$ ($p < 0.05$) non-continuous LTPA $R = 0.33$ ($p < 0.05$)	fetal continuous LTPA $R = 0.31$ (n.s.) non-continuous LTPA $R = 0.04$ (n.s.)	—
May, Scholtz, [39]	Difference in infant HRV between exercise and control group	infant exercise: 38.8 ± 10.8 control: 34.8 ± 14.6 (n.s.)	infant[a] exercise: 1.03 ± 0.14 control: 0.87 ± 0.21 ($p = 0.01$)	—
Gustafson, [42]	Difference in fetal HRV between exercise and control group adjusted for fetal breathing	—	fetal[a] estimate: 0.34; SE: 0.14 (n.s.)	fetal[a] estimate: 1.06; SE: 0.36 (n.s.)
May, [38]	Correlation between maternal LTPA (intensity, duration) and fetal HRV Regression to predict fetal heart measures	fetal intensity[b] $R = 0.28$ ($p < 0.05$) duration[c] $R = 0.44$ ($p < 0.005$) positively predicted by intensity ($p = 0.033$)	fetal intensity[b] $R = 0.27$ (n.s.) duration[c] $R = 0.39$ ($p < 0.01$) positively predicted by duration ($p = 0.005$)	—
Stutzman [43]	Within and between group changes from pre (gw20) to post (gw36) for each of the four groups; results are only presented for the HRV outcomes measured in supine position	—	—	maternal exercise – NW: gw20: 777.1 ± 1072 gw36: 787.8 ± 1042 (n.s.) exercise – OaO: gw20: 523.2 ± 621 gw36: 231.9 ± 203.5 (n.s.) control – NW: gw20: 746.3 ± 667 gw36: 461.3 ± 583 (n.s.) control – OaO: gw20: 652.1 ± 984 gw36: 326.1 ± 506 (sig.)*
May, [40]	Changes in fetal HRV between exercise and control groups depending on fetal state (active vs. passive) at gw28, gw32, and gw36	fetal[a,e] gw28: exercise: 3.1 ± 0.3 control 2.9 ± 0.2 (n.s.) gw32: exercise: 3.2 ± 0.3 control: 3.1 ± 0.3 (n.s.)	fetal[a,e] gw28: exercise: 1.8 ± 0.3 control 1.6 ± 0.3 (n.s.) gw32: exercise: 1.8 ± 0.3 control: 1.6 ± 0.3 (n.s.)	—

Table 3 Outcome measurements of each study *(Continued)*

		gw36: exercise: 3.4 ± 0.3 control: 3.1 ± 0.3 ($p = 0.03$)	gw36: exercise: 2.0 ± 0.5 control: 1.7 ± 0.3 ($p = 0.03$)	
Satyapriya [36]	Changes in maternal HRV pre and during exercise session and pre and post exercise session (acute effects) at gw20 and gw36 (effects over time) Important: differences between maternal HRV measurements at gw20 and gw36 (effects over time) were not reported to be tested for significance	—	—	—

(*F* fetal, *gw* gestational week, *HRV* heart rate variability, *LTPA* leisure-time physical activity, *M* maternal, *ms* millisecond, *NW* normal weight; *n.s* not significant, *OaO* overweight and obese, *RMSSD* root mean square of successive difference, *SE* standard error, *sig* significant, *SDNN* standard deviation of normal-to-normal intervals, *TP* total power)

*p-values were not provided

[a]data were log transformed to fulfill Gaussian distribution

[b]$kcal \cdot min^{-1}$

[c]minutes during third trimester

[d]level of significance was defined as $p \leq 0.05$ for all analyzes performed by Van Leeuwen et al. [41]

[e]measurements are only presented for active fetal state. Note that sample size is reduced at all time points (GA weeks 28 ($n = 39$), 32 ($n = 37$), 36 ($N = 29$)); results for quiet fetal state are not presented in this table because sample size is very small in this group

non-continuous maternal LTPA. VLF, LF, and HF were significantly correlated with continuous but not with non-continuous maternal LTPA. RMSSD did not significantly correlate with continuous nor did it correlate with non-continuous maternal LTPA. Gustafson et al. [42] estimated the difference of fetal HRV exercise in periods of fetal breathing and periods of no-fetal breathing of women who exercised for a minimum of 30 min on three or more days a week (exercise group) compared to the control group who did less exercise. RMSSD, TP, VLF, and LF were not significantly different between the exercise and control group, regardless of fetal breathing or not, but showed trends of significance ($p = 0.08$, $p = 0.06$, $p = 0.06$, and $p = 0.07$ respectively). The intermediate frequency (IntF) as well as the HF were significantly increased in fetuses of the exercise group compared to fetuses of the control group. May et al. [38] assessed whether fetal HRV is correlated with intensity (kilocalories per minute) and duration (minutes of PA during third trimester) of maternal PA performed in the third trimester of pregnancy. SDNN and VLF significantly correlated with both intensity as well as duration. The RMSSD, LF, HF, and IntF significantly correlated with duration but not with intensity. Finally, May et al. [40] assessed the difference of fetal HRV of fetuses in women who exercised for a minimum of 30 min on three or more days a week (exercise group) compared fetuses in women of the control group who did less exercise, depending on fetal state at three different time points (weeks of gestation 28, 32, and 36) in pregnancy. In active fetal state, at gestational week 36 all assessed parameters of HRV (SDNN, RMSSD, VLF, LF, IntF, HF) were significantly higher in fetuses of women in the exercise group compared to fetuses of women in the control group. At gestational week 28 and gestational week 32 differences were not significant for any of these parameters (Tables 3, 4, and 5).

Infant outcomes

Only one article referred to the influence of regular maternal PA on *infant* HRV [39]. The authors showed that RMSSD, LF and HF were significant higher in infants born of women who performed a minimum of 30 min of exercise three times a week (exercise group) compared to women who did less exercise (control group). SDNN and LF/HF were not significantly different between these groups (Tables 3, 4, and 5).

Quality assessment

Using the standardized QATQS, the overall rating of the two articles referring to the intervention studies was strong [36, 43], the articles of May, Scholtz et al. [39] and May et al. [38] was moderate, and the articles of May et al. [47], Van Leeuwen et al. [41], May, Suminski et al. [37], Gustafson et al. [42], and May et al. [40] was weak (Table 6). The longitudinal study by May et al. [40] and related articles were rated weak for 'representativeness' since the authors provided inconsistent reporting of the sample size without providing reasons for dropouts. In consequence, the readers of the articles are not able to retrace whether the samples of the articles are representative of the target population or not. In the intervention study performed by Satyapriya et al. [36], trainers and participants could not be blinded, but the team who did the assessments and statistics was blinded.

Discussion

This systematic review of scientific literature on the influence of maternal PA on maternal, fetal or infant HRV identified nine articles. A summary of all findings is

Table 4 Outcome measurements of each study

First author, year	Type of analyses	VLF (ms^2)	LF (ms^2)	HF (ms^2)	IntF (ms^2)
May, [47]	Difference in maternal HRV between exercise and control group at gw28, gw32, and gw36	maternal gw28: exercise: 1082.6 ± 1135.6 control: 558.9 ± 392.0 ($p = 0.03$)	maternal gw28: exercise: 436.8 ± 614.0 control: 263.7 ± 213.0 (n.s.)	maternal gw28: exercise: 1402.3 ± 2990.0 contro:l 431.1 ± 395.4 (n.s.)	—
		gw32: exercise: 1237.2 ± 942.5 control: 669.1 ± 513.1 ($p = 0.008$)	gw32: exercise: 377.2 ± 473.7 control: 186.3 ± 135.9 ($p = 0.05$)[d]	gw32: exercise: 911.2 ± 1334.8 control: 363.5 ± 365.0 ($p = 0.048$)	
		gw36: exercise: 1529.4 ± 1325.8 control: 1097.2 ± 701.9 (n.s.)	gw36: exercise: 368.6 ± 394.1 control: 201.2 ± 163.3 (n.s.)	gw36: exercise: 805.6 ± 1165.5 control: 322.4 ± 387.4 (n.s.)	
Van Leeuwen, [41]	Difference in maternal and fetal HRV between exercise and control group	—	—	—	—
May, Suminski, [37]	Correlation between continuous and non-continuous maternal LTPA and fetal HRV	fetal continuous LTPA $R = 0.45$ ($p < 0.005$)	fetal continuous LTPA $R = 0.34$ ($p < 0.05$)	fetal continuous LTPA $R = 0.4$ ($p < 0.05$)	—
		non-continuous LTPA $R = 0.06$ (n.s.)	non-continuous LTPA $R = 0.29$ (n.s.)	non-continuous LTPA $R = 0.03$ (n.s.)	
May, Scholtz, [39]	Difference in infant HRV between exercise and control group	—	infant[a] exercise: 2.38 ± 0.2 control: 2.06 ± 0.36 ($p = 0.002$)	infant[a] exercise: 1.72 ± 0.27 control: 1.38 ± 0.39 ($p = 0.004$)	—
Gustafson, [42]	Difference in fetal HRV between exercise and control group adjusted for fetal breathing	fetal[a] estimate: 1.25; SE: 0.45 (n.s.)	fetal[a] estimate: 1.01 SE: 0.46 (n.s.)	fetal[a] estimate: 0.81; SE: 0.25 ($p = 0.03$)	fetal[a] estimate: 1.22; SE: 0.42 ($p = 0.03$)
May, [38]	Correlation between maternal LTPA (intensity, duration) and fetal HRV Regression to predict fetal heart measures	fetal intensity[b] $R = 0.29$ ($p < 0.05$)	fetal intensity[b] $R = 0.20$ (n.s.)	fetal intensity[b] $R = 0.24$ (n.s.)	fetal intensity[b] $R = 0.27$ (n.s.)
		duration[c] $R = 0.34$ ($p < 0.05$)	duration[c] $R = 0.32$ ($p < 0.05$)	duration[c] $R = 0.38$ ($p < 0.01$)	duration[c] $R = 0.32$ ($p < 0.05$)
		positively predicted by duration ($p = 0.007$)	positively predicted by duration ($p = 0.014$)	positively predicted by duration ($p = 0.003$)	—
Stutzman [43]	Within and between group changes from pre (gw20) to post (gw36) for each of the four groups; results are only presented for the HRV outcomes measured in supine position	—	maternal exercise – NW: gw20: 194.4 ± 242 gw36: 116.2 ± 148 (n.s.)	maternal exercise – NW: gw20: 278.9 ± 504 gw36: 290.8 ± 606 (n.s.)	—
			exercise – OaO: gw20: 126.6 ± 143.7 gw36: 37.8 ± 15 (n.s.)	exercise – OaO: gw20: 101.1 ± 99.7 gw36: 25.4 ± 23.8 (n.s.)	
			control – NW: gw20: 184.2 ± 176 gw36: 83.4 ± 76 (sig.)*	control – NW: gw20: 361.9 ± 370 gw36: 111.8 ± 161 (n.s.)	
			control – OaO: gw20: 141.1 ± 181 gw36: 107.5 ± 202.1 (sig.)*	control – OaO: gw20: 376.1 ± 723 gw36: 122.2 ± 265.7 (n.s.)	

Table 4 Outcome measurements of each study *(Continued)*

May, [40]	Changes in fetal HRV between exercise and control groups depending on fetal state (active vs. passive) at gw28, gw32, and gw36	fetal[a,e] gw28: exercise: 4.2 ± 0.5 control 3.9 ± 0.5 (n.s.) gw32: exercise: 4.6 ± 0.6 control: 4.1 ± 0.5 (n.s.) gw36: exercise: 4.8 ± 0.6 control: 4.2 ± 0.6 ($p = 0.04$)	fetal[a,e] gw28: exercise: 4.2 ± 0.5 control 3.9 ± 0.5 (n.s.) gw32: exercise: 4.6 ± 0.6 control: 4.1 ± 0.5 (n.s.) gw36: exercise: 4.8 ± 0.6 control: 4.2 ± 0.6 ($p = 0.03$)	fetal[a,e] gw28: exercise: 2.2 ± 0.5 control 1.8 ± 0.5 (n.s.) gw32: exercise: 2.2 ± 0.6 control: 1.9 ± 0.5 (n.s.) gw36: exercise: 2.6 ± 0.8 control: 2.0 ± 0.4 ($p = 0.01$)	fetal[a,e] gw28: exercise: 2.3 ± 0.6 control 1.7 ± 0.9 (n.s.) gw32: exercise: 1.9 ± 0.8 control: 1.3 ± 0.6 (n.s.) gw36: exercise: 2.3 ± 0.9 control: 1.4 ± 0.7 ($p = 0.02$)
Satyapriya [36]	Changes in maternal HRV pre and during exercise session and pre and post exercise session (acute effects) at gw20 and gw36 (effects over time) Important: differences between maternal HRV measurements at gw20 and gw36 (effects over time) were not reported to be tested for significance		maternal pre (gw20) and post (gw36) intervention gw20: exercise pre session: 74.8 ± 5.9 post session: 74.1 ± 6.6 (n.s.) control pre session: 73.3 ± 8.0 post session: 70.5 ± 11.6 (n.s.) gw36: exercise pre session: 76.3 ± 4.9 post session: 72.5 ± 6.0 ($p = 0.001$) control pre session: 74.2 ± 9.5 post session: 70.9 ± 7.4 (n.s.)	maternal pre (gw20) and post (gw36) intervention gw20: exercise pre session: 25.2 ± 5.9 post session: 26.0 ± 6.6 (n.s.) control pre session: 26.7 ± 8.0 post session: 29.4 ± 11.6 (n.s.) gw36: exercise pre session: 23.2 ± 4.9 post session: 27.5 ± 6.0 ($p = 0.001$) control pre session: 25.0 ± 7.2 post session: 29.1 ± 7.4 ($p = 0.006$)	—

(*F* fetal, *gw* gestational week, *HF* high frequency, *HRV* heart rate variability, *IntF* intermediate frequency, *LF* low frequency, *LTPA* leisure-time physical activity, *M* maternal, *ms* millisecond, *NW* normal weight, *n.s* not significant, *OaO* overweight and obese, *SE* standard error, *sig* significant, *VLF* very low frequency)

[*] *p*-values were not provided

[a] data were log transformed to fulfil Gaussian distribution

[b] $kcal \cdot min^{-1}$

[c] minutes during third trimester

[d] level of significance was defined as $p \leq 0.05$ for all analyzes performed by Van Leeuwen et al. [41]

[e] measurements are only presented for active fetal state. Note that sample size is reduced at all time points (GA weeks 28 ($n = 39$), 32 ($n = 37$), 36 ($N = 29$)); results for quiet fetal state are not presented in this table because sample size is very small in this group

given in Table 7. Overall, the four articles that included maternal HRV as an outcome showed inconsistent results [36, 41, 43, 47]. Of the five articles that referred to the influence of maternal PA on fetal HRV, all the articles showed increases in fetal HRV depending on maternal PA on most parameters [37, 38, 40–42].

The inconsistency of findings with regard to maternal HRV might be due to differences in PA intensity, timing in pregnancy, or due to differences in weight status of the participants. One article showed trends of increased HRV (moderate intensity exercise, small sample size) [41], one showed decreased HRV (OaO pregnant women) [43], another showed increased HRV (moderate intensity exercise) [47], and one article showed no changes on HRV (low intensity exercise group) [36]., Both, increased BMI and progressing pregnancy cause increased sympathetic control resulting in altered HRV outcomes [15–20]. It is expected that based on both of these scenarios the OaO pregnant women will have a different exercise HRV adaptation and therefore, the study performed by Stutzman et al. [43] found a decreased HRV compared to the other studies that investigated normal weight pregnant women. Additionally, moderate intensity PA was found to be associated with a significant increase [47] or a trend of increased HRV [41] whereas low intensity PA was not associated with changes in HRV [36]. This, however may lead to the conclusion that regularly performed maternal PA of moderate intensity may be more effective to improve maternal HRV than low intensity PA. To verify this hypothesis, more studies, including different intensities of maternal PA and its influence on maternal HRV, should be performed.

Results of the five articles on fetal HRV were more consistent, but the association of maternal PA with fetal HRV might change over time. The significant increases of different fetal HRV parameters presented in the article of May et al. [40] were only significant at gestational

Table 5 Outcome measurements of each study

First author, year	Type of analyses	LF/HF (ms^2)	HF/TP (ms^2)	VLF/LF (ms^2)	VLF/HF (ms^2)
May, [47]	Difference in maternal HRV between exercise and control group at gw28, gw32, and gw36	maternal gw28: exercise: 0.6 ± 0.4 control: 0.85 ± 0.6 (n.s.) gw32: exercise: 1.05 ± 0.9 control: 0.77 ± 0.5 (n.s.) gw36: exercise: 1.07 ± 1.5 control: 1.2 ± 1.1 (n.s.)	—	—	—
Van Leeuwen, [41]	Difference in maternal and fetal HRV between exercise and control group	—	—	—	—
May, Suminski, [37]	Correlation between continuous and non-continuous maternal LTPA and fetal HRV	—	—	—	—
May, Scholtz, [39]	Difference in infant HRV between exercise and control group	infant exercise: 5.02 ± 2.16 control: 5.23 ± 2.24 (n.s.)	—	—	—
Gustafson, [42]	Difference in fetal HRV between exercise and control group adjusted for fetal breathing	fetal[a] estimate: 0.20; SE: 0.37 (n.s.)	—	fetal[a] estimate: 0.24; SE: 0.41 (n.s.)	fetal[a] estimate: 0.59; SE: 0.46 (n.s.)
May, [38]	Correlation between maternal LTPA (intensity, duration) and fetal HRV Regression to predict fetal heart measures	—	—	—	
Stutzman [43]	Within and between group changes from pre (gw20) to post (gw36) for each of the four groups; results are only presented for the HRV outcomes measured in supine position	maternal exercise – NW: gw20: 2.02 ± 1.6 gw36: 3.51 ± 3.16 (n.s.) exercise – OaO: gw20: 1.66 ± 1.1 gw36: 2.08 ± 1.3 (n.s.) control – NW: gw20: 0.97 ± 0.92 gw36: 2.26 ± 2.1 (n.s.) control – OaO: gw20: 1.3 ± 1.7 gw36: 2.18 ± 1.3 (n.s.)	maternal exercise – NW: gw20: 0.217 ± 0.15 gw36: 0.187 ± 0.22 (n.s.) exercise – OaO: gw20: 0.207 ± 0.12 gw36: 0.120 ± 0.06 (n.s.) control – NW: gw20: 0.396 ± 0.16 gw36: 0.175 ± 0.09 (n.s.) control – OaO: gw20: 0.365 ± 0.19 gw36: 0.188 ± 0.19 (n.s.)	—	—
May, [40]	Changes in fetal HRV between exercise and control groups depending on fetal state (active vs. passive) at gw28, gw32, and gw36	—	—	—	—
Satyapriya [36]	Changes in maternal HRV pre and during exercise session and pre and post exercise session (acute effects) at gw20 and gw36 (effects over time) Important: differences between maternal HRV measurements at gw20 and gw36 (effects over time) were not reported to be tested for significance	maternal pre (gw20) and post (gw36) intervention gw20: exercise pre session: 3.5 ± 0.2 post session: 3.1 ± 1.0 (n.s.) control pre session: 2.9 ± 0.8 post session: 2.8 ± 1.2 (n.s.)	—	—	—

Table 5 Outcome measurements of each study *(Continued)*

	gw36: exercise pre session: 3.5 ± 0.8 post session: 2.8 ± 0.3 ($p = 0.001$) control pre session: 3.2 ± 0.9 post session: 2.6 ± 0.9 ($p = 0.001$)	

(*F* fetal, *gw* gestational week, *HF* high frequency, *HRV* heart rate variability, *LF* low frequency, *LTPA* leisure-time physical activity, *M* maternal, *ms* millisecond, *NW* normal weight, *n.s* not significant, *OaO* overweight and obese, *sig* significant, *SE* standard error, *TP* total power, *VLF* very low frequency)
[a]data were log transformed to fulfil Gaussian distribution
[b]measurements are only presented for active fetal state. Note that sample size is reduced at all time points (GA weeks 28 ($n = 39$), 32 ($n = 37$), 36 ($N = 29$)); results for quiet fetal state are not presented in this table because sample size is very small in this group

week 36 but not at weeks of gestation 28 and 32. The only article that referred to the influence of maternal PA on infant HRV reported significant increases in most of the HRV parameters [39]. Therefore, the overall consistency of the findings is high reflecting that maternal PA may increase fetal HRV, especially in late pregnancy. Nevertheless, since quality of four of five articles assessing fetal HRV was weak, and were based on only one study, level of evidence has to be rated as low.

The overall global rating for the standardized quality assessment of the articles is moderate to weak (Table 6). Only the two intervention studies were of strong quality [36, 43]. However, these articles only reported data on maternal and not on fetal or infant HRV. Furthermore, they reported inconsistent results showing decreases as well as increases of maternal HRV depending on the type of maternal exercise. In addition, Satyapriya et al. [36] compared maternal HRV between women of an exercise group that performed yoga and women of a control group that performed standard prenatal exercise. Since both groups, the exercise as well as the control group, were physically active, it is unclear whether the changes in HRV depends on PA alone or on for example pregnancy induced cardiovascular adaptations. Therefore, future intervention studies in pregnant women assessing HRV measurements depending on maternal PA should include a physically non-active control group.

Seven articles originated from the same study and sample carried out by May et al. [40]. Although the authors highlight in each article that respective data are post-hoc analyses of a subset of the original longitudinal study, it is unclear why the number of participants differs among these articles (Table 1). In the original article the authors report that 61 women were enrolled into the study and state that not all women participated in all three visits due to non-compliance or delivery prior to 36 weeks of gestation. However, the reasons for the different sample sizes reported in the studies, as well as for participant drop-out, were unclear. For studies assessing PA in participants, especially in pregnant women, it is of utter importance to clarify why participants were excluded or dropped out of a study to ensure that the reason for drop-out was not potential complications as a result of PA. Only one article [40] took fetal state (active

Table 6 Quality assessment of the included articles according to the EPHPP tool

First author, year	Representativeness	Design	Confounders	Blinding[b]	Methods	Drop-outs	Global rating[a]
May, [47]	Weak	Moderate	Strong	NA	Strong	Weak	Weak
Van Leeuwen, [41]	Weak	Moderate	Weak	NA	Strong	Weak	Weak
May, Suminski, [37]	Weak	Moderate	Strong	NA	Strong	Weak	Weak
May, Scholtz, [39]	Weak	Moderate	Strong	NA	Strong	Strong	Moderate
Gustafson, [42]	Weak	Moderate	Weak	NA	Strong	Weak	Weak
May, [38]	Weak	Moderate	Strong	NA	Strong	Strong	Moderate
Stutzman [43]	Moderate	Strong	Strong	NA	Strong	Strong	Strong
May, [40]	Weak	Moderate	Weak	NA	Strong	Weak	Weak
Satyapriya [36]	Moderate	Strong	Strong	NA	Moderate	Moderate	Strong

(*EPHPP* Effective Public Health Practice Project, *NA* not applicable)
[a]Strong, no weak component rating; moderate, one weak component rating; weak, two or more weak component ratings
[b]The component 'blinding of outcome assessors and participants' has been considered not applicable for observational and interventional studies. The reason for considering blinding not applicable for intervention studies in this case is that in studies with physical activity intervention the assessors (i.e. researchers) and the participants are very likely to know the outcome of the randomization [51]

Table 7 Summary of study results concerning the influence of maternal PA on HRV

Finding	First author, year	SDNN	RMSSD	TP	HF	HF/TP	IntF	LF	VLF	VLF/HF	VLF/LF	LF/HF
Maternal	May, [47]	↑	↑[a]	-	↑[a]	-	-	↑[a]	↑[a]	-	-	n.s.
	Van Leeuwen, [41]	n.s.	n.s.	-	-	-	-	-	-	-	-	-
	Stutzman [43]	-	-	(↑)	n.s.	n.s.	-	(↑)	-	-	-	n.s.
	Satyapriya [36]	-	-	-	↑	-	-	↓	-	-	-	↓
Fetal	Van Leeuwen, [41]	↑	↑	-	-	-	-	-	-	-	-	-
	May, Suminski, [37]	↑	n.s.	-	↑	-	-	↑	↑	-	-	-
	Gustafson, [42]	-	n.s.	n.s.	↑	-	↑	n.s.	n.s.	n.s.	n.s.	n.s.
	May, [38]	↑	↑	-	↑	-	↑	↑	↑	-	-	-
	May, [40]	↑[a]	↑[a]	-	↑[a]	-	↑[a]	↑[a]	↑[a]	-	-	-
Infant	May, Scholtz, [39]	n.s.	↑	-	↑	-	-	↑	-	-	-	-

(*HF* high frequency, *HRV* heart rate variability, *IntF* intermediate frequency, *LF* low frequency, *n.s. RMSSD* root mean square of successive difference, *SDNN* standard deviation of normal-to-normal intervals, *TP* total power, *VLF* very low frequency)

↑, increase; ↓, decrease; -, variable not assessed

(↑), HRV parameters were decreased from gw20 to gw36 in all 4 groups but these decreases were only significant in the control groups. In consequence, there was a relative increase of maternal HRV parameters in the exercise groups compared to the control groups namely that the decrease of HRV was smaller in the exercise groups. Therefore, we used this symbol (↑) to illustrate relative increase

[a]significant changes in HRV between exercise and control group have been found but not at all time-points of measuring (gw28, gw32, gw36)

vs. quiet) into account when assessing the influence of maternal PA on fetal HRV depending on fetal state (active vs. quiet). Since fetal heart measurements are mediated by fetal behavior [52, 53], future studies should consider this aspect. Without taking fetal state into account, interpretations of fetal HRV data are impossible. Furthermore, the authors used the MPAQ to retrospectively assess self-reported LTPA performed during the nine months of pregnancy plus three months before pregnancy. Since objective measurements of PA delivers more valid results than self-reported (subjective) measurements [54, 55], future studies assessing PA in pregnancy should use objective devices such as accelerometers, or use an exercise intervention (randomized design).

Conclusions

Based on the current evidence available and the inconsistency of the study results, our overall conclusion is that the hypothesis that maternal PA influences maternal HRV cannot be supported. Nonetheless, some studies showed a trend that maternal HRV may be improved, especially after regularly performed maternal PA of moderate intensity.

Given that most of the articles referring to fetal HRV showed positive effects, we also conclude that there is a trend that maternal PA might increase fetal HRV. Only one study assessed infant HRV, and therefore no conclusion can be drawn as yet. As a consequence, we are not able to provide a clinical conclusion at this time but moderate intensity maternal PA might be more beneficial to improve HRV compared to low intensity maternal PA. Since HRV is a noninvasive and surrogate marker to determine fetal overall health and the development of fetal ANS, more evidence is needed to clarify whether this highly relevant marker during pregnancy can be influenced by maternal PA. Therefore, we recommend that future studies on the influence of maternal PA on HRV should consider exercise intensity, maternal overweight and obesity, progression of gestation as well as fetal state. Additionally, future studies should include well-designed intervention studies with a physically inactive control group or longitudinal studies objectively measuring maternal PA.

Appendix 1 Complete search term for Pubmed

("Motor Activity"[Mesh:NoExp] OR "Exercise"[Mesh] OR "Sports"[Mesh] OR "Physical Exertion"[Mesh] OR "Early Ambulation"[Mesh] OR "Exercise Therapy"[Mesh] OR "Exercise Movement Techniques"[Mesh] OR "Motor Activit*"[tiab] OR "Physical Activit*"[tiab] OR "Locomotor Activit*"[tiab] OR Exercis*[tiab] OR "Physical Exercis*"[tiab] OR "Isometric Exercis*"[tiab] OR "Aerobic Exercis*"[tiab] OR Training[tiab] OR Stretching[tiab] OR "Physical Condition*"[tiab] OR "Physical Fitness"[tiab] OR "Physical Endurance"[tiab] OR "Movement Therap*"[tiab] OR "Fitness Training"[tiab] OR Plyometric[tiab] OR Stretch-Shortening[tiab] OR Weight-Lifting[tiab] OR Weight-Bearing[tiab] OR Running[tiab] OR Jogging[tiab] OR Walk*[tiab] OR Bicycle[tiab] OR Cycle[tiab] OR Bicycling[tiab] OR Cycling[tiab] OR Rowing[tiab] OR Swim*[tiab] OR Ambulation[tiab] OR Mobil*[tiab] OR Pilates[tiab] OR Yoga[tiab]) AND (Pregnancy[Mesh] OR Gravidity[Mesh] OR "Pregnant Women"[Mesh] OR Pregnan*[tiab] OR Gravid*[tiab] OR Gestation*[tiab] OR "Pregnant Wom#n"[tiab] OR Childbearing[tiab] OR Matern*[tiab] OR Fetal[tiab]) AND ("Heart Rate Variability"[Mesh] OR "Heart Rate Variability"[tw] OR "Heart Outcome"[tiab] OR "Heart Measurement"[tiab]

OR "Cardiovascular Outcome"[tiab] OR "Cardiovascular Measurement"[tiab] OR "Cardiovascular Adaptation"[tiab] OR "Autonomic Nervous System"[tiab] OR "Parasympathetic Nervous System"[tiab] OR "Sympathetic Nervous System"[tiab] OR "Vagus Nerve"[tiab]).

Abbreviations

ANS: autonomic nervous system; C: control group; E: exercise group; ECG: electrocardiograph; EPHPP: Effective Public Health Practice Project; F: fetal; gw: gestational week; HF: high frequency; HRV: heart rate variability; I: infant; IntF: intermediate frequency; LF: low frequency; LTPA: leisure-time physical activity; M: maternal; MCG: magnetocardiogram; MPAQ: Modifiable Physical Activity Questionnaire; NA: not applicable; NN: normal-to-normal; NW: normal weight; OaO: overweight and obese; RMSSD: root mean square of successive difference; SDNN: standard deviation of normal-to-normal intervals; SE: standard error; TP: total power; VLF: very low frequency

Acknowledgements

None.

Funding

None.

Authors' contributions

PD and MvP contributed substantially to concept and design of the review, acquisition of data as well as to analysis and interpretation of data. ST contributed substantially to acquisition of data as well as to analysis and interpretation of data. EW, MS, and WR contributed substantially to data analysis and interpretation. All authors drafted the article and approved the final version.

Competing interests

The authors declare that they have no competing interests.

Author details

[1]Department of Physical Activity and Public Health, Institute of Sports Science, University of Graz, Mozartgasse 14, Graz 8010, Austria. [2]Centre for Exercise Science and Sports Medicine, School of Therapeutic Sciences, Faculty of Health Sciences, University of Witwatersrand, Private Bag 3, Johannesburg 2050, South Africa. [3]Department of Public and Occupational Health, EMGO Institute for Health and Care Research, VU University Medical Centre, Van der Boechorststraat 7, Amsterdam 1081 BT, The Netherlands.

References

1. Weissgerber TL, Wolfe LA. Physiological adaptation in early human pregnancy: adaptation to balance maternal-fetal demands. Appl Physiol Nutr Metab. 2006;31:1–11. doi:10.1139/h05-003.
2. Chapman AB, Abraham WT, Zamudio S, Coffin C, Merouani A, Young D, et al. Temporal relationships between hormonal and hemodynamic changes in early human pregnancy. Kidney Int. 1998;54:2056–63. doi:10.1046/j.1523-1755.1998.00217.x.
3. Capeless EL, Clapp JF. Cardiovascular changes in early phase of pregnancy. Am J Obstet Gynecol. 1989;161:1449–53.
4. Norwitz ER, Schust DJ, Fisher SJ. Implantation and the survival of early pregnancy. N Engl J Med. 2001;345:1400–8. doi:10.1056/NEJMra000763.
5. Johansson S, Norman M, Legnevall L, Dalmaz Y, Lagercrantz H, Vanpée M. Increased catecholamines and heart rate in children with low birth weight: perinatal contributions to sympathoadrenal overactivity. J Intern Med. 2007;261:480–7. doi:10.1111/j.1365-2796.2007.01776.x.
6. Wadhwa PD, Culhane JF, Rauh V, Barve SS. Stress and preterm birth: neuroendocrine, immune/inflammatory, and vascular mechanisms. Matern Child Health J. 2001;5:119–25.
7. Satpathy HK, Fleming A, Frey D, Barsoom M, Satpathy C, Khandalavala J. Maternal obesity and pregnancy. Postgrad Med. 2008;120:9. doi:10.3810/pgm.2008.09.1920.
8. Phillips DIW. External influences on the fetus and their long-term consequences. Lupus. 2006;15:794–800.
9. Schobel HP, Fischer T, Heuszer K, Geiger H, Schmieder RE. Preeclampsia – a state of sympathetic overactivity. N Engl J Med. 1996;335:1480–5. doi:10.1056/NEJM199611143352002.
10. National Institute of Child Health and Human Development Research Planning Workshop. Electronic fetal heart rate monitoring: research guidelines for interpretation. National Institute of Child Health and Human Development Research Planning Workshop. Am J Obstet Gynecol. 1997;177:1385–90.
11. Malik M. Heart rate variability. Curr Opin Cardiol. 1998;13:36–44.
12. Raczak G, Daniłowicz-Szymanowicz L, Kobuszewska-Chwirot M, Ratkowski W, Figura-Chmielewska M, Szwoch M. Long-term exercise training improves autonomic nervous system profile in professional runners. Kardiol Pol. 2006;64:135–40. discussion 141-2.
13. Mandigout S, Melin A, Fauchier L, N'Guyen LD, Courteix D, Obert P. Physical training increases heart rate variability in healthy prepubertal children. Eur J Clin Invest. 2002;32:479–87.
14. Sandercock GRH, Bromley PD, Brodie DA. Effects of exercise on heart rate variability: inferences from meta-analysis. Med Sci Sports Exerc. 2005;37:433–9.
15. Felber Dietrich D, Schindler C, Schwartz J, Barthelemy J-C, Tschopp J-M, Roche F, et al. Heart rate variability in an ageing population and its association with lifestyle and cardiovascular risk factors: results of the SAPALDIA study. Europace. 2006;8:521–9. doi:10.1093/europace/eul063.
16. Arone LJ, Mackintosh R, Rosenbaum M, Leibel RL, Hirsch J. Autonomic nervous system activity in weight gain and weight loss. Am J Physiol. 1995;269:R222–5.
17. Arrone LJ, Mackintosh R, Rosenbaum M, Leibel RL, Hirsch J. Cardiac autonomic nervous system activity in obese and never-obese young men. Obes Res. 1997;5:354–9.
18. Spraul M, Ravussin E, Fontvieille AM, Rising R, Larson DE, Anderson EA. Reduced sympathetic nervous activity. A potential mechanism predisposing to body weight gain. J Clin Invest. 1993;92:1730–5. doi:10.1172/JCI116760.
19. Felber Dietrich D, Ackermann-Liebrich U, Schindler C, Barthelemy J-C, Brandli O, Gold DR, et al. Effect of physical activity on heart rate variability in normal weight, overweight and obese subjects: results from the SAPALDIA study. Eur J Appl Physiol. 2008;104:557–65. doi:10.1007/s00421-008-0800-0.
20. Stein PK, Hagley MT, Cole PL, Domitrovich PP, Kleiger RE, Rottman JN. Changes in 24-hour heart rate variability during normal pregnancy. Am J Obstet Gynecol. 1999;180:978–85.
21. Henje Blom E, Olsson EM, Serlachius E, Ericson M, Ingvar M. Heart rate variability (HRV) in adolescent females with anxiety disorders and major depressive disorder. Acta Paediatr. 2010;99:604–11. doi:10.1111/j.1651-2227.2009.01657.x.
22. DiPietro JA, Bornstein MH, Hahn C-S, Costigan K, Achy-Brou A. Fetal heart rate and variability: stability and prediction to developmental outcomes in early childhood. Child Dev. 2007;78:1788–98. doi:10.1111/j.1467-8624.2007.01099.x.
23. Graça LM, Cardoso CG, Clode N, Calhaz-Jorge C. Acute effects of maternal cigarette smoking on fetal heart rate and fetal body movements felt by the mother. J Perinat Med. 1991;19:385–90.
24. Halmesmäki E, Ylikorkala O. The effect of maternal ethanol intoxication on fetal cardiotocography: a report of four cases. Br J Obstet Gynaecol. 1986;93:203–5.
25. Caspersen CJ, Powell KE, Christenson GM. Physical activity, exercise, and physical fitness: definitions and distinctions for health-related research. Public Health Rep. 1985;100:126–31.
26. Clapp JF. The effects of maternal exercise on fetal oxygenation and feto-placental growth. Eur J Obstet Gynecol Reprod Biol. 2003;110(Suppl):80–5. doi:10.1016/S0301-2115(03)00176-3.
27. Clapp JF, Kiess W. Effects of pregnancy and exercise on concentrations of the metabolic markers tumor necrosis factor alpha and leptin. Am J Obstet Gynecol. 2000;182:300–6.
28. Clapp JF. Effects of Diet and Exercise on Insulin Resistance during Pregnancy. Metab Syndr Relat Disord. 2006;4:84–90. doi:10.1089/met.2006.4.84.

29. Dye TD, Knox KL, Artal R, Aubry RH, Wojtowycz MA. Physical activity, obesity, and diabetes in pregnancy. Am J Epidemiol. 1997;146:961–5.
30. Bung P, Artal R. Gestational diabetes and exercise: a survey. Semin Perinatol. 1996;20:328–33.
31. Downs DS, DiNallo JM, Kirner TL. Determinants of pregnancy and postpartum depression: prospective influences of depressive symptoms, body image satisfaction, and exercise behavior. Ann Behav Med. 2008;36: 54–63. doi:10.1007/s12160-008-9044-9.
32. Carter JB, Banister EW, Blaber AP. Effect of Endurance Exercise on Autonomic Control of Heart Rate. Sports Med. 2003;33:33–46. doi:10.2165/00007256-200333010-00003.
33. Okazaki K, Iwasaki K-i, Prasad A, Palmer MD, Martini ER, Fu Q, et al. Dose-response relationship of endurance training for autonomic circulatory control in healthy seniors. J Appl Physiol. 2005;99:1041–9. doi:10.1152/japplphysiol.00085.2005.
34. D'Silva LA, Davies RE, Emery SJ, Lewis MJ. Influence of somatic state on cardiovascular measurements in pregnancy. Physiol Meas. 2014;35:15–29. doi:10.1088/0967-3334/35/1/15.
35. Routledge FS, Campbell TS, McFetridge-Durdle JA, Bacon SL. Improvements in heart rate variability with exercise therapy. Can J Cardiol. 2010;26:303–12.
36. Satyapriya M, Nagendra HR, Nagarathna R, Padmalatha V. Effect of integrated yoga on stress and heart rate variability in pregnant women. Int J Gynaecol Obstet. 2009;104:218–22. doi:10.1016/j.ijgo.2008.11.013.
37. May LE, Suminski RR, Berry A, Langaker MD, Gustafson KM. Maternal physical activity mode and fetal heart outcome. Early Hum Dev. 2014;90:365–9. doi:10.1016/j.earlhumdev.2014.04.009.
38. May LE, Suminski RR, Langaker MD, Yeh H-W, Gustafson KM. Regular maternal exercise dose and fetal heart outcome. Med Sci Sports Exerc. 2012; 44:1252–8. doi:10.1249/MSS.0b013e318247b324.
39. May LE, Scholtz SA, Suminski R, Gustafson KM. Aerobic exercise during pregnancy influences infant heart rate variability at one month of age. Early Hum Dev. 2014;90:33–8. doi:10.1016/j.earlhumdev.2013.11.001.
40. May LE, Glaros A, Yeh H-W, Clapp JF, Gustafson KM. Aerobic exercise during pregnancy influences fetal cardiac autonomic control of heart rate and heart rate variability. Early Hum Dev. 2010;86:213–7. doi:10.1016/j.earlhumdev.2010.03.002.
41. van Leeuwen P, Gustafson KM, Cysarz D, Geue D, May LE, Grönemeyer D. Aerobic exercise during pregnancy and presence of fetal-maternal heart rate synchronization. PLoS One. 2014;9, e106036. doi:10.1371/journal.pone.0106036.
42. Gustafson KM, May LE, Yeh H-W, Million SK, Allen JJB. Fetal cardiac autonomic control during breathing and non-breathing epochs: the effect of maternal exercise. Early Hum Dev. 2012;88:539–46. doi:10.1016/j.earlhumdev.2011.12.017.
43. Stutzman SS, Brown CA, Hains SMJ, Godwin M, Smith GN, Parlow JL, Kisilevsky BS. The effects of exercise conditioning in normal and overweight pregnant women on blood pressure and heart rate variability. Biol Res Nurs. 2010;12:137–48. doi:10.1177/1099800410375979.
44. Avery ND, Wolfe LA, Amara CE, Davies GA, McGrath MJ. Effects of human pregnancy on cardiac autonomic function above and below the ventilatory threshold. J Appl Physiol. 2001;90:321–8.
45. Carpenter RE, D'Silva LA, Emery SJ, Uzun O, Rassi D, Lewis MJ. Changes in heart rate variability and QT variability during the first trimester of pregnancy. Physiol Meas. 2015;36:531–45. doi:10.1088/0967-3334/36/3/531.
46. Siepmann M, Hennig U-D, Siepmann T, Nitzsche K, Mück-Weymann M, Petrowski K, Weidner K. The effects of heart rate variability biofeedback in patients with preterm labour. Appl Psychophysiol Biofeedback. 2014;39:27–35. doi:10.1007/s10484-013-9238-1.
47. May LE, Knowlton J, Hanson J, Suminski R, Paynter C, Fang X, Gustafson KM. Effects of Exercise During Pregnancy on Maternal Heart Rate and Heart Rate Variability. PM R. 2016;8:611–7. doi:10.1016/j.pmrj.2015.11.006.
48. Effective Public Health Practice Project. Quality Assessment Tool for Quantitative Studies. 2008. http://www.ephpp.ca/tools.html. Accessed 30 Aug 2016.
49. Armijo-Olivo S, Stiles CR, Hagen NA, Biondo PD, Cummings GG. Assessment of study quality for systematic reviews: a comparison of the Cochrane Collaboration Risk of Bias Tool and the Effective Public Health Practice Project Quality Assessment Tool: methodological research. J Eval Clin Pract. 2012;18:12–8. doi:10.1111/j.1365-2753.2010.01516.x.
50. Thomas BH, Ciliska D, Dobbins M, Micucci S. A process for systematically reviewing the literature: providing the research evidence for public health nursing interventions. Worldviews Evid Based Nurs. 2004;1:176–84. doi:10.1111/j.1524-475X.2004.04006.x.
51. Oja P, Titze S, Bauman A, de Geus B, Krenn P, Reger-Nash B, Kohlberger T. Health benefits of cycling: a systematic review. Scand J Med Sci Sports. 2011;21:496–509. doi:10.1111/j.1600-0838.2011.01299.x.
52. Davidson SR, Rankin JH, Martin CB, Reid DL. Fetal heart rate variability and behavioral state: analysis by power spectrum. Am J Obstet Gynecol. 1992; 167:717–22.
53. Einspieler C. Fetal Behaviour: A Neurodevelopmental Approach. London: Mac Keith Press; 2012.
54. Rousham EK, Clarke PE, Gross H. Significant changes in physical activity among pregnant women in the UK as assessed by accelerometry and self-reported activity. Eur J Clin Nutr. 2006;60:393–400. doi:10.1038/sj.ejcn.1602329.
55. Brett KE, Wilson S, Ferraro ZM, Adamo KB. Self-report Pregnancy Physical Activity Questionnaire overestimates physical activity. Can J Public Health. 2015;106:302. doi:10.17269/cjph.106.4938.

19

eRegistries: governance for electronic maternal and child health registries

Sonja L. Myhre[1*], Jane Kaye[2], Lee A. Bygrave[3], Margunn Aanestad[4], Buthaina Ghanem[5], Patricia Mechael[6,7] and J. Frederik Frøen[1,8]

Abstract

Background: The limited availability of maternal and child health data has limited progress in reducing mortality and morbidity among pregnant women and children. Global health agencies, leaders, and funders are prioritizing strategies that focus on acquiring high quality health data. Electronic maternal and child health registries (eRegistries) offer a systematic data collection and management approach that can serve as an entry point for preventive, curative and promotive health services. Due to the highly sensitive nature of reproductive health information, careful consideration must be accorded to privacy, access, and data security. In the third paper of the eRegistries Series, we report on the current landscape of ethical and legal governance for maternal and child health registries in developing countries.

Methods: This research utilizes findings from two web-based surveys, completed in 2015 that targeted public health officials and health care providers in 76 countries with high global maternal and child mortality burden. A sample of 298 public health officials from 64 countries and 490 health care providers from 59 countries completed the online survey. Based on formative research in the development of the eRegistries Governance Guidance Toolkit, the surveys were designed to investigate topics related to maternal and child health registries including ethical and legal issues.

Results: According to survey respondents, the prevailing legal landscape is characterized by inadequate data security safeguards and weak support for core privacy principles. Respondents from the majority of countries indicated that health information from medical records is typically protected by legislation although legislation dealing specifically or comprehensively with data privacy may not be in place. Health care provider trust in the privacy of health data at their own facilities is associated with the presence of security safeguards.

Conclusion: Addressing legal requirements and ensuring that privacy and data security of women's and children's health information is protected is an ethical responsibility that must not be ignored or postponed, particularly where the need is greatest. Not only are the potential harm and unintended consequences of inaction serious for individuals, but they could impact public trust in health registries leading to decreased participation and compromised data integrity.

Keywords: Ethics, Law, Data privacy, Security, Governance, Registry, Maternal and child health

* Correspondence: sonja.myhre@fhi.no
[1]Department of International Public Health, Norwegian Institute of Public Health, P.O. Box 4404, Nydalen N-0403, Oslo, Norway
Full list of author information is available at the end of the article

Background

At the 2014 Maternal and Child Health Summit, World Bank Group President Jim Yong Kim proclaimed, "Our vision is to register every single pregnancy and every single birth by 2030" [1]. As the Millennium Development Goal (MDG) era draws to a close and the Sustainable Development Goals (SDG) are ushered in, a shift towards long-term investments, sustainable strategies, and infrastructure development have emerged as new priorities [2, 3]. Growing support for strengthening civil registration and vital statistics [4–6] and the call for more and better maternal health data in 2010 by leadership in eight global health agencies [7] all point to the need to improve data collection strategies in low and middle income countries (LMIC). Against this backdrop, in June 2015 the World Health Organization (WHO), the United States Agency for International Development (USAID), and the World Bank released *The Roadmap for Measurement and Accountability* and Post-2015 *5-Point Call to Action* that highlight strategies for improving data collection, analysis, access, and use [8]. The dearth of timely and accurate maternal and child health data has limited countries' ability to measure progress in reducing maternal and child deaths worldwide but has galvanized leaders [9–11] and funders [12, 13] to prioritize strategies to acquire high quality maternal and child health data.

Electronic health registries (eRegistries) for maternal and child programs provide a unique approach given their potential to support both clinical and public health decision-making, enhance health care coverage, and improve health outcomes by providing individual data along the continuum of care that can pinpoint when, where, and why women encounter health problems [14–16]. Field studies and research applying the registry concept to maternal health have demonstrated promise [17, 18] in contrast with ad hoc, resource-intense surveys and statistical estimates of maternal mortality (i.e., MMR) that have been criticized for their inability to accurately assess MDG progress [19]. The burgeoning focus on measurement, monitoring and infrastructure and universal health coverage and equity are consistent with registry methodology that involves ongoing, population-based data collection that strengthens data availability, quality and use [16, 20].

While electronic maternal and child health registries compile comprehensive individual health data [14, 15, 21] Frost et al, personal communication, 2016, the highly sensitive nature of reproductive health information and the vulnerability of women and children living in LMICs demand careful consideration of privacy, confidentiality, and data security. The pace of the data revolution has outstripped the ability of existing laws and traditional approaches to address concerns introduced by digital technology [22–25]. Electronic health data, for example, are susceptible to intentional or inadvertent breaches of security with serious implications for individuals' privacy that did not exist in the 'paper era.' The transition from paper to electronic records, thus, demands contemporary strategies that ensure patient privacy, confidentiality, and data security [26].

The *Principles for Digital Development*, an initiative involving WHO, the World Bank, USAID, the Bill and Melinda Gates Foundation, and a host of other international agencies, provide guidance on how to integrate best practices in ICT projects and specifically highlights the need to address privacy and security in their eighth principle [27]. Responsible data stewardship practices among communities [28] and ethical checklists for use in humanitarian operations [29] are two recent examples of guidance tools. However, despite the proliferation of health registries around the world, few publications provide an overarching framework or discuss approaches to ethical or governance issues specifically for registries [30–32]. To address this gap, the eRegistry Governance Guidance Toolkit (Frame 1) was developed to provide an overview of the ethical and legal issues pertaining to electronic registries and identify best practices that protect women and children's health data in LMICs [33].

The research literature on ethical and governance issues in LMICs suggests that these countries face additional challenges compared to developed countries and may need to address different ethical and legal issues concerning electronic health registries due to a lack of capacity, training, and ICT expertise, along with low literacy rates, limited infrastructure and weak governance [34–36]. The WHO's Global Observatory for eHealth series, for example, notes that LMICs face unique challenges in monitoring and managing eHealth data [37, 38] while a TrustLaw report on mHealth data privacy and security issues underscores the importance of culture and context [39]. A lack of clear policies, governance, and legislation has also been observed by researchers in LMIC countries [40, 41]. Ideally, local capacity is needed in public health, medical informatics, law, medical ethics, and privacy protection to address privacy and security issues.

Physical infrastructure limitations such as lack of rooms, partitions, or curtains may also negatively influence patient privacy in the context of health service provision. Resource-constrained settings may negatively impact attitudes and perspectives regarding medical confidentiality practices, particularly with respect to illiterate or poor populations [42, 43]. The concept of confidentiality in a medical context, for example, may also be understood and practiced differently depending on the setting due to differing cultural and social expectations regarding privacy [44].

The consequences of neglecting to address privacy or security issues that pertain to a maternal and child health registry in LMICs have the potential to compromise public trust. As a 'public health good,' a registry relies on trust, which is achieved and maintained by appropriate measures to protect individual privacy. Reproductive health data demand the highest level of care given that it may contain information on HIV status, pregnancy terminations, or other highly stigmatizing information [45]. Privacy breaches for health registries are particularly concerning given the sensitivity of this type of personal health data. Theft or internal disclosure, for example, may result in personal information being divulged for profit, intelligence, defamation, or embarrassment resulting in stigma, discrimination, exclusion, or persecution [46]. Privacy protections are regarded as a basic human right that can only be abrogated in cases where there is ample justification [47, 48].

Privacy protections need to consider both internal (e.g., negligent or malicious actions by health care providers), and external threats (e.g. hackers) to ensure that personal health data are only used for the intended purpose and accessed or disclosed to authorized personnel under strict controls. For example, a judgment issued by the European Court of Human Rights, (I v Finland, 2009), concluded that Finland had violated the European Convention on Human Rights, Article 8 given that hospital authorities had failed to adequately implement technological measures to ensure confidentiality of a patient's medical data [49]. A report prepared by the International Telecommunications Union on cybersecurity in LMICs also emphasized the importance of security policies that are customized, continually optimized, and adapted to the stakeholders and the local environment in which they are implemented [50]. "Privacy by design" is one strategy that proactively incorporates security measures throughout the design of software or information systems via technological means such as access controls, passwords, and encryption [51].

Governance mechanisms also assume an important role [52]. Borrowing from the biobank literature, governance is defined by formal oversight mechanisms (i.e., regulatory bodies, legal instruments) and informal mechanisms (i.e., advisory boards, policies, guidance, professional values, and culture) that together guide decision-making, compliance, and policy development [53]. Governance may be developed to address a range of issues including accountability, transparency, redress, purpose specification, data collection limitations, secondary use of data,, security breach notifications, and data quality and integrity [46].

To assess the current perceptions and status of legal, privacy, and data security issues, public health officials and health care providers residing in 76 countries were invited to complete an online survey. Seventy-five of these countries, according to the Commission on Information and Accountability for Women's and Children's Health (CoIA), shoulder the greatest burden of maternal and child mortality [54] while the occupied Palestinian territory was included given the challenges related to healthcare access and political instability [55].

Methods

This paper is based on findings from two web-based surveys that targeted public health officials and health care providers (i.e., midwives, nurses and doctors in reproductive, maternal, and child health). Based on formative research conducted in the development of the eRegistries Governance Guidance Toolkit (Frame 1), the aim of the surveys was to assess the current status of legal, privacy and security issues relevant to maternal and child health registries in LMICs.

Frame 1: The eRegistries Governance Guidance Toolkit

The eRegistries Governance Guidance Toolkit [56] was developed to advise countries on how to proceed with the establishment, operation, use, and maintenance of an eRegistry for maternal and child health that is lawful and compliant with existing legal requirements, protective of women's rights and privacy, and supportive of the public health aims of the registry. Formative research undertaken in the development of this toolkit involved an extensive review of standards, methods, and procedures established by health registry systems (i.e., cancer, chronic disease, diabetes, and clinical) and vital statistics (i.e., birth registration). The Toolkit was reviewed by experts in registry law, informatics, and public health.

The Toolkit identifies best practices, discusses benefits of legislation, regulations, and guidelines, and provides guidance for countries that can be adapted to local contexts. The Toolkit outlines the essential governance components including: purpose specification, legal, fiscal, and operational responsibility, reporting requirements and enforceability, data quality, data security, confidentiality policies, and data access, and public engagement. The Toolkit considers relevant international instruments, conventions, and declarations that focus on human rights, privacy, data protection, and data security as these may provide useful information, particularly for LMICs that lack national legislation or enforcement bodies.

eRegistries for maternal and child health must function within the legal framework where they operate which can involve legal requirements pertaining to medical research, public health, women's and children's rights, and information law (i.e., data protection law, ethical use of data). One challenge of developing governance guidance in a global context is the inherent diversity in how countries approach law, ethics, and health. Social and cultural differences in how privacy, confidentiality, and security are managed may influence laws, policies and protocols. The Toolkit encourages country level adaptation and advises against transplanting legal language or documents from one country to another. Instead, country level policies should be rooted in their own institutional fabric. Translated adaptations, for example, often fail to embrace subtle social or cultural mores that may affect acceptance.

Survey methods

The survey recruitment strategy consisted of individualized email invitations to reproductive, maternal, newborn and child health (RMNCH) medical and health organizations, Ministries of Health, Institutes of Public Health, and other related government offices (e.g., statistics bureaus, RMNCH departments, etc.) working in any of the 75 countries identified as the highest burden countries by CoIA and the occupied Palestinian territory, collectively called CoIA countries in this paper. Surveys and invitations were available in English, French and Portuguese. (The surveys are available upon request from the first author.)

The public health official survey sample consists of 298 individuals from 64 countries (84 % of the invited countries). A total of 470 health care providers from 59 countries (78 % of invited countries) participated in the health care provider survey. Among public health officials, approximately two-thirds worked at the national or regional level in a Ministry or public health institute or agency. Among health care providers, the professional breakdown included 170 (37 %) doctors, 66 14 %) nurses, 149 (32 %) midwives and 81 (17 %) other RMNCH professionals. Eighty percent ($n = 341$) of the health care providers worked in urban or suburban areas while one- fifth (88) were in rural or isolated areas. Among the health care providers, 198 (44 %) reported working at a public or private hospital, 46 (10 %) worked at a district facility, community health post or maternity home, 91 (20 %) were employed at a public health organization, 62 (14 %) were employed at a MoH, and 49 (11 %) selected 'other.'

A breakdown of the public health official survey respondents by the six WHO regions found that 37 of 42 CoIA countries (88 %) were represented from the African region (88 %), 4 out of 6 (67 %) in the America region, 2 out of 5 (40 %) CoIA countries in the European region, 5 out of 6 (83 %) CoIA countries in the South-East Asian region, 6 out of 7 countries (86 %) in the Western Pacific region, and all ten CoIA countries in the Eastern Mediterranean region (100 %). Among health care provider survey respondents in CoIA countries, 32 out of 42 (76 %) countries were represented in the African region, 8 out of 10 (80 %) countries in the Eastern Mediterranean region, 2 out of 5 (40 %) European countries, 4 out of 6 (67 %) of the South-East Asian countries, and all countries in the America (6/6) and Western Pacific region (7/7) were represented. The personalized invitations contained live links to the online surveys and requested that individuals participate and share the survey with peers, colleagues and professional networks (i.e., a snowball sampling recruitment method) in order to boost the sample size via a referral strategy. Paper-based surveys were made available in some circumstances. Launched in November 2013, responses were accepted until February 2015. Repeated efforts were attempted for all non-responsive countries.

Thematic areas measured by the survey included national registry infrastructure, legal and ethical issues, data security, health care service provision, reporting and dissemination practices, data quality, and data usage. This paper focuses on the ethical and legal domains while results concerning the other topics are reported elsewhere [14, 15, 57] Frost et al, personal communication, 2016. The public health official and health care provider surveys contained overlap of core thematic content but also included questions adapted specifically to the different target groups in order to capture their unique professional and workplace perspectives. The public health official survey, for example, included detailed questions on civil registration systems and data utilization whereas the health care provider survey contained specific items on service provision and data reporting from a health care provider perspective.

Ethical review

The survey was reviewed by the Regional Committees for Medical and Health Research Ethics in Norway and received a letter of exemption given that all information collected was fully anonymous (Reference number: IRB 0000 1870). All respondents were informed that their answers were completely anonymous and that they could withdraw from the survey at any time.

Data analysis

Descriptive statistics were used to present most findings while generalized linear models (PROC GLM) were used to assess more complex associations. Exact confidence intervals were generated from tables. All analyses were done using SAS 9.4. Responses from the public health officials were collapsed to the country level while health care providers were analyzed on the individual level. This strategy was specifically chosen to avoid masking the inherent variability among health care provider settings while facilitating national level assessments with public health official responses.

With regard to data security measures, the surveys asked about physical, technical, and administrative safeguards for protecting electronic registry medical records. Due to missing data among health care provider responses, only public health official data are reported. With regard to the question on level of trust that health care providers have in their own facility's security, respondents were asked to rate how comfortable they would be having their own data stored at their work facility using a five-item Likert scale ranging from very comfortable to very uncomfortable.

Results

This paper describes the perceptions and perspectives of health care providers and public health officials from 76 LMICs with respect to privacy, access, and data security of personal health information.

Current legal privacy protections

Human rights generally and the right to privacy specifically are usually enshrined in legislation or regulations that are passed by legislative bodies and can be readily enforced. Survey respondents were asked if their country had laws or regulations that protect a person's privacy or confidentiality concerning their personal health data (i.e., information or medical records). Public health officials from 69 % of the 61 responding countries ($n = 42$; 95 % CI: 56–80) reported that their country had legislation protecting individual privacy.

Access

The survey explored different forms of access ranging from individual-level access by women to access among health care professionals or others directly or indirectly involved in a patient's care. In the majority of countries ($n = 48$; 79 %; 95 % CI: 66–88), public health officials indicated that individuals have the right to access their own medical records.

Access by others was assessed by asking respondents, *"Aside from health professionals directly involved in a patient's care, who else has access to patient medical records without patient consent?"* Health care providers indicated that many actors within and outside the health system have access to medical records without patient consent. The survey results found that health care providers working in diverse settings indicated that access to data by actors not directly involved with the patient included: other health care providers not directly involved with the patient's care ($n = 174$; 45 %; 95 % CI: 40–51), administrative staff ($n = 163$; 43 %; 95 % CI: 38–48), financial staff ($n = 82$; 21 %; 95 % CI: 17–26), government ($n = 111$; 29 %: 95 % CI: 25–34), school ($n = 25$; 7 %; 95 % CI: 4–10), employers ($n = 28$; 7 %; 95 % CI: 5–10), researchers ($n = 137$; 36 %: 95 % CI: 21–41), and family members ($n = 26$; 7 %; 95 % CI: 4–10) (Fig. 1). In circumstances in which patients are asked to provide consent to share health information, health care providers mentioned multiple methods such as written ($n = 256$; 67 %; 95 % CI: 62–72), verbal ($n = 160$; 42 %; 95 % CI: 37–47) and biometric approval ($n = 46$; 12 %; 95 % CI: 9–16).

Respondents were asked about the secondary use of registry data for research purposes. Ninety-four percent of countries ($n = 46$; 95 % CI: 83–99), according to public health officials, indicated that researchers could request access to the data whereas only 63 % ($n = 31$; 95 % CI: 18–45) reported that internal health personnel could obtain access. In 61 % ($n = 30$) of countries (95 % CI: 46–75), the general public could apply to use national health data for research purposes.

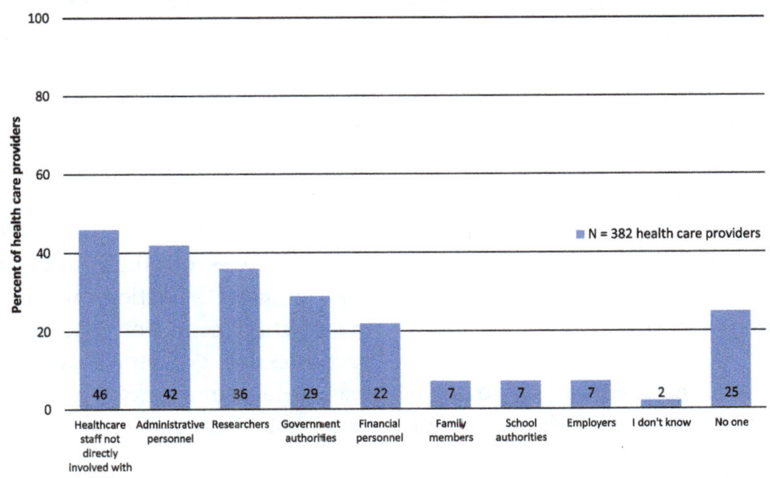

Fig. 1 Access to patient health records without patient consent. Legend: Percent of responding health care providers indicating access to patient health care records without consent, by category

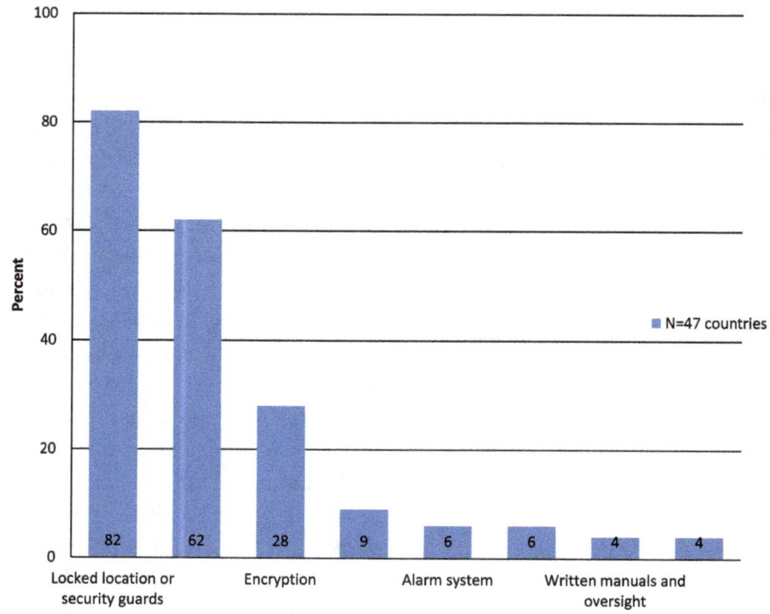

Fig. 2 Data security safeguards. Legend: Percent of countries, based on public health official survey

Data security

Security measures designed to protect health information are categorized as physical, technical, or administrative safeguards. Data security questions in the public health official survey were only answered by individuals indicating that they worked in data management by using a skip logic question before this section ($n = 47$). According to their responses, most countries still rely on traditional physical safeguards typically used for paper systems such as locked buildings and security guards (Fig. 2). Alarm systems were reported by very few countries ($n = 3$; 6 %; 95 % CI: 1–18)). Nine percent of countries ($n = 4$; 95 % CI: 2–20) have no physical safeguards at all. The use of passwords to access data and files was the most commonly reported technical safeguard noted by public health officials in 62 % of the countries ($n = 29$; 95 % CI: 46–75). Encryption - a method of protecting data in transit that converts data into another form that can only be understood by authorized parties - was reported in use by 27 % of countries ($n = 13$; 95 % CI: 16–43). Restricted access, considered an administrative security measure, was reported in 89 % of countries ($n = 42$; 95 % CI: 79–98). Very few countries reported the use of written security manuals or monitoring committees.

Another strategy to ensure data security is to store health data separately from unique identifier codes or numbers. According to public health officials, among countries that stored individual level data ($n = 37$), approximately half ($n = 18$; 49 %; 95 % CI: 32–66)) indicated that data and codes were stored together, 35 % stored data and codes separately ($n = 13$; 95 % CI: 20–53), and 16 % reported that they did not know how data was stored ($n = 6$; 95 % CI: 6–32).

Among health care providers, 63 % ($n = 236$; 95 % CI: 58–68) indicated that they were comfortable with the privacy and security of storing their own health records at the facility in which they worked, one-quarter reported feeling very comfortable and 20 % ($n = 73$; 95 % CI: 16–24) reported feeling very or slightly uncomfortable. Upon closer examination, individual comfort level was associated with the presence of security safeguards such as locked buildings or security guards ($p < .0001$) and password protection ($p < .0028$). Of note, Rwanda stood out as an exemplary country given that all 20 respondents selected the highest level of comfort with regard to storing their personal health information at their work facility.

Discussion

Privacy

The majority of countries have national constitutions that address individual privacy [38] and, similarly, medical professional codes of ethics, international instruments (i.e., the Helsinki Declaration) and the Hippocratic oath embrace patient confidentiality. In addition, a regulation impact assessment of ten African countries documented that many legal frameworks recognize and protect an individual's right to privacy [58]. Data privacy law, for example, may fall under both civil codes and telecommunication legislation.

Although the survey questions did not specify data privacy legislation, a comparison of the respondents answering that their country had general privacy legislation indicates that a much smaller fraction have actually passed comprehensive data privacy legislation, i.e., legislation that specifically regulates various stages of the processing of personal data with the principal object of safeguarding privacy (57). Data privacy legislation has been passed in more than 100 countries worldwide based on numerous sources including books [59], reports [58, 60], published articles [61, 62], online web pages [63] and international law directories [64–66], but further analysis reveals that only 21 % of these countries are among the 75 high burden countries identified by CoIA countries. In other words, of the 106 countries that have successfully passed data privacy laws, 22 are among those with the highest burden. Pending data privacy legislation is currently under consideration in ten additional high burden countries signifying a growing trend [58, 61].

In addition to the importance of the adoption of data privacy laws in high burden countries, data privacy is a process that involves data protection regimes and enforcement bodies to regulate compliance [67]. Although neither survey addressed this issue, it is worth noting that there is pressure from Europe to introduce data privacy regimes that meet the adequacy standards set by the European Data Protection Directive 95/46/EC. Thus, data privacy law is part of a larger process requiring attention to enforcement by data protection authorities. Given that this survey only assessed one aspect of data privacy, a more thorough evaluation is needed of the impact of data privacy legislation on public health officials' and health care providers' experiences.

Access

The high proportion of the 76 high burden countries reporting individual access to their own personal health data suggests that many of these countries have legally enshrined their value of patients' rights and autonomy. Findings concerning access to patient records, however, indicate that a substantial number of actors outside of the health system have access to medical records without patient consent. In particular, access to patient medical records by government authorities, for example, may have significant privacy implications for women. Access to registry data by government authorities, law enforcement, and or the judicial system may threaten women's privacy and hinder registry participation for fear of self-incrimination as discussed in Frame 2 on Brazil's pregnancy registration law. The potential violation of confidentiality, considered the core of the physician-patient privilege, may prompt women to avoid formal health systems in favor of less regulated options.

Frame 2: Brazil's pregnancy registration law

The Brazilian Ministry of Health's enactment of a health law establishing a national pregnancy registration system raises important lessons regarding issues that can seriously impact public trust. The presumed impetus for Brazil's registry law was the 2011 case, *Alyne v Brazil* that was brought before the UN Committee on the Elimination of Discrimination against Women Committee by the Center for Reproductive Health Rights and Advocacia Cidadã pelos Direitos Humanos on behalf of the Brazilian woman's family that died during childbirth due to allegedly inadequate maternal health care [68]. Ruling in favor of the deceased's family, Brazil was found in violation of international obligations to provide adequate access to maternal health care and urged to take steps to remedy their system.

On December 26, 2011, Brazil's president passed an emergency Provisional Measure 557, the 'National System for Registration, Surveillance and Monitoring of Pregnant and Postpartum Women for the Prevention of Maternal Mortality.' The timing sidestepped congressional approval suggesting anticipated opposition. The stated aim of the statute was to improve access, coverage, and quality of maternal health care in order to reduce Brazil's high number of maternal deaths.

The main point of contention is the obligatory nature of participation combined with the potential for self- incrimination if a pregnant woman elects to terminate her pregnancy [69]. Brazil's restrictive abortion law only allows abortions when the mother's life is in danger, the pregnancy is the result of rape, or severe genetic abnormalities are detected. Consequently, a woman is subject to prosecution if she terminates her pregnancy. The discord between Brazil's abortion law with mandatory universal pregnancy registration poses obvious challenges given that the legal parameters of the pregnancy registry include compulsory participation without informed consent or opt-out options [70]. While it may be argued that health registries legitimately perform best with universal participation and implied consent, the obligatory nature of Brazil's system is not counterbalanced by legal provisions that protect a woman from incrimination or ensure optimal health care.

One solution is to restrict the use of registry data aside from the intended purpose for public health. This can be achieved by clearly stating the registry purpose in a legal mandate with parameters that prevent personal health information from being used to incriminate participants in a court of law. Despite the proclaimed intention of MP 557 to reduce maternal deaths, the unintended consequence may be an increase in maternal deaths due to avoidance of early prenatal care or an increase in unsafe abortion procedures. The structure of MP 557 ultimately erodes the essential trust between women and health care providers.

Consequently, women may choose to not seek medical care in order to avoid being registered. Thus, not protecting women's privacy undermines public trust and may result in reduced public support for health registries.

Security

Security is defined as strategies such as safeguards, policies, or protocols through which access or sharing of patient health information by stakeholders is controlled and protected from intentional or unintentional disclosure to unauthorized persons, and from loss, destruction or alternation [40]. Security controls applied to electronic data can take many forms including anonymity techniques, encryption, authentication systems, access control models, access policies, user roles, audit logs, and education and training of employees [71].

As reported by public health officials, the physical, administrative, and technical data security safeguards currently in use do not appear to adequately safeguard women's and children's highly sensitive health information. A common assumption is that since electronic information systems are in a nascent stage in many LMICs [72], the skills to access systems unlawfully are similarly underdeveloped. Yet, this discounts potential threats from outside a country [73]. Such general skepticism of potential threats may reflect an overall lack of concern and subsequent inaction by many e- and mHealth projects in LMICs. Moreover, data and information security is maintained differently in resource-constrained countries given the limited ICT capacity, training, and resources. As a result, privacy and security issues have not received the same attention in countries with emerging electronic health systems. In addition, a workforce inexperienced or untrained in safe data practices may not fully appreciate the far-reaching implications of security breaches.

Another rationale for not prioritizing security issues is the notion that health needs outweigh privacy concerns in LMIC countries [46]. Moreover, there may be a presumption that it is too premature to address these issues prior to security legislation or regulation being adopted. The potential for harm and unintended consequences of ignoring legal and ethical issues, however, is considerable on both an individual and societal level. Compromising the privacy of an individual's sensitive health information can have devastating consequences for the individual and his/her family and on a larger scale, could undermine trust in electronic health information systems in general thereby undercutting efforts to improve health.

Implications for practice and future research

Initiating eRegistries for women and children into countries with the greatest need necessitates due diligence to ensure that the ethical and legal considerations are attended to in order to protect women and children's health data. The current gaps in protections for privacy and data security suggest that internal governance should be crafted to address these issues. Future research should continue to investigate the influence of culture, literacy rates, privacy, infrastructure and capacity in LMICs [36]. A notable challenge of developing guidance in a global context is the inherent diversity in how countries approach law, ethics, and health. Cultural beliefs and religious practices may significantly influence approaches to confidentiality, privacy, and security [67].

A country's legal, ethical, and cultural parameters will also affect the processes, priorities, and policies that are developed as noted in the Palestine experience in Frame 3 [74]. Thus, it is essential to carefully evaluate and assess the legal, regulatory, ethical, social, and cultural environment and adapt guidance accordingly. Transplanting legal language or documentation from one country to another can be problematic. Country-level policies should be rooted in their own social and institutional fabric as translated adaptations are typically not able to embrace subtle social and cultural mores that can negatively impact acceptance and compliance.

Frame 3: Mapping Palestine's legal landscape for an MCH eRegistry

Presently, Palestine is in the process of establishing and implementing an eRegistry for maternal and child health in the absence of formal legislation or presidential decree. Due to the unresolved and unpredictable political situation and historically overlapping legal traditions, navigating the Palestinian legal system is complicated. The Palestinian Basic Law (passed in 2002 and amended in 2003 and 2005) functions as a temporary constitution while the Palestinian Legislative Council (i.e., Parliament) is the legislative branch with limited ability to act or govern.

Mapping the legal, regulatory, and ethical landscape using a global situation analysis tool tailored for the Palestinian context was the first step taken to identify gaps and actions necessary to ensure an ethical and lawful framework for an eRegistry for maternal and child health. The mapping exercise revealed that Palestine has limited legislation relevant to health registries. Palestine's civil registration law enacted in 1966 and amended in 2001, according to a UN technical report, for example, is relevant to health registries.

Palestine does not have a specific data privacy law although provisions in the Penal Law No. 16 of 1960 indicate that disclosing confidential information is unlawful and can result in imprisonment for up to three years. As well, there is mention of honoring data confidentiality and individuals' privacy in Article 4 of the General Statistics Law (2000) [66]. Although there are no health registry laws in place, the Public Health Law (2004) does address general maternal and child health issues in Articles 4 and 5 [75].

Ensuring that data security, data protection and women's privacy are fully protected in the eRegistry poses challenges given this legal environment but also provides opportunities to recommend comprehensive governance structures accompanied by robust national protocols and guidelines. Technical solutions embedded in the eRegistry platform, like the 'privacy by design' framework developed in Canada [51] ensure privacy through de-identification strategies as well as regulate access through authorization protocols, encrypt health information to assure anonymity, and address insider threats to data privacy via auditing strategies. Local and customary patient-provider practices and relationships as well as social norms must also be considered in order to develop culturally competent approaches.

Conceptually, these efforts have recently been described in terms of data stewardship that contribute to a 'chain of trust' [76] that can facilitate good will and public trust. Depicting this process as a successive set of steps reinforces the importance of maintaining communication with stakeholders regarding the responsibilities of data stewardship of women's health information.

Strengths and limitations

There are advantages and challenges inherent to web-based surveys. Advantages include timeliness, cost, and viability of obtaining responses from a global target group. Web-based recruitment strategies facilitated achieving a large number of responses from a diverse set of countries which is one strength of the study. Variability in the number of responses from each country, however, limits generalizability. Given that survey participation relied on internet access, some individuals may not have participated due to poor or unavailable internet connectivity thus limiting representativeness. Survey responses with a high proportion of missing values were not included in the analysis. Finally, external validation of survey items was challenging due to the evolving state of data privacy policies and regulations in LMICs. Despite these limitations, the study explores compelling issues that merit further inquiry.

Conclusion

Reflecting on the essential elements for health registries, one researcher commented that the "confidentiality and ethical issues can often decide the success of the registry [77]." Privacy and security woven into health registry systems must bolster public trust, promote adoption, and maintain individual confidentiality. Data should not be used in a way that compromises a patient's rights to confidentiality and privacy. Given the value, opportunity, and potential of maternal and child health registry data to contribute to improved maternal and child health, it is imperative to address privacy by building in core principles and protocols combined with oversight and accountability mechanisms [51]. This research hopes to shed light on the challenge of balancing individual privacy without deterring responsible data use. The field must invest in better defining and understanding risk while at the same time not losing sight of the public good and practical potential of maximizing health data analysis. The transition from the MDG to the SDGs, learning from early experiences in implementing eRegistries, and a maturing approach to protecting privacy and security in a digital age, provides a unique opportunity for both vision and responsible engagement. Underlying efforts to leverage innovation and new technology, as in all other movements to improve health, is the responsibility to respect universal human rights.

Abbreviations

CoIA: Commission on Information and Accountability for Women's and Children's Health; ICT: Information and communication technology; LMIC: Low and middle income country; MCH: Maternal and child health; MDG Millennium Development Goal; MMR: Maternal mortality ratio; RMNCH: Reproductive, maternal, newborn, and child health; SDG: Sustainable Development Goal; UN: United Nations; USAID: United States Agency for International Development; WHO: World Health Organization

Acknowledgements

The authors wish to express their appreciation for Ingrid K. Friberg's contribution to the data analysis and Jagrati Jani-Bølstad's editorial comments throughout the manuscript editing process. We also are grateful for Steve French and Ameha Dammena Wudie's significant contributions to the survey development and recruitment process. Finally, the authors express their gratitude to the survey participants for providing valuable input for this paper. The views expressed in this article do not necessarily represent the decisions, policy, or views of the authors' affiliations.

Funding

The Norwegian Agency for Development Cooperation (Norad) funded the harmonized Reproductive Health Registries project (GLO-4279 QZA 12/0355 harmonized Reproductive Health Registries) that led to the eRegistries Initiative (QZA-14/0022 Every Mother and Child Counts). This was led in partnership by the Norwegian Institute of Public Health and the WHO Department for Reproductive Health and Research, with Queensland University (Australia), the University of Oxford (UK), and the Health Information Systems Program (Vietnam).
The contribution by JFF was supported in part by the Centre for Intervention Science in Maternal and Child Health (CISMAC; project number 223269), which is funded by the Research Council of Norway through its Centers of Excellence scheme and the University of Bergen, Norway.

Authors' contributions

SM led the survey design and recruitment and contributed to the conception, design, and drafting of the paper. JK was involved in the design and revision of the manuscript. All authors contributed to the content of the paper, read, and approved the final version.

Competing interests

The authors declare that they have no competing interests.

Author details
[1]Department of International Public Health, Norwegian Institute of Public Health, P.O. Box 4404, Nydalen N-0403, Oslo, Norway. [2]Centre for Health, Law and Emerging Technologies, Nuffield Department of Population Health, University of Oxford, Rosemary Rue Building, Old Road Campus, Headington, Oxford OX3 7LF, UK. [3]Department of Private Law, Faculty of Law, University of Oslo, Postboks 6706St Olavs plass, 0130 Oslo, Norway. [4]Department of Informatics, University of Oslo, Gaustadalléen 23 B, N-0373 Oslo, Norway. [5]Palestinian National Institute of Public Health, Qaddoura Street, Ministry of Health Building, 1st Floor, Postbox 54812, Ramallah, Palestine. [6]School of Advanced International Studies, Johns Hopkins University, 1717 Massachusetts Ave, NW, Washington, DC 20036, USA. [7]HealthEnabled, Unit D11, Westlake Square, Westlake Drive, Westlake, Cape Town, South Africa7945. [8]Centre for Intervention Science in Maternal and Child Health, University of Bergen, Postbox 780005020 Bergen, Norway.

References

1. By Counting Every Life, Every Life Counts. [http://www.worldbank.org/en/news/feature/2014/06/23/by-counting-every-life-every-life-counts]. Accessed 15 Sept 2015.
2. Lu Y, Nakicenovic N, Visbeck M, Stevence A. Five priorities for the UN sustainable development goals. Nature. 2015;520.
3. Handley K, Boerma T, Victora C, Evans TG. An inflection point for country health data. Lancet Global Health. 2015;3(8):e437–8.
4. AbouZahr C, de Savigny D, Mikkelsen L, Setel PW, Lozano R, Lopez AD. Towards universal civil registration and vital statistics systems: the time is now. Lancet. 2015;386(10001):1407–18.
5. AbouZahr C, de Savigny D, Mikkelsen L, Setel PW, Lozano R, Nichols E, Notzon F, Lopez AD. Civil registration and vital statistics: progress in the data revolution for counting and accountability. Lancet. 2015;386(10001):1373–85.
6. The Lancet. CRVS systems: a cornerstone of sustainable development. Lancet. 2015;385(9981):1917.
7. Chan MKM, Lob-Levyt J, Obaid T, Schweizer J, Sidibe M, et al. Meeting the demand for results and accountability: a call for action on health data from eight global health agencies. PLoS Med. 2010;7(1):e1000223.
8. USAID, World Bank Group, WHO. The Roadmap for Health Measurement and Accountability. Washington, DC: MA4Health; 2015.
9. Chan M. From new estimates to better data. Lancet. 2012;380(9859):2054.
10. Kim JY. Data for better health—and to help end poverty. Lancet. 2012; 380(9859):2055.
11. United Nations. A World that Counts: Mobilising the data revolution for sustainable development. New York: United Nations; 2014. http://www.undatarevolution.org/wpcontent/uploads/2014/11/A-World-That-Counts.pdf. Accessed 15 Sept 2015.
12. Gates M. Measure for measure: we can make dramatic progress in lowering maternal mortality – but we need better data, and more of it. In: Foreign policy. 2013.
13. Gates M. Bridging the gender gap: how big data can improve the lives of a billion women and girls. In: Foreign policy. 2013.
14. Frøen JF, Myhre SL, Frost MJ, Chou D, Mehl G, Say L, Chang S, Fjeldheim I, Friberg IK, French SD et al. eRegistries: electronic registries for maternal and child health. BMC Pregnancy Childbirth. 2015;16(1).
15. Flenady V, Wojcieszek AM, Fjeldheim I, Friberg IK, Nankabirwa V, Jani-Bølstad J, Myhre S, Middleton P, Crowther C, Ellwood D et al. eRegistries: indicators for the WHO essential interventions for reproductive, maternal, newborn and child health. BMC Pregnancy Childbirth. 2016; (accepted).
16. Kendall T, Langer A. Critical maternal health knowledge gaps in low- and middle-income countries for the post-2015 era. Reprod Health. 2015;12:55.
17. Labrique AB, Pereira S, Christian P, Murthy N, Bartlett L, Mehl G. Pregnancy registration systems can enhance health systems, increase accountability and reduce mortality. Reprod Health Matters. 2012;20(39):113–7.
18. Goudar SS, Carlo WA, McClure EM, Pasha O, Patel A, Esamai F, Chomba E, Garces A, Althabe F, Kodkany B, et al. The maternal and newborn health registry study of the global network for women's and children's health research. Int J Gynaecol Obstet. 2012;118(3):190–3.
19. Attaran A. An immeasurable crisis? A criticism of the millennium development goals and why they cannot be measured. PLoS Med. 2005;2(10):e318.
20. Vega J. Universal health coverage: the post-2015 development agenda. Lancet. 2013;381(9862):179–80.
21. Dreyer N, Garner S. Registries for robust evidence. JAMA. 2009;302(7):790–1.
22. Hodge J, Gostin LO, Jacobsen PD. Legal issues concerning electronic health information: privacy, quality, and liability. JAMA. 1999;282(15):1466–71.
23. Barrows RC, Clayton PD. Privacy, confidentiality, and electronic medical records. J Am Med Inform Assoc. 1996;3(2):139–48.
24. Ozair FFJN, Sharma A, Aggarwal P. Ethical issues in electronic health records: a general overview. Perspect Clin Res. 2015;73–6.
25. Spriggs M, Arnold MV, Pearce CM, Fry C. Ethical questions must be considered for electronic health records. J Med Ethics. 2012;38(9):535–9.
26. Williamson OD, Cameron PA, McNeil JJ. Medical registry governance and patient privacy. Med J Aust. 2004;181(3):125–6.
27. Principles for digital development [http://digitalprinciples.org/]. Accessed 1 Sept 2015.
28. National Committee on Vital and Health Statistics. Toolkit for communities using health data: How to collect, use, protect, and share data responsibly. Hyattsville, Maryland, 2015.
29. Data Collection in Humanitarian Response: A guide for incorporating protection [http://pqdl.care.org/Practice/Data%20Collection%20in%20Humanitarian%20Response,%20A%20Guide%20for%20Incorporating%20Protection.pdf]. Accessed 1 Sept 2015.
30. Gliklich R, Dreyer N, Leavy M, editors. Registries for evaluating patient outcomes: a user's guide (3rd edition). Rockville: Agency for Healthcare Research and Quality; 2014.
31. Aymé S, Kole A, Rodwell C. Rare Diseases Task Force Report on Patient registries the field of rare diseases: overview of the issues surrounding the establishment, governance and financing of academic registries. 2011. [http://www.eucerd.eu/?post_type=document&p=1218]. Accessed 1 Sept 2015.
32. de Abajo Iglesias F, Grande Feito L, Júdez Gutiérrez J, Concepción M, Arribas M, Terracini B, Pampols Ros T, Campos Castelló J, Martín Uranga A, Abascal Alonso M, et al. Ethical guidelines governing the creation and use of registries for biomedical research purposes. 2007;1–52. [http://www.isciii.es/ISCIII/es/contenidos/fd-el-instituto/fdorganizacion/fd-estructura-directiva/fd-subdireccion-general-servicios-aplicados-formacion-investigacion/fd-centros-unidades/fd-instituto-investigacion-enfermedadesraras/Directrices_Registros_web.pdf]. Accessed 1 Sept 2015.
33. The eRegistries Governance Guidance Toolkit. [https://www.fhi.no/globalassets/dokumenterfiler/eeregistries/eregistries-lp-3-eregistries-governance-guidance-toolkit-06.08.16.pdf]. Accessed 16 Aug 2016.
34. Tovi MD, Muthama MN, Mutua NM. Addressing the challenges of data protection in developing countries. Eur J Comput Sci Inf Technol. 2013;1(2):1–9.
35. Lucas H. Information and communications technology for future health systems in developing countries. Soc Sci Med. 2008;66(10):2122–32.
36. Were MC, Meslin EM. Ethics of implementing electronic health records in developing countries: points to consider. AMIA Annu Symp Proc. 2011;2011: 1499–505.
37. WHO and ITU. eHealth and Innovation in Women's and Children's Health: a baseline review based on the findings of the 2013 survey of CoIA countries. Geneva: World Health Organization; 2014.
38. WHO. Legal frameworks for eHealth: based on the findings of the second global survey on eHealth. Global observatory for eHealth series, vol. 5. Geneva: World Health Organization; 2012.
39. mHealth Alliance, TrustLaw Connect. Patient privacy in a mobile world: a framework to address privacy law issues in mobile health. London: Thomson Reuters Foundation; 2014. [http://www.trust.org/contentAsset/raw-data/03172beb-0f11-438e-94be-e02978de3036/file]. Accessed 1 Sept 2015.
40. Omary Z, Lupiana D, Mtenzi F, Wu B. Analysis of the challenges affecting e-healthcare adoption in developing countries: a case study of Tanzania. Int J Inf Stud. 2010;2(1):38–50.
41. Juma K, Nahason M, Apollo W, Gregory W, Patrick O. Current status of e-health in Kenya and emerging global research trends. Int J Inf Commun Technol Res. 2012;2(1):50–4.
42. Privacy International. Privacy and human rights: an international survey of privacy laws and practice. 2010. [http://gilc.org/privacy/survey/]. Accessed 1 Sept 2015.
43. Makulilo AB. Privacy and data protection in Africa: a state of the art. Int Data Privacy Law. 2012;2(3):163–78.
44. Norman ID, Aikins MK, Binka FN. Ethics and electronic health information

technology: challenges for evidence-based medicine and the physician-patient relationship. Ghana Med J. 2011;45(3):115–24.
45. Hosein G, Nyst C. Aiding surveillance: an exploration of how development and humanitarian aid initiatives are enabling surveillance in developing countries. In: Social Science Electronic Publishing. 2013.
46. Policy Engagement Network. Electronic health privacy and security in developing countries and humanitarian operations. In: Protecting medical information in eHealth projects. London: London School of Economics and Political Science; 2010. p. 1–28.
47. UN General Assembly, Universal Declaration of Human Rights, 10 December 1948, 217A (III), 3rd Sess, Supp No 13, UN Doc A/810 at 71. [http://www.refworld.org/docid/3ae6b3712c.html]. Accessed 1 Sept 2015.
48. UN General Assembly, International Covenant on Civil and Political Rights. 16 December 1966, United Nations, Treaty Series, vol. 999, p. 171. [http://www.refworld.org/docid/3ae6b3aa0.html]. Accessed 1 Sept 2015.
49. European Court of Human Rights. I v Finland no. 20511/03. In: Edited by The European Court of Human Rights; 17 July 2008.
50. Cybersecurity guide for developing countries. Geneva: International Telecommunication Union, 2007. [http://www.itu.int/ITU-D/cyb/publications/2007/cgdc-2007-e.pdf]. Accessed 1 Sept 2015.
51. Pencarrick Hertzman C, Meagher N, McGrail KM. Privacy by design at population data BC: a case study describing the technical, administrative, and physical controls for privacy-sensitive secondary use of personal information for research in the public interest. J Am Med Inform Assoc. 2013;20(1):25–8.
52. Kaye J. From single biobanks to international networks: developing e-governance. Hum Genet. 2011;1–6.
53. European Commission. Biobanks for Europe - a challenge for governance. Luxembourg: Publications Office of the European Union; 2012.
54. Commission on Information and Accountability in Maternal and Child Health. Keeping promises, measuring results. Geneva: World Health Organization; 2011.
55. Rahim HFA, Wick L, Halileh S, Hassan-Bitar S, Chekir H, Watt G, Khawaja M. Maternal and child health in the occupied Palestinian territory. Lancet. 2009; 373(9667):967–77.
56. Kaye J, Myhre S, Bell J, Mitchell M, Phillips A. The eRegistries governance guidance toolkit. 2015. Retrieved on 18 August 2016 from https://www.fhi.no/globalassets/dokumenterfiler/eregistries/eregistries-lp-3-eregistries-governance-guidance-toolkit_06.08.16.pdf.
57. Myhre SL, Jani-Bølstad J, Friberg IK, Frøen JF. The status of maternal, and child health registries in high burden countries. Retrieved on 1 Sept 2015 from www.eregistries.org.
58. Townsend B. mHealth regulation impact assessment Africa. In: GSM Association, editor. Mobile for development mHealth. 2015.
59. Bygrave L. Data privacy law: an international perspective. Oxford: Oxford University Press; 2014.
60. Rich C. Privacy laws in Africa and the Middle East. In: The Bureau of National Affairs, editor. Privacy and security law report. Bloomberg: BNA; 2014.
61. Greenleaf G. Sheherezade and the 101 data privacy laws: origins, significance and global trajectories. J Law Inf Sci. 2014;23(1):EAP1–46.
62. Greenleaf G. China's incremental data privacy law: MIIT 'user data protection' regulations. In: Privacy laws & business international report, UNSW law research paper No 2014–07. 2013.
63. Data Privacy Law: Internet, Policy and Information Law from Latin America. Retrieved on 1 Sept 2015 from [http://www.dataprivacylaws.com.ar/data-protectionagencies/].
64. DLA Piper. Data Protection Laws of the World Handbook, Third Edition [https://www.dlapiper.com/en/global/insights/publications/2014/01/data-protection-laws-of-theworld-handbook/]. Accessed 10 Sept 2015.
65. International Compendium of Data Privacy Laws. Retrieved 10 Sept 2015 from [http://www.bakerlaw.com/files/Uploads/Documents/Data%20Breach%20documents/International-Compendium-of-Data-Privacy-Laws.pdf].
66. Global Data Privacy Directory. Retrieved 1 Sept 2015 from [http://www.nortonrosefulbright.com/files/global-data-privacy-directory-52687.pdf]
67. Makulilo AB. Data protection regimes in Africa: too far from the European 'adequacy' standard? Int Data Privacy Law. 2013;3(1):42–50.
68. Chilton A, Gorlach I. Recent developments in health law. J Law Med Ethics. 2012;40(3):696–704.
69. Kane G. Brazil's insidious new pregnancy registration law violates the privacy of women. In: Slate. January 6, 2012. Retrieved 1 Sept 2015 from http://www.slate.com/blogs/xx_factor/2012/01/06/brazilian_pm_557_how_the_pregnancy_registration_law_violates_the_privacy_of_women.html
70. Wells M. Pregnant and desperate in evangelical Brazil. In: Foreign policy. February 18, 2015. Retrieved 1 Sept 2015 from http://foreignpolicy.com/2015/02/18/brazilabortion-dilma-catholic/.
71. Fernández-Alemán JL, Señor IC, Lozoya PÁO, Toval A. Security and privacy in electronic health records: a systematic literature review. J Biomed Inform. 2013;46(3):541–62.
72. Vital Wave Consulting. Health Information Systems in Developing Countries. Palo Alto, California: Vital Wave Consulting; 2009. [http://www.minsa.gob.pe/ogei/conferenciaops/recursos/43.pdf]. Accessed 10 Sept 2015.
73. Hosein G. Privacy and developing countries. Privacy research papers. Canada: Office of the Privacy Commissioner of Canada; 2011. p. 1–21.
74. Luna D, Otero C, Marcelo A. Health informatics in developing countries: systematic review of reviews. Contribution of the IMIA working group health informatics for development. Yearb Med Inform. 2013;8(1):28–33.
75. Palestinian Legislative Council. Public health law. Palestine, April 23, 2005. Retrieved on 1 Sept 2015 from http://www.hdip.org/public%20health%20law%20English.pdf.
76. Bloomrosen M, Detmer D. Advancing the framework: use of health data—a report of a working conference of the American medical informatics association. J Am Med Inform Assoc. 2008;15(6):715–22.
77. Evatt B. World federation of hemophilia guide to developing a national patient registry. Montreal: World Federation of Hemophilia; 2005.

Does mobile phone ownership predict better utilization of maternal and newborn health services?

Juan Nie[1,2,3,5], Jennifer Anna Unger[3,4], Susan Thompson[3,5], Marisa Hofstee[3], Jing Gu[1,2*] and Mary Anne Mercer[3,5]

Abstract

Background: Increasingly popular mobile health (mHealth) programs have been proposed to promote better utilization of maternal, newborn and child health services. However, women who lack access to a mobile phone are often left out of both mHealth programs and research. In this study, we determine whether household mobile phone ownership is an independent predictor of utilization of maternal and newborn health services in Timor-Leste.

Methods: The study included 581 women aged 15–49 years with a child under the age of two years from the districts of Manufahi and Ainaro in Timor-Leste. Participants were interviewed via a structured survey of knowledge, practices, and coverage of maternal and child health services, with additional questions related to ownership and utilization of mobile phones. Mobile phone ownership was the exposure variable, and the dependent variables included having at least four antenatal care visits, skilled birth attendance, health facility delivery, a postnatal checkup within 24 h, and a neonatal checkup within 24 h for their youngest child. Logistic regression models were applied to assess for associations.

Results: Sixty-seven percent of women reported having at least one mobile phone in the family. Women who had a mobile phone were significantly more likely to be of higher socioeconomic status and to utilize maternal and newborn health services. However, after adjusting socioeconomic factors, household mobile phone ownership was not independently associated with any of the dependent variables.

Conclusion: Evaluations of the effects of mHealth programs on health in a population need to consider the likelihood of socioeconomic differentials indicated by mobile phone ownership.

Keywords: mHealth, Mobile phone ownership, Maternal, newborn, and child health, Health services

Abbreviations: ANC, Antenatal Care; CATCH, Core Assessment Tool on Child Health; DHS, Demographic and Health Survey; HAI, Health Alliance International; KPC, Knowledge, Practices and Coverage; LMIC, Low and Middle Income Countries; MDG, Millennium Development Goal; mHealth, Mobile Health; MMR, Maternal Mortality Ratio; MNCH, Maternal, Newborn, and Child Health; NNC, Neonatal Care; PCA, Principal Component Analysis; PNC, Postnatal Care; SBA, Skilled Birth Attendants; SDG, Sustainable Development Goal; USAID, United States Agency for International Development

* Correspondence: gujing5@mail.sysu.edu.cn
[1]School of Public Health, Sun Yat-sen University, No. 74 Zhongshan 2nd Road, Guangzhou 510080, People's Republic of China
[2]Sun Yat-sen Global Health Institute, Sun Yat-sen University, No. 74 Zhongshan 2nd Road, Guangzhou 510080, People's Republic of China
Full list of author information is available at the end of the article

Background

Maternal, newborn, and child health (MNCH) has recently attracted increased global attention. United Nations Millennium Development Goal (MDG) 4 focused on reducing the mortality of children under 5, while MDG 5 advocated global involvement in reducing the maternal mortality ratio [1, 2]. The subsequent Sustainable Development Goal for health targeted specific reductions in maternal, newborn and child health [3]. Although recent evidence indicates steady progress is being made towards these goals, maternal and neonatal mortality remain global challenges [4]. It is estimated that almost 300,000 women died of pregnancy, delivery, or postnatal complications in 2013 worldwide, with 99 % of these deaths occurring in low to middle income countries (LMIC) [5]. Annually there are approximately 3 million neonatal deaths, the majority of which occur in LMICs [6]. Although there are many factors contributing to these deaths, inadequate utilization of maternal and newborn health services remains a barrier to reducing maternal morbidity and improving newborn health. In 2012, nearly 40 million births were not attended by skilled birth personnel and only fifty-two percent of pregnant women received the recommended minimum of four antenatal care visits in developing regions [5]. Thus, additional strategies are needed to promote better utilization of health services related to pregnancy and childbirth.

The penetration of mobile phone services has provided health workers and health systems access to populations that have been difficult to reach by traditional approaches [7]. According to the International Telecommunications Union, the number of mobile cellular subscriptions will reach seven billion globally by the year of 2014, with more than three quarters of those in the developing world [8]. Mobile health (mHealth), which represents a variety of health programs utilizing mobile phones, has been increasingly applied in LMIC countries to achieve better health outcomes.

With the emergence of mHealth programs, health workers have seized opportunities to utilize mobile phones to connect health systems with pregnant women. Text messaging, as a low cost, accessible, and convenient tool for health education, medical reminders, and communication, is playing a role in promoting mutual interaction between women of reproductive age and health care providers [9]. mHealth via text messaging has also been a means of delivering health information and direct health services [10]. Recent evaluations of mHealth programs have demonstrated that various forms of text messaging can increase the utilization of antenatal care, skilled birth attendance and postnatal health services while improving customer satisfaction [11–16].

Despite the rapid development and early benefits of mHealth programs, most of these interventions focus on the population who already have mobile phones, leaving non- mobile phone owners without similar support and investigation. Although mHealth interventions have been shown to reach people in rural and remote areas [17], inequities in mobile phone access still remain [18–21]. Effective program development requires an understanding of populations without access to a mobile phone, including their health care utilization. In this study, we aim to investigate socioeconomic factors and the utilization of maternal and newborn health services among a population of postpartum women with and without access to mobile phones in rural Timor-Leste. We also explore the association between access to mobile phones and the utilization of health services related to pregnancy and childbirth among women in this setting.

Methods

Study setting

According to the 2009/2010 Demographic and Health Survey (DHS) [22], Timor-Leste has one of the highest Maternal Mortality Ratios (MMR) in the world, 557 deaths per 100,000 live births. Despite 86 % attendance by pregnant women for at least one antenatal care visit ($ANC1^+$), only 55 % complete the recommended four ANC visits ($ANC4^+$) during pregnancy [22]. Approximately 30 % of women utilize skilled birth attendants (SBA) for their delivery, and one in five births are delivered in a health facility. The majority of women (68 %) do not receive any postnatal check [22]. Mobile phones are increasingly popular among women in Timor-Leste, where in 2009 only 40 % of households owned a mobile phone [22], and by 2012 in Manufahi and Ainaro districts, where our study took place, 69 and 66 % of women respectively had a household mobile phone.

Study design

A baseline survey was conducted in February and March, 2012, in Ainaro and Manufahi districts prior to the launch of the *Liga Inan* mobile phone project of Health Alliance International (HAI) to assess the level of knowledge, practices, and health service coverage related to maternal health, and to collect information about mobile phone ownership and usage patterns in both districts. This study is a secondary data analysis of data from that baseline survey.

Data sources

Institutional Review Board approval for the study was obtained from the University of Washington Human Subjects Division, as well as from the Cabinet for Health Research and Development, an institution overseeing ethical review of all health research in Timor-Leste. Approval for a waiver of written consent was obtained because a number of women were expected to be unable to sign their names. Interviewers approached eligible women to explain the survey and ask them if they would participate, and then documented their informed consent prior to the interview (please see Additional file 1). If participants under the age of 17 were unmarried, consent from a parent/guardian was obtained. If participants under the age of 17 were married, consents were provided by themselves, as married girls between 15 or 16 were considered emancipated according to the Timor-Leste Civil Code.

The survey questionnaire was developed from the USAID's Rapid CATCH (Core Assessment Tool on Child Health) Survey [23], combined with questions retrieved from a Demographic and Health survey (DHS) that was conducted in Timor-Leste [24]. Additional questions about mobile phone use were developed by HAI project staff and tested extensively in the field. Data were collected on demographic characteristics; number and timing of antenatal care visits, birthing practices, postnatal care, and neonatal care; and ownership and utilization of mobile phones. The English questionnaire was translated into the local language of Tetun, and interviews were conducted in Tetun.

Participants

Women aged 15–49 years old with a child up to 24 months of age were eligible for the baseline survey, conducted in February and March 2012 in Ainaro and Manufahi districts. The survey employed stratified cluster sampling. In each of the 8 total subdistricts, 8 clusters of 9 households, totaling 72 households per subdistrict, were included using a standard formula for cluster survey sampling [25]. If there were two women in the household, the mother with the youngest child was interviewed. If women who met the selection criteria were absent from the house, the study team would return if possible. Sixteen eligible women were excluded from the study because they were not at home and not expected to return. If the original selected village did not contain enough participants, researchers found substitute participants from the nearest village. Seventy-two participants were enrolled in each subdistrict except for the subdistrict of Turiscai, which had 77 participants. In total, 581 women were interviewed.

Variables

Socio-demographic characteristics, mobile phone ownership, and selected maternal and newborn health services were characterized using descriptive statistics. We included demographic characteristics (age, years of schooling, household commodities, materials of the roof and floor, literacy), number of births, number of children, and travel time to the nearest health facility in the analysis. Household ownership of mobile phones was the exposure variable of interest. We coded our exposure variable as *mobile phone owners* and *non-mobile phone owners*, defined as women who did or did not have access to a mobile phone in their household. Outcome variables included *ANC4+* (defined as had antenatal care visits four or more times during last pregnancy), *SBA* (had a skilled birth attendant, such as a midwife or a doctor, deliver their last baby), *health facility delivery* (delivered their last baby at a health facility), *early postnatal care* (had a postnatal checkup by a health worker within 24 h after delivery either at a health facility, home or other location), *and early neonatal care* (had their newborn baby checked by a health worker within 24 h after the baby was born).

Original continuous data such as age, years of school, number of children, and travel time to the nearest health facility were classified into categories. Based on the methods introduced in DHS [26–29], we calculated the wealth index by compositely measuring the cumulative living standards based on household assets: electricity, radio, television, bicycle, car or truck, horse or other animal powered transport, type of roofing, and type of flooring. Principal Component Analysis (PCA) was applied to assess the factor weight of each asset. The wealth index, which is a continuous variable, was then divided into five indices, which are Highest, Fourth, Middle, Second, and Lowest levels [29].

Statistical methods

Demographic characteristics of women with a mobile phone and those who did not have a mobile phone were described by the frequency and percentage, and were compared using the chi-square test for categorical data. The chi-square test was also used in bivariate analysis to explore the relationship of independent variables, including mobile phone ownership, with utilization of maternal and newborn health services. We included independent variables that could be potential confounders to the outcomes into the logistic model, including the covariates of age, education, parity, wealth index, travel time to the nearest health facility, and literacy. Variables are selected stepwise by backward elimination from the original list, with variables that have p values less than 0.20 removed from the model. Odds ratios (OR) and 95 % confidence intervals (CI) are reported.

Data entry and sample size calculation were completed with Epi Info 7.0. We used STATA version 12.0 (StataCorp, Texas) to conduct data analysis, and set 0.05 as the significance level (alpha). The *svyset STATA* command was used to adjust cluster effects of our data collection. We weighted the results of the survey to accommodate for the difference in the population size or sample size between clusters, subdistricts, and the two program districts.

Results

Participants

A total of 581 participants from Manufahi and Ainaro districts were enrolled in the study. Three hundred and sixty four (67 %) participant households owned at least one mobile phone. Baseline characteristics of participants are shown in Table 1. The mean age of participants was 27.8 years [SD = 0.39, 95 % CI: 27.0–28.6]. About half of women (52 %) had received secondary or above education while two-thirds were capable of reading and/or writing. The majority of the women (70 %) lived within one hour of the nearest health facility, and half (49 %) had at least four children. Less than half the women, 46 %, attended their first visit before the gestational age of 3 months, and 95 % before 6 months.

Demographics and mobile phone ownership

Table 1 compares the demographic characteristics of participants according to household ownership of mobile phones. In comparison to participants without mobile phones, those with mobile phones were significantly more likely to be educated ($p = 0.000$), wealthy ($p = 0.000$), and more capable of reading and/or writing ($p = 0.000$). Women with mobile phones were also more likely to be located closer to health facilities, with a relationship of borderline significance ($p = 0.060$),

Utilization of maternal and newborn health services and mobile phone ownership

We examined the utilization of maternal and newborn health services among survey participants: ANC 4+, SBA, health facility delivery, and postnatal and neonatal care within 24 h of delivery. A majority of the participants (72 %) achieved ANC 4+. Less than half (43 %) of participants reported SBA at their last delivery, and only one-third (31 %) delivered their last baby at a health facility. Approximately one-third (31 %) of women reported receiving a postnatal checkup by a health worker within 24 h of the delivery, and 34 % reported having a postnatal checkup after 24 h of the delivery. A quarter reported bringing their baby in for a neonatal checkup within 24 h of delivery, and 39 % more than 24 h after delivery.

The unadjusted utilization rates for women who had a household mobile phone as compared to those without a phone were significantly higher for ANC 4+ (OR = 1.92; 95 % CI: 1.23–3.00; $p = 0.005$), delivering with a skilled birth attendant (OR = 2.45; 95 % CI: 1.55–3.86; $p = 0.000$), having health facility delivery (OR = 2.68; 95 % CI: 1.61–4.44; $p = 0.000$), and receiving a postnatal checkup within 24 h after delivery (OR = 2.11; 95 % CI: 1.43–3.14; $p = 0.000$) and neonatal checkup within 24 h after delivery (OR = 1.74; 95 % CI: 1.05–2.90; $p = 0.032$) (Table 2).

Table 1 Demographic characteristics of study participants

Variables	N (%) of the participants			p***
	Mobile phone owners 67 % ($N = 364$)	Non mobile phone owners 33 % ($N = 217$)	Total ($N = 581$)	
Age				0.240
≤20	47(13)	30(14)	77(13)	
21–24	69(21)	46(19)	115(20)	
25–29	121(32)	48(24)	169(29)	
30–34	66(18)	41(20)	107(19)	
≥35	61(16)	52(24)	113(19)	
Mean (year) (SD)	27.5(0.44)	28.3(0.66)	27.8(0.39)	
Education level				0.000
No	51(16)	75(39)	126(23)	
Primary	84(22)	65(28)	149(24)	
Secondary or above	229(62)	77(33)	306(52)	
Wealth Index				0.000
Lowest	45(12)	73(33)	118(19)	
Fourth	52(12)	68(34)	120(19)	
Middle	74(22)	45(20)	119(22)	
Second	92(26)	15 (6)	107(19)	
Highest	101(28)	16(6)	117(21)	
Parity				0.360
1	57(15)	33(14)	90(15)	
2–3	128(38)	74(32)	202(36)	
≥4	179(46)	110(53)	289(49)	
Health facility travel time[a]				0.060
0–60 min	261(74)	139(62)	400(70)	
>60 min	103(26)	77(38)	180(30)	
Literacy				0.000
Cannot read and write	81(25)	105(54)	186(34)	
Can read or write	283(75)	112(46)	395(66)	
District				0.640
Manufahi	172(51)	121(48)	293(50)	
Ainaro	192(49)	96(52)	288(50)	
Gestational months at 1st ANC visit[b]	345	188	533	0.090
1–3	175(48)	94(42)	269(46)	
4–6	162(49)	82(50)	244(49)	
7–9	8(3)	12(8)	20(5)	

[a] One data point is missing
[b] 533 women had at least 1 ANC visit when they had their last child
*** All p-values are produced using Chi-square test, adjusted for cluster effect

Table 2 Association between mobile phone ownership and health services related to pregnancy and childbirth

Variable	Mobile phone owners ($N = 364$)	Non mobile phone owners ($N = 217$)	Unadjusted OR 95 % CI	P	Adjusted OR 95 % CI[a]	P^{**}
Antenatal care				0.005		0.133
ANC ≥4	264(76)	136(63)	1.92(1.23,3.00)		0.74(0.51,1.09)	
ANC <4	100(24)	81(37)	Ref.		Ref.	
Skilled birth attendance				0.000		0.100
Yes	174(50)	61(29)	2.45(1.55,3.86)		1.29(0.67,2.51)	
No	190(50)	156(71)	Ref.		Ref.	
Health Facility Delivery				0.000		0.115
Yes	113(37)	33(18)	2.68(1.61,4.44)		1.13(0.56,2.28)	
No	251(63)	184(82)	Ref.		Ref.	
PNC within 24 h				0.000		—
Yes	128(36)	45(21)	2.11(1.43,3.14)		—	—
No	236(64)	172(79)	Ref.		Ref.	—
NNC within 24 h				0.032		—
Yes	100(29)	140(19)	1.74(1.05,2.90)		—	
No	264(71)	177(81)	Ref.		Ref.	

[a]Adjusted for cluster effect, and factors related to the outcomes. Factors include age, education, wealth index, parity, travel time to the nearest health facility, and literacy

[**]All p-value are produced using the maximum likelihood ratio test

The multivariate model for mobile phone ownership included parity as well as the socioeconomic variables for age of mother, education level, wealth index, travel time to the nearest health facility, and literacy. Adjusting for those variables, the relationship between mobile phone ownership and ANC4+ was not statistically significant (aOR = 0.74; 95 % CI: 0.51–1.09; $p = 0.133$), nor was there a significant association between mobile phone ownership and skilled birth attendance (aOR = 1.29; 95 % CI: 0.67–2.51; $p = 0.100$) or health facility delivery (aOR = 1.13; 95 % CI: 0.56–2.28; $p = 0.115$). In multivariate regression for early postnatal care and early neonatal care, after including all the significant covariates identified in bivariate analysis, mobile phone ownership is removed from the regression model, with a p value larger than 0.20. No significant associations were found between mobile phone ownership and early neonatal and postnatal care.

Discussion

Our findings demonstrate that women with household ownership of a mobile phone were more likely to utilize maternal and newborn health services. However, when adjusting for socioeconomic status, mobile phone ownership was not an independent predictor for antenatal care attendance, uptake of skilled birth attendance, health facility delivery, early postnatal or early neonatal care.

Women with a household mobile phone had higher socioeconomic status than those in homes without a phone. Mobile phone ownership may in fact serve as a surrogate for higher socioeconomic status, with low ownership in rural communities and among poor people [18, 20], and women with higher socioeconomic status are also more likely to utilize health services [30, 31]. Hence, women who had a mobile phone are *a priori* more likely to have greater access to health services. The 33 % of women in our study who did not have access to a mobile phone were less likely to utilize health services, and were thus most in need of the intervention.

Increasingly mHealth programs focus on the effects of interventions such as text messaging to disseminate health promotion information. Very few studies analyzed the limitations associated with unequal mobile phone access. Our findings indicate inequities related to socioeconomic status in use of maternal and newborn health services between mobile phone owners and those without a mobile phone. This is extremely important for the implementation of mHealth programs in low- or middle-income countries where unequal access to mobile phones still exists. As most mHealth programs focus on those with mobile phones, these findings support the concern that the populations without a mobile phone who are left out in the benefits of mHealth programs are actually the most in need of interventions. Even in some programs where women were given phone credit, they still could not fully benefit from the text messaging health education, or text reminders [11, 15]. Finally, supplying phones during mHealth programs or research studies is unlikely to be a sustainable approach once countries try to scale programs.

For maximum impact on the health of the general population, mHealth efforts should be integrated with other strategies to reach women who do not have access to mobile phones, such as household or community level health promotion. Strategies such as women's groups, for example, could help those without a mobile phone access health information or contact health providers using the mobile phones of their group members. Collecting information on all women including those not enrolled in mHealth programs will help to better understand the populations not eligible for these efforts.

This study also suggests that the influence of mobile phones, even for women who have them, may not be sufficient to overcome the barriers to skilled delivery care that arise from structural factors such as lack of emergency transport, inadequate financial preparation for delivery, and deficiencies in quality of obstetric health services. In this study from Timor-Leste, mobile phone ownership was not independently associated with skilled birth attendance. One of the likely reasons for that finding is that emergency transport was not widely available in Timor-Leste. The power of mobile phones to help facilitate skilled birth attendance and health facility delivery may not be adequate to overcome greater barriers such as inadequate emergency obstetric transport, long distances from a facility, and other factors such as cultural or social influences. Hence, mHealth programs need to work in parallel with other interventions to improve the quality of care and to construct well-functioning emergency obstetric transport and referral systems.

Limitations of the Study

This is the first study of which we are aware to address the inequity in maternal and newborn health services utilization among populations with and without access to a mobile phone. There are, however, limitations in our study. The survey on which the study is based did not involve questions related to the purposes of mobile phone usage, which makes it hard to explore whether these women had used their mobile phones to contact health providers, transport, or other women with experience of ANC or SBA. Another limitation lies in using mobile phone ownership as the independent variable, instead of mobile phone use. Among women in our study who reported having access to a mobile phone, only 82 % of the women reported it was their own phone, the rest using their family mobile phones. We did not examine these two groups independently and thus may not have accurately assessed the regular use of mobile phones by this population. The survey was conducted during the rainy season, and selection bias probably existed when researchers had to eliminate a few of the clusters in remote areas that were isolated by rivers and substitute some that were more accessible. In addition, interviewers did not check health care records to verify the reported care, and there was a higher level of postnatal and neonatal care reported in the survey than seen in other sources of district data.

Further studies would be useful to assess the effect of mobile phones on utilization of services, so as to better understand the mechanisms by which phone access may facilitate uptake. Additionally, qualitative research could investigate women's views on how mobile phones could help them in contacting health providers, obtaining health knowledge related to pregnancy and childbirth, or building up social connection with women who have more experiences in delivery at health facilities or with skilled birth personnel. Further study would be helpful to assess the needs of the population that is not eligible for mHealth interventions and explore available methods to reach them.

Conclusions

This study provides evidence that socioeconomic factors may be important barriers to the success of mHealth programs that focus exclusively on women having access to a mobile phone. Programs with an mHealth component will be most effective if they integrate with other interventions to also reach those who have limited or no access to mobile phones.

Acknowledgement
We would like to express our gratitude to Judith N. Wasserheit for her contribution to the conception and design of this study. Special thanks are given to staff of Health Alliance International and Catalpa International who designed and implemented the Liga Inan project in Timor-Leste. Special thanks are also given to Charles Mock, who provided professional biostatistics support in data analysis. The Liga Inan project in Manufahi and Ainaro districts is funded by the U.S. Agency for International Development.

Authors' contributions
JN performed the statistical analysis and drafted the manuscript. JU helped to draft the manuscript and revised the manuscript critically for intellectual content. ST participated in the design of the study and interpretation of the results. MH developed the questionnaire, implemented the survey, and provided critical review of the manuscript. JG formed the research questions and provided statistics methods solution for the article. MAM contributed to the conception and design of the research, interpretation of the results, and revision of the manuscript. All authors read and approved the final manuscript.

Competing interest
The authors declare that they have no competing interests.

Author details
[1]School of Public Health, Sun Yat-sen University, No. 74 Zhongshan 2nd Road, Guangzhou 510080, People's Republic of China. [2]Sun Yat-sen Global Health Institute, Sun Yat-sen University, No. 74 Zhongshan 2nd Road, Guangzhou 510080, People's Republic of China. [3]Department of Global Health, University of Washington, 1510 N.E. San Juan Road, Seattle, WA 98195-7965, USA. [4]Department of Obstetrics & Gynecology, University of Washington, Harborview Medical Center, 325 Ninth Ave, Box 359865, Seattle, WA 98104, USA. [5]Health Alliance International, 1107 NE 45th Street, Suite 350, Seattle, WA 98105, USA.

References

1. We can end poverty: United Nations Millennium Development Goals and beyond 2015. Goal 4:REDUCE CHILD MORTALITY. http://www.un.org/millenniumgoals/childhealth.shtml. Accessed 2013.
2. We can end poverty United Nations Millennium Goals and beyond 2015: GOAL 5: IMPROVE MATERNAL HEALTH. http://www.un.org/millenniumgoals/maternal.shtml; 2013.
3. United Nations A/RES/71. Transforming Our World: the 2030 Agenda for Sustainable Development. United Nations; 2015. https://sustainabledevelopment.un.org/content/documents/21252030%20Agenda%20for%20Sustainable%20Development%20web.pdf.
4. Lozano R, Wang H, Foreman KJ, Rajaratnam JK, Naghavi M, Marcus JR, Dwyer-Lindgren L, Lofgren KT, Phillips D, Atkinson C, et al. Progress towards Millennium Development Goals 4 and 5 on maternal and child mortality: an updated systematic analysis. Lancet. 2011;378(9797):1139–65.
5. Nations U. The Millennium Development Goals Report 2014. 2014. http://www.un.org/millenniumgoals/2014%20MDG%20report/MDG%202014%20English%20web.pdf. Accessed 2014.
6. Liu L, Johnson HL, Cousens S, Perin J, Scott S, Lawn JE, Rudan I, Campbell H, Cibulskis R, Li M, et al. Global, regional, and national causes of child mortality: an updated systematic analysis for 2010 with time trends since 2000. Lancet. 2012;379(9832):2151–61.
7. mHealth for development. The Opportunity of Mobile Technology for Healthcare in the Developing World. 2014. http://www.unfoundation.org/news-and-media/publications-and-speeches/mhealth-for-development-1.html. Accessed 2014.
8. Union IT. ICT facts and figures: The world in 2014. Geneva: International Telecommunications Union. 2014. http://www.itu.int/en/ITU-D/Statistics/Documents/facts/ICTFactsFigures2014-e.pdf. Accessed 2014.
9. Gentles SJ, Lokker C, McKibbon KA. Health information technology to facilitate communication involving health care providers, caregivers, and pediatric patients: a scoping review. J Med Internet Res. 2010;12(2):e22.
10. HealthyPeople.gov. 2012. Health Communication and Health Information Technology. http://www.healthypeople.gov/2020/topicsobjectives2020/overview.aspx?topicid=18. Accessed 2013.
11. Lund S, Nielsen BB, Hemed M, Boas IM, Said A, Said K, Makungu MH, Rasch V. Mobile phones improve antenatal care attendance in Zanzibar: a cluster randomized controlled trial. BMC Pregnancy Childbirth. 2014;14:29.
12. Jareethum R, Titapant V, Chantra T, Sommai V, Chuenwattana P, Jirawan C. Satisfaction of healthy pregnant women receiving short message service via mobile phone for prenatal support: A randomized controlled trial. J Med Assoc Thai. 2008;91(4):458–63.
13. Kaewkungwal J, Singhasivanon P, Khamsiriwatchara A, Sawang S, Meankaew P, Wechsart A. Application of smart phone in "Better Border Healthcare Program": a module for mother and child care. BMC Med Inform Decis Mak. 2010;10:69.
14. Tesfaye S, Barry D, Gobezayehu AG, Frew AH, Stover KE, Tessema H, Alamineh L, Sibley LM. Improving Coverage of Postnatal Care in Rural Ethiopia Using A Community-based, Collaborative Quality Improvement Approach. J Midwifery Womens Health. 2014;59 Suppl 1:S55–64.
15. Lund S, Hemed M, Nielsen BB, Said A, Said K, Makungu MH, Rasch V. Mobile phones as a health communication tool to improve skilled attendance at delivery in Zanzibar: a cluster-randomised controlled trial. Bjog. 2012;119(10):1256–64.
16. Desta BF, Mohammed H, Barry D, Frew AH, Hepburn K, Claypoole C. Use of mobile video show for community behavior change on maternal and newborn health in rural Ethiopia. Journal of Midwifery and Women's Health. 2014;59(SUPPL1):S65–72.
17. Cole-Lewis H, Kershaw T. Text messaging as a tool for behavior change in disease prevention and management. Epidemiol Rev. 2010;32(1):56–69.
18. Lester RT, Ritvo P, Mills EJ, Kariri A, Karanja S, Chung MH, Jack W, Habyarimana J, Sadatsafavi M, Najafzadeh M, et al. Effects of a mobile phone short message service on antiretroviral treatment adherence in Kenya (WelTel Kenya1): a randomised trial. Lancet. 2010;376(9755):1838–45.
19. Kaplan WA. Can the ubiquitous power of mobile phones be used to improve health outcomes in developing countries? Global Health. 2006;2:9.
20. Wesolowski A, Eagle N, Noor AM, Snow RW, Buckee CO. Heterogeneous mobile phone ownership and usage patterns in Kenya. PLoS One. 2012;7(4):e35319.
21. Forestiera E, Graceb J, Kenn C. Can information and communication technologies be pro-poor. Telecommun Policy. 2002;26:623–46.
22. National Statistics Directorate (NSD) [Timor-Leste], Ministry of Finance [Timor-Leste], and ICF Macro. 2010. Timor-Leste Demographic and Health Survey 2009-10. Dili, Timor-Leste: NSD [Timor-Leste] and ICF Macro. http://dhsprogram.com/pubs/pdf/FR235/FR235.pdf.
23. Knowledge, Practices, and Coverage Survey 2000. Rapid Core Assessment Tool on Child Health (CATCH). http://pdf.usaid.gov/pdf_docs/PNACK209.pdf. Accessed Oct 2000.
24. USAID. Questionnaires:Household, Woman's, and Man's Demographic and Health Surveys Methodology. http://dhsprogram.com/pubs/pdf/FR235/FR235.pdf. Accessed Dec 2010.
25. Bennett S, Woods T, Liyanage WM, Smith DL. A simplified general method for cluster-sample surveys of health in developing countries. World Health Stat Q. 1991;44(3):98–106.
26. Filmer D, Pritchett LH. Estimating wealth effects without expenditure data– or tears: an application to educational enrollments in states of India. Demography. 2001;38(1):115–32.
27. McKenzie JD. Measuring Inequality with Asset Indicators. J Popul Econ. 2005;18(2):229–60.
28. Vyass S, Kumaranayake L. Constructing socioeconomic status indexes: How to use principal component analysis. Health Policy Plan. 2006;21(6):459–68.
29. Mbuagbaw LC, Gofin R. A new measurement for optimal antenatal care: determinants and outcomes in Cameroon. Matern Child Health J. 2011;15(8):1427–34.
30. Barros AJ, Victora CG. Measuring coverage in MNCH: determining and interpreting inequalities in coverage of maternal, newborn, and child health interventions. PLoS Med. 2013;10(5):e1001390.
31. de Graaf JP, Steegers EA, Bonsel GJ. Inequalities in perinatal and maternal health. Curr Opin Obstet Gynecol. 2013;25(2):98–108.

21

Determinants of use of supervised delivery care under Ghana's fee exemption policy for maternal healthcare

Henrietta Asante-Sarpong[1*], Adobea Yaa Owusu[1], Sheela Saravanan[2], Ernest Appiah[1] and Mumuni Abu[3]

Abstract

Background: Improving access to supervised and emergency obstetric care resources through fee reduction/exemption maternity care initiatives has been touted as one major strategy to avoiding preventable maternal deaths. Evaluations on the effect of Ghana's fee exemption policy for maternal healthcare have largely focused on how it has influenced health outcomes and patterns of use of supervised care with little attention to understanding the main factors influencing use. This study therefore sought to explore the main individual and health system factors influencing use of delivery care services under the policy initiative in the Central Region.

Methods: A cross-sectional study was conducted using 412 mothers with children aged less than one year in one largely rural and another largely urban districts in the Central Region of Ghana from September to December 2013. Data were collected using a questionnaire survey on the socio-demographic characteristics of mothers, their knowledge and use of care under the fee free policy. Chi-square and Binary Logistic Regression tests were used to evaluate the main determinants of delivery care use under the policy.

Results: Out of the 412 mothers interviewed, 268 (65 %) reported having delivered their most recent birth under the fee exemption policy even though awareness about the policy was almost universal 401 (97.3 %) among respondents. Utilization however differed for the two study districts. Respondents in the Cape Coast Metropolis (largely urban) used delivery service more (75.7 %) than those in the largely rural Assin North Municipal area (54.4 %). Binary logistic regression results identified maternal age, parity, religion, place of residence, awareness and knowledge about the fee exemption policy for maternal healthcare as significantly associated with the likelihood of delivery care use under the policy. The likelihood of using supervised delivery care under the policy was lower for mothers aged 20–29 compared to those in the age bracket of 40–49 (Odds ratio (OR) = 0.069, $p = 0.003$). For their index (last child), mothers who already had 1, 2 or 3 births were more likely to deliver under the policy than those with five or more births.

Mothers living in urban areas were 3.79 times more likely to use delivery services under the policy than those living in rural areas (OR = 3.793, $p = 0.000$). The likelihood of using delivery services under the policy was higher for mothers who were aware and had full knowledge of the total benefit package of the policy (OR = 13.820, $p = 0.022$ and OR = 2.985, $p = 0.001$ for awareness and full knowledge respectively).

(Continued on next page)

* Correspondence: h.asarpong@arhr.org.gh; boatemaa23@yahoo.com; myboatemaa23@gmail.com
[1]Institute of Statistical Social and Economic Research, University of Ghana, P.O. Box LG 74, Legon, Accra, Ghana
Full list of author information is available at the end of the article

(Continued from previous page)

Conclusions: Delivery service use under the free maternal healthcare policy is relatively low (65 %) when compared with nearly universal awareness (97.3 %) about the policy. Factors influencing delivery service use under the policy operate at both individual and policy implementation levels. Effective interventions to improve delivery service use under the policy should target the underlying individual and health policy implementation factors identified in the study.

Keywords: Maternal deaths, Supervised care, Fee exemption policy for maternity care, Maternal healthcare

Background

Maternal mortality is a major public health problem globally but most especially in sub-Saharan Africa [1]. In Ghana, maternal mortality continues to be pervasive and improvements have been rather slow. The country's Maternal Mortality Ratio (MMR) is estimated to be 350 per 100,000 live births [1]. Investments in supervised and emergency obstetric care resources have been noted as being critical to avoiding these deaths as most deaths, occur around delivery and are caused by haemorrhage [2].

Multiple challenges however confront women's quest to access supervised care. These challenges include poor or inadequate health infrastructure, limited or unavailable medical supplies [3], adherence to negative socio-cultural beliefs and practices about pregnancy and child birth [4] and bad or non-existent transportation infrastructure to the nearest health facilities [5]. Financial challenges to accessing care have been particularly highlighted as critical to the use of supervised care [6, 7].

To address the financial challenges to accessing supervised care at birth, several counties including Ghana have adopted innovative financing mechanisms to address financial challenges to seeking care. The mechanisms introduced include fee exemptions, cash assistance, voluntary service contributions and public-private partnerships [8].

Studies on the effect of these financing mechanisms in low-and middle-income countries have focused on demand for obstetric services and healthcare expenditures. Ir, Souk and Van Damme [9] assessed the effectiveness of a Voucher Scheme introduced by the Cambodian Government in 2007 to improve access to skilled attendance for poor women in three rural health districts. The authors noted that even though the scheme had strong potential for reducing financial barriers to accessing skilled care at birth, other interventions for improving the supply of sufficient quality maternity services was necessary for the scheme to achieve its full potential [9]. In Burkina Faso Ridde, Kouanda, Bado, Bado & Haddad [10] assessed the effect of a national maternal healthcare subsidy policy on household spending on facility-based deliveries and found that the policy was very effective in reducing household costs for delivery care [10]. Ridde and Diarra [11] have also expressed the need for further attention to be given to sustainable financing mechanisms for the effective implementation of fee-exemption initiatives [11].

In 2003, the government of Ghana introduced a delivery fee exemption policy that exempts all pregnant women from paying for delivery care in public, mission and some private facilities. Otherwise known as the "free delivery policy", the policy exempts all pregnant women from paying for all normal deliveries and the management of all assisted deliveries including caesarean sections. Under the policy, women are also exempted from paying for the management of medical and surgical complications arising out of deliveries, including the repair of vesico-vaginal and recto-vaginal fistulae [12].

Similar to other studies that have been undertaken in low- and middle- income countries on maternal healthcare financing mechanisms, previous studies in Ghana have largely examined the delivery fee exemption policy in terms of how it has influenced utilisation patterns [13, 14] and healthcare expenditures [15]. Less attention has been given to understanding the driving factors influencing use within local contexts. This study therefore sought to explore the key individual and health policy implementation factors influencing use of delivery care services under Ghana's free delivery policy.

Methods

Study setting

The Central Region was selected for the study based on the following reasons: (i) the region was selected among the first four pilot regions in which the fee exemption policy for maternal deliveries was implemented in 2003. (ii) compared to the three other pilot regions (Northern, Upper East and Upper West), the Central Region has not witnessed improvements in skilled attendance rate particularly between 2008 and 2012 when services under the policy was administered through the NHIS. (iii) Contrastingly the region also has a Maternal Mortality Ratio of 520/100,000 live births [16] a ratio which is far higher than the national average of 350/100,000 live births [1].

Two districts (Cape Coast Metropolitan Area and Assin North Municipal Area) in the Central Region were purposively selected from the seventeen districts of the region for the study. The two districts compared to the others have the highest maternal mortality ratios [17]. Cape Coast Metro is also largely urban whereas Assin North is largely rural [16] a scenario that provides an opportunity to assess differences in care received under the policy within rural and urban settings.

Study participants

The primary study population was mothers of reproductive age (15–49 years) with children under one year of age. The choice of women with these characteristics was based on the study goal that aims to examine factors influencing delivery service use under the 'free maternal healthcare' policy. The target population largely serves as the potential users and benefactors of services under the policy. Secondly, mothers whose most recent birth occurred 12 months prior to the survey are most likely to recall and give a better account of their experiences.

A total of 412 mothers were selected from the study districts (Cape Coast, $n = 206$; Assin North, $n = 206$) using a combined multi-staged, stratified and simple random sampling techniques. The sample size was determined with recourse to Kish [18] since the population under study was homogeneous and the total population of mothers with at least a child under one is not known [18]. The study participants were selected from eight different localities (4 rural and 4 urban) identified from a list of all rural and urban localities in the study areas through a simple random approach. The calculated sample populations for rural and urban areas from the total sample was shared equally across the study localities as the study population was homogeneous and therefore likely to share similar views and experiences.

This was followed by the identification of households in each locality from which women were interviewed. The identification of households began with a surveillance exercise that was undertaken by the research assistants through the help of local opinion leaders and healthcare volunteers in the respective localities. Having identified households in which mothers eligible for the interviews reside, a list/sampling frame of these mothers was produced for each locality. From the sampling frame of mothers produced for each locality, a simple random approach (writing the names of each eligible respondent on pieces of papers, shaking them arbitrarily and selecting required number from the whole) was later employed to select the total number of respondents earmarked for each settlement or locality.

Data generation

Data were collected through the administration of a standardized questionnaire. The data collection exercise was undertaken concurrently in the two study districts between the months of September to December 2013. The questionnaire was administered to all 412 mothers and consisted of sections that asked questions related to their background characteristics such as age, marital status, education, religion and ethnicity, place of residence, employment status and parity.

Similar questions were asked for the background information of their spouses/partners. The other sections had questions related to their obstetric history, their knowledge and perceived need of services provided under the free delivery policy; and experiences with use of delivery care under the delivery fee exemption policy.

Study variables

The dependent variable is use of delivery services under the fee exemption policy. It was derived from the question, "Did you deliver for free under the 'free delivery policy' or you paid for delivery services?" The dependent variable was measured by using the labels 1 and 2 with 1 being 'Delivery for free' and 2, 'Delivery not for free.

The independent variables were selected with reference to what has been used in previous studies. They comprised of those related to the socio-demographic characteristics of women as well as their partners and others on the free delivery policy. The variables selected on the socio-demographic characteristics of women and their husbands/partners included age, religion, level of education, employment status, marital status, parity, place of residence and ethnicity. The variables were defined and measured as follows.

Education was defined as completed educational status and was ranked from 1 to 5 with label 1 for No formal education, 2 for primary education, 3 for Middle/Junior High School (JHS), 4 for Secondary/Senior High School (SHS)/Technical education, 5 for higher than secondary. Employment status was defined as the category of work respondents were engaged in and was ranked from 1 to 5 with 1 for 'unemployed', 2 (Self-employed), 3 (Paid employee), 4 (Paid informal worker) and 5 (Other forms of employment mostly seasonal employment). Parity referred to the total number of live births a woman had and was ranked from 1 to 5 with 1 for parity one, 2 for parity two, 3 for parity three, 4 for parity 4 and 5 for parity five and above. Place of residence was ranked 1 and 2 with 1 being Urban and 2, Rural. The marital status of respondents was ranked into three categories. Those who were currently married or cohabiting were assigned rank 1, formerly married, rank 2 and single, never married women given rank 3.

The variables for the free delivery policy were awareness about the 'free delivery' policy and knowledge about benefit package for the 'free delivery' policy. Awareness of the free delivery policy was defined as having heard about the existence of the policy and ranked 1 for a 'Yes' and 2 for a 'No'. Knowledge about the policy was also ranked as 1 and 2 with 1 referring to answering yes to having knowledge about the full benefit package of the policy and 2 for answering no to having knowledge about the policy.

Statistical analysis

The Statistical Package for the Social Sciences (SPSS) software version 20.0 was used to analyze the quantitative data. Descriptive statistics were used for frequency counts and percentage distribution of background characteristics of respondents as well as prevalence of use of delivery services under the free maternal healthcare policy. The Chi-Square test was used to test for the statistical associations between use of delivery care and other independent variables. The binary-logistic regression model was used for identifying the main determinants of use of delivery care under the fee exemption policy.

Three models containing variables of interest were fitted for the outcome variable (use of delivery care). The first model contained variables on the socio-demographic characteristics of mothers. This model was used to assess the association between their socio-demographic characteristics and use of delivery services. The second model contained variables on the demographic characteristics of the selected mothers and that of their husbands/partners. This helped to assess whether the husband's/partner's characteristics influenced the association between the background characteristics of the woman and the outcome variable. A third model containing variables on the socio-demographic characteristics of the woman as well as that of their husbands/partners and the free delivery policy was also estimated. The final model (Model 3) was used to estimate whether health policy and husbands'/partners' socio- demographic characteristic factors moderate the association between mothers' socio-demographic characteristics and delivery care use.

Results

Socio-demographic characteristics of respondents

Information collected on the socio-demographic characteristics of mothers interviewed included their age, level of education, marital status, parity, employment status, place of residence, religion and ethnicity. As shown in Table 1, majority of the mothers were within the age bracket of 20–29 years (58 %) with only 4.4 % in the age bracket of 40–49 years. A significant proportion of the respondents were married or cohabiting (87.7 %), had had some level of education (85.4 %) with those with Middle/JHS level education in the majority (39.6 %). Only 2.4 % had received tertiary level education.

In terms of ethnicity, 78.4 % of the total respondents were Akans with majority from the Fante ethnic group. The other Akan ethnic groups mentioned were Asante, Akyem and Bono. This finding was not surprising as most residents of the Central Region belong to the Fante ethnic group. Ewes were the second largest ethnic group (16 %) with mothers from other ethnic groups mostly of northern Ghana decent (Nanumba, Dagomba and Hausa) forming 3.9 % of the sample. The mothers were mostly Christians (83.6 %) with the majority (35.7 %) affiliated to Pentecostal or Charismatic churches as is the trend nationally. A greater proportion of the respondents were self-employed (58 %) and engaged mostly in trading activities with only 5.8 % engaged in formal employment. A little over half of the mothers (58.5 %) resided in urban areas with 41.5 % residing in rural localities which also reflect the national trend of increasing urban residence in Ghana. The proportion of Ghanaians living in urban areas has increased from 43.8 % in the year 2000 to 50.9 % in 2010 [16].

Determinants of delivery service use

Three binary logistic regression models were used to identify the determinants of delivery care use under the fee exemption policy. Chi-square tests were also used to assess the statistical associations between utilization and selected independent variables. More than half (65 %) of mothers interviewed delivered their most recent birth with the policy. Comparing the two districts, utilization of delivery services was rather low for the Assin North Municipal Area 54.4 % ($n = 112$) compared with 75.7 % ($n = 156$) in Cape Coast Metropolis).

From the Chi-square test results, religion (0.000), place of residence (rural/urban) (0.000), parity (0.003) and marital status (0.010) had a statistically significant association with delivery care use. Comparing the two districts, the variables that had a statistically significant relationship with utilization of delivery services in the Cape Coast Metropolis were education, marital Status, religion and parity. Religion and place of residence were significantly related to the use of delivery services in the Assin North municipal area. Maternal age, education, employment status, place of delivery and attendant at delivery did not have a statistically significant relationship with utilization of delivery care.

The results of the three binary logistic regression models are presented in Table 2. Model 1 which contains variables on the socio-demographic characteristics of the woman confirmed parity, religion, marital status and place of residence as significantly related to delivery care use under the free maternal healthcare policy.

In model 1, at $p \leq 0.05$, mothers aged 20–29 and 30–39 were 0.178 and 0.421 respectively less likely to use delivery services than those aged 40–49. The likelihood of using delivery care under the policy was lower for mothers who were married or co-habiting and mothers who were either widowed, divorced/separated compared to those who were single. Mothers who resided in urban areas were 3.57 times more likely to use delivery services under the policy than those in rural areas. Mothers with 1, 2 and 3 births had higher odds of delivering with the policy than those with five or more births. Orthodox Christians and other Christians of the Seventh Day Adventist (SDA) group and Jehovah's Witnesses were less likely to deliver

Table 1 Percentage distribution of background characteristics of respondents

Background Characteristics	Frequency	Percent
Age Group		
20–29	239	58.0
30–39	155	37.6
40–49	18	4.4
Total	412	100
Highest level of education		
Pre-school	22	5.3
Primary	108	26.2
Middle/JSS/JHS	163	39.6
Secondary/SSS/SHS/Tech/Voc	49	11.9
Higher than secondary	10	2.4
Don't know	6	1.5
No education	54	13.1
Total	412	100.0
Marital status		
Married or cohabiting	355	87.7
Divorced/separated	14	3.5
Widowed	2	0.5
Never married/never cohabited	34	8.4
Total	405	100
Religious affiliation		
Catholic	42	10.2
Anglican	4	1.0
Methodist	54	13.1
Presbyterian	16	3.9
Pentecostal/charismatics	147	35.7
Other Christian	81	19.7
Moslem	45	10.9
Traditional	4	1.0
Spiritualist	6	1.5
No religion	11	2.7
Other	2	0.5
Total	412	100.0
Employment status		
Unpaid family worker/farmer	60	16
Unemployed	5	1.3
Self-employed	218	58
Employee - formal work (paid)	42	11.2
Informal work (paid)	31	8.2
Others	20	5.3
Total	376	100.0

Table 1 Percentage distribution of background characteristics of respondents *(Continued)*

Parity		
1	125	30.3
2	109	26.5
3	65	15.8
4	35	8.5
5 and above	78	18.9
Total	412	100.0

with the policy compared to Muslims. The relationship between mother's education, ethnicity and employment status and delivery care use was not significant statistically.

Model 2 contained variables on the socio-demographic characteristics of mothers as well as that of their partners. In model 2, all the background characteristics of mothers identified as predictors of delivery service use in model 1 still remained statistically significant except for the marital status of the mother. The variables on husbands'/partners' characteristics introduced (age, education and employment status) were not statistically significant predictors of delivery service use. The introduction of the husbands'/partners' variables was however important as it helped to increase the adjusted coefficient of determination (R^2) from (0.302) in model 1 to (0.380).

Model 3 contained variables on the socio-demographic characteristics of the woman and that of the husband or partner as well as variables on the free delivery policy. The results identified religion, parity, place of residence and maternal age as statistically significant predictors of delivery service use. In addition, awareness and full knowledge about the free maternal healthcare policy were also found to be statistically significant predictors of delivery service use. Maternal education, ethnicity and employment status were not observed as statistically significant predictors of delivery service use under the policy.

The odds of delivering with the policy was 2.985 times higher for mothers who had full knowledge about the policy relative to those who did not have full knowledge about the policy. Similarly, mothers who were aware of the existence of the free maternal healthcare policy were 13.820 times more likely to have delivery services under the policy than those who were not aware of the policy.

The likelihood of using delivery care under the policy was lower for mothers aged 20–29 compared to those in the age bracket of 40–49 (Odds ratio (OR) = 0.069, $p = 0.003$). Mothers who already had 1, 2 or 3 children were more likely to deliver their index child under the policy than those with five or more births. Mothers living in urban areas were 3.793 times more likely to use delivery services under the policy than those living in rural areas (OR = 3.793, $p = 0.000$).

Table 2 Binary logistic regression results of predictors of delivery care use using individual, husband/partner and health policy factors

Variable	Model 1 Individual variables	Model 2 Individual/ Partner variables	Model 3 Individual/Partner/ Health Policy variables
	Odds Ratio	Odds Ratio	Odds Ratio
Age Group (RC = 40–49)			
20–29	0.178	0.088**	0.069**
30–39	0.421	0.271	0.247
Parity (RC = 5 and above)			
1	3.405**	4.998**	5.283**
2	3.974***	5.338**	6.390***
3	4.171**	4.675**	5.713**
4	2.146	3.248	3.087
Religion (RC = Muslim)			
Christian (Catholic)	0.719	0.584	0.527
Christian (Orthodox)	0.146***	0.110***	0.077***
Other Christian (SDA, Jehovah's Witnesses)	0.344*	0.305	0.283
Christian (Pentecostal/Charismatic)	0.581	0.751	0.847
Other (Traditional/Spiritual/No religion)	0.299	0.613	0.636
Education (RC = Other – Vocational, Technical)			
No Education	1.019	0.788	0.968
Primary	1.006	0.450	0.427
Middle/JHS	1.771	1.214	1.141
Secondary/SHS/Technical	2.403	2.343	2.634
Higher than Secondary	3.226	0.263	0.217
Ethnicity (RC = Other (Ga-Adangme, Guan, Hausa))			
Akan	1.531	2.873	2.905
Ewe	2.049	3.151	2.724
Marital Status (RC = Single (Never married, Never-cohabited)			
Married/cohabiting	0.316*	0.124	0.094
Formerly in union (Widowed, Divorced/Sep)	0.114**	0.178	0.098
Residence (RC = Rural)			
Urban	3.566***	3.188***	3.793***
Employment Status (RC = Other – seasonal work)			
Unemployed	2.151	2.969	4.714
Self-employed	1.416	1.448	1.809
Employee (Paid)	0.994	4.691	13.629
Informal work (paid)	2.896	3.891	4.673
Husband/Partner Education (RC = Other- Vocational, Technical)			
No education		0.791	0.652
Primary		4.297	5.177
Middle/JHS		4.740	6.222
Secondary/SHS/Technical		2.336	2.925
Higher than Secondary		7.573	8.317
Husband Employment Status (RC = Other – seasonal work)			
Unpaid Family worker		1.317	1.227
Unemployed		3.075	3.150

Table 2 Binary logistic regression results of predictors of delivery care use using individual, husband/partner and health policy factors *(Continued)*

Self-employed		1.889	1.784
Employee (Formal work paid)		3.654	6.386
Informal work (paid)		3.096	3.320
Age of husband		1.024	1.022
Awareness about policy (RC = No)			
Awareness about policy (Yes)			13.820*
Full knowledge about policy (RC = No)			
Full Knowledge (Yes)			2.985***
Constant	2.723	0.532	0.020
Nagelkerke R^2	0.302	0.380	0.433

Note: For significance levels
RC reference category
$^{*}p < 0.05$; $^{**}p < 0.01$; $^{***}p < 0.001$

The introduction of variables on the fee exemption policy (awareness and full knowledge of the free delivery's benefit package) was relevant as those variables were also significant in explaining delivery care use under the policy. Additionally, model 3 was an improvement over models 1 and 2 as the adjusted coefficient of determination (R^2) increased further to close to 45 % (0.433) compared to 0.302 for model 1 and 0.380 for model 2.

Discussion

In this study we found that over two-thirds of mothers who participated in the study used supervised delivery services under the fee exemption policy for maternal healthcare for their most recent birth. Utilization was however lower for mothers in the largely rural district than those from urban districts. A little over 7 out of 10 mothers in urban areas delivered for free under the policy compared to approximately 5 in 10 for mothers in rural areas. The findings is in line with an earlier study that has confirmed a possibility of marked variations in utilization of maternal healthcare services under given healthcare financing mechanism due to challenges in the design and/or implementation of the policy or initiative [19].

The study also found the major determinants of delivery care use under the policy as, age, religion, marital status, parity, place of residence, awareness and knowledge about the fee exemption policy.

The likelihood of using delivery care under the policy was lower for younger mothers aged 20–29 compared to older mothers in the age bracket of 40–49. The finding is inconsistent with previous studies [20] and at the same time consistent with others [21, 22]. The relatively lower use of the free delivery services by younger mothers could be partly attributed to concerns of the quality of maternity care received under the policy. The Central region has been particularly noted as one region with a very low uptake of care provided under the National Health Insurance Scheme (NHIS) which includes free maternity care and lack of confidence in the programme has been noted as one major reason [23]. Younger mothers who most likely will be having their first births will most likely be very enthusiastic about receiving the most efficient care and may therefore choose to pay for maternity services which many consider to be of a better quality than services provided for free. Older mothers particularly those who already have many children on the other hand may have varied expenditures to deal with and would therefore not prefer to add that of an additional birth if they can receive care at no cost.

The study also found that mothers with lower parity had higher odds of delivering with the policy than those with higher parity. Previous studies have also confirmed a strong association between lower parity and use of maternal healthcare services [22, 24]. Within the study setting usage of free care was lower for mothers with higher parities relative to those with lower parities partly because ordinarily, women with many children have been exposed to a number of childbearing episodes and therefore will not be too enthusiastic and religious to seek for supervised care even when it comes at no cost.

On religion, the results showed that orthodox Christians and other Christian religious groups as the Seventh Day Adventists (SDA) and Jehovah's Witnesses had a lower likelihood of delivering with the policy than Muslim women. There was no significant relationship between supervised care use under the policy and religion among mothers who were Traditionalist/Spiritualist. The finding on religion may suggest differences in religious ideologies in seeking for supervised/facility-based services during pregnancy and childbirth among different religious groups. Previous studies [21, 25, 26] have confirmed a strong association between religion and health-seeking behaviours during pregnancy, delivery and the post-partum period.

Place of residence has been found to constitute a major determinant of healthcare use as it shapes individual opportunities and exposure to healthcare resources [22, 27]. It is therefore not surprising that place of residence was highly significant in predicting delivery care use under the policy. Similar to what has been reported in earlier studies [22, 27, 28], mothers residing in rural areas were 3.79 times less likely to use delivery services under the free delivery policy than those living in urban areas. These studies have shown that urban settlements in Ghana and other developing economies receive a better share of healthcare resources including supervised maternity services. Additionally, well-known community-level barriers including poor transportation networks and distance to available healthcare facilities could partly explain variations in access to services between women in rural and urban areas [20].

Most rural communities are disadvantaged when it comes to the distribution of health infrastructure, human and medical resources and the availability of transportation infrastructure to the nearest health facility. The findings suggest the need for increased attention to improving healthcare resources in rural areas to ensure that resources are equitably distributed across rural and urban areas. Mothers will be willing and happy with using supervised care during pregnancy and childbirth if a good facility is available and accessible to them.

The study also introduced variables on health policy in the regression analysis as it has become imperative to look beyond individual- and community-level factors in addressing challenges to accessing supervised care at birth. Addressing challenges associated with accessing care under a given healthcare policy is largely beyond the remit of the individual woman. The variables introduced (awareness and knowledge about the fee exemption policy) were statistically significant in explaining delivery care use under the policy.

Some of the findings of the study were not consistent with certain hypotheses explaining maternal healthcare service use. For instance maternal education which has often been identified as a catalyst to empowering women and exposing them to better use of healthcare services [20, 24, 27] was not statistically associated with delivery care use in the study setting. This could be attributed to the general low level of education of most indigenous inhabitants of the Central region. The region has been classified among the poorest regions in Ghana with majority of its inhabitants not highly educated [23]. Education could therefore not be critical in influencing women's delivery decisions in this study.

The study acknowledges some limitations which should be considered in the interpretation of the results. First, even though the study was undertaken in a pilot region in which the fee exemption policy was implemented, the findings cannot be generalized for the entire region since only 2 districts out of the nineteen (19) existing districts were selected. Secondly, the findings can best inform decisions regarding effective implementation of the delivery fee exemption policy at only the micro level. Furthermore, the study was cross-sectional and employed the use of a structured questionnaire to collect primary data. Information collected from the questionnaire survey was largely reliable in answering the study's objective of identifying factors that influences women's use of supervised care at birth. A questionnaire survey is however limited in so far as it does not allow for probing to understand further and provide meanings to the study's findings. Even though useful, the present study was not intended to provide qualitative insights into how the factors identified influence women's use of supervised delivery care under the policy.

Conclusions

The study identified place of residence (rural/urban) as one of the strongest determinants of supervised care use under the free maternal healthcare policy with mothers residing in rural areas less likely to use the services than those in urban areas. The results on place of residence have very useful implications for effective implementation of the free delivery policy with regards to improving equitable access to care for both rural and urban inhabitants. The finding suggests that efforts at improving access to supervised care under the "free delivery" policy should not only target disadvantaged individuals but also disadvantaged localities in which many poor and disadvantaged women live.

Additionally individual and policy level factors affecting delivery service use such as maternal age, parity, marital status, awareness and knowledge about the free delivery policy have been identified in the study. Service improvement interventions that take cognisance of these factors are likely to have an impact on utilisation of supervised care under the delivery fee exemption policy.

Overall, the findings of this study have policy implications for addressing some unfinished business of Millennium Development Goal (MDG) 5 on improving maternal health under the Sustainable Development Goals (SDGs). In particular, the findings from this study provide useful lessons for realizing targets for improving maternal and child health (targets 3.1, 3.2 and 3.8) under SDG 3 which seeks to ensure healthy lives and promotes well-being for all at all ages. A realistic and achievable inter-sectorial intervention programmes aimed at addressing both individual and policy implementation bottlenecks should be put in place to improve maternal health during the post MDG period especially for rural localities.

Abbreviations

ADDRF, African Doctoral Dissertation Research Fellowship; APHRC, African Population and Health Research Centre; DAAD, Deutscher Akademischer Austausch Dienst/German Academic Exchange Service; DHMT, District Health Management Team; IDRC, International Development Research Centre; IRB, Institutional Review Board; ISSER, Institute of Statistical Social and Economic Research; MDG, Millennium Development Goal; NHIS, National Health Insurance Scheme; NMIMR, Noguchi Memorial Institute for Medical Research; SDA, Seventh Day Adventist; SDGs, Sustainable Development Goals; SPSS, Statistical Package for the Social Sciences

Acknowledgements

The research received financial support from the German Academic Exchange Service (DAAD) through the PhD in Development Studies programme offered by the Institute of Statistical Social and Economic Research, University of Ghana. The research was also partially funded by an African Doctoral Dissertation Research Fellowship award offered by the African Population and Health Research Center (APHRC) in partnership with the International Development Research Centre (IDRC).
The authors are also grateful to Barbara English, Master Editor at Wordsmiths English Consultancy for reviewing and providing useful inputs into the initial draft of the manuscript.

Funding

The data collection and management for this study was funded by the Deutscher Akademischer Austausch Dienst (DAAD)/German Academic Exchange Service and an African Doctoral Dissertation Research Fellowship (ADDRF) award received by the lead author. The ADDRF award was offered by the African Population and Health Research Center in partnership with the International Development Research Centre (IDRC). The data analysis and write-up did not receive any financial support.

Authors' contributions

HAS is the principal author and was involved in developing the research concept, conception of the methodology, data collection, data analysis, interpretation of results and writing of manuscript. AYO contributed to developing the research concept, the conception of the methodology, interpretation of the results and review of manuscript. SS supported in developing the research concept, conception of the research methodology and review of manuscript. EA contributed to the research concept, review of data collection instruments, supervision of data collection and review of manuscript. MA participated in the conception of the methodology, supervised the statistical analysis and edited the manuscript. All authors read and approved the final manuscript.

Authors' information

HAS is a Doctoral Fellow of the Institute of Statistical Social and Economic Research (ISSER), University of Ghana (UG). AYO is a Senior Research Fellow, ISSER, UG. SS is a Senior Researcher, South Asia Institute. EA is Research Fellow, ISSER. MA is a lecturer at the Regional Institute for Population Studies, UG.

Competing interests

The authors declare that they have no competing interests.

Ethics approval and consent to participate

Ethical clearance for undertaking the study was sought from the Institutional Review Board (IRB) of the Noguchi Memorial Institute for Medical Research, University of Ghana. The study protocol and respondent consent forms were reviewed, and approved by the board with an ethical approval code NMIMR–IRB CPN 113/12-13. The Central Regional Directorate of the Ghana Health Service and the District Health Management Teams (DHMT) offices of the selected districts as well as the local government authorities in the respective districts were also consulted for approval before the commencement of data collection exercise. Participants for the interviews were provided with all the relevant study information to assess their willingness to participate in the study. They were informed that the information to be collected was strictly for academic purposes (thesis and publications) and their participation was voluntary. The study participants were therefore interviewed only after they had agreed to do so. Respondents who agreed to participate in the study were requested to sign or thumb-print a consent form.

Author details

[1]Institute of Statistical Social and Economic Research, University of Ghana, P.O. Box LG 74, Legon, Accra, Ghana. [2]South Asia Institute, Im Neuenheimer Feld 330, 69120 Heidelberg, Germany. [3]Regional Institute for Population Studies, University of Ghana, P.O. Box LG 96, Legon, Accra, Ghana.

References

1. Chou D, Inoue M, Mathers C, Oestergaard M, Say, Mills S, Suzuki E, Wilmoth J. Trends in maternal mortality: 1990 to 2008. Estimates developed by WHO UNICEF UNFPA and The World Bank. Geneva: World Health Organization; 2010.
2. Campbell OMR, Graham WJ. Strategies for reducing maternal mortality: getting on with what works. Lancet. 2006;368(9543):1284–99.
3. Cham M, Sundby J, Vangen S. Availability and quality of emergency obstetric care in Gambia's main referral hospital: women-users' testimonies. Reprod Health. 2009;6(1):5–12.
4. Kyomuhendo GB. Low use of rural maternity services in Uganda: impact of women's status, traditional beliefs and limited resources. Reprod Health Matters. 2003;11(21):16–26.
5. Wagle R, Sabroe S, Nielsen B. Socioeconomic and physical distance to the maternity hospital as predictors for place of delivery: an observation study from Nepal. BMC Pregnancy Childbirth. 2004;4(1):8–17.
6. Bazzano AN, Kirkwood B, Tawiah-Agyemang C, Owusu-Agyei S, Adongo P. Social costs of skilled attendance at birth in rural Ghana. Int J Gynecol Obstet. 2008;102(1):91–4.
7. Levin A, Dmytraczenko T, McEuen M, Ssengooba F, Mangani R, Van Dyck G. Costs of maternal health care services in three anglophone African countries. Int J Health Plann Manage. 2003;18(1):3–22.
8. Devadasan N, Elias MA, John D, Grahacharya S, Ralte L. A conditional cash assistance programme for promoting institutional deliveries among the poor in India: process evaluation results. In: Fabienne R, Sophie W, Vincent D, editors. Reducing financial barriers to obstetric care in low-income countries. Antwerp: Studies in health services organisation and policy; 2008. p. 167–98.
9. Ir DH, Souk N, Van Damme W. Using targeted vouchers and health equity funds to improve access to skilled birth attendants for poor women: a case study in three rural health districts in Cambodia. BMC Pregnancy Childbirth. 2010;10(1):1–11.
10. Ridde V, Kouanda S, Bado A, Bado N, Haddad S. Reducing the medical cost of deliveries in Burkina Faso is good for everyone, including the poor. Plos One. 2012;3(7):1–8.
11. Ridde V, Diarra A. A process evaluation of user fees abolition for pregnant women and children under five years in two districts in Niger (West Africa). BMC Health Serv Res. 2009;9(1):89–104.
12. Ofori-Adjei D. Ghana's free delivery care policy. Ghana Med J. 2007;41(3):94–5.
13. Ansong-Tornui J, Armar-Klemesu M, Arhinful D, Penfold S, Hussein J. Hospital based maternity care in Ghana-findings of a confidential enquiry into maternal deaths. Ghana Med J. 2007;3(41):125–32.
14. Witter S, Adjei S, Armar-Klemesu M, Graham W. Providing free maternal health care: ten lessons from an evaluation of the national delivery exemption policy in Ghana. Glob Health Action. 2009;2:1–5.
15. Asante FA, Chikwama C, Daniels A, Armar-Klemesu M. Evaluating the economic outcomes of the policy of fee exemption for maternal delivery care in Ghana. Ghana Med J. 2007;3(41):110–7.

16. Ghana Statistical Service. 2010 Population and housing census: Summary report of final results. Accra: Ghana Statistical Service; 2012.
17. Ghana Health Service. Central regional annual report 2012. Accra: Ghana Health Service; 2013.
18. Kish L. Survey sampling. New York: Wiley-Interscience; 1965.
19. Powell-Jackson T, Morrison J, Tiwari S, Neupane B, Costello A. The experiences of districts in implementing a national incentive programme to promote safe delivery in Nepal. BMC Health Serv Res. 2009;9(1):97–107.
20. Ononokpono DN, Odimegwu CO, Imasiku EN, Adedini SA. Does it really matter where women live? A multilevel analysis of the determinants of postnatal care in Nigeria. Matern Child Health J. 2013;17 Suppl 1:1–10.
21. Doku D, Neupane S, Doku PN. Factors associated with reproductive health care utilization among Ghanaian women. BMC Int Health Hum Rights. 2012; 12:29–36.
22. Gabrysch S, Campbell OMR. Still too far to walk: Literature review of the determinants of delivery service use. BMC Pregnancy Childbirth. 2009;9(1): 34–51.
23. Ghana Statistical Service Ghana Living Standards Survey. Report of the Fifth Round (GLSS 5). Accra: GSS; 2008.
24. Overbosch G, Nsowah-Nuamah N, Van Den Boom G, Damnyag L. Determinants of antenatal care use in Ghana. J Afr Econ. 2004;13(2):277–301.
25. Gyimah SO, Takyi BK, Addai I. Challenges to the reproductive-health needs of African women: on religion and maternal health utilization in Ghana. Soc Sci Med. 2006;62(12):2930–44.
26. Hazarika I. Factors that determine the use of skilled care during delivery in India: implications for achievement of MDG-5 targets. Matern Child Health J. 2010;15(8):1381–8.
27. Fotso JC, Ezeh A, Oronje R. Provision and use of maternal health services among urban poor women in Kenya: what do we know and what can we do? J Urban Health. 2008;85(3):428–42.
28. Gething PW, Amoako Johnson F, Frempong-Ainguah F, Nyarko P, Baschieri A, Aboagye P, Falkingham J, Matthews Z, Atkinson PM. Geographical access to care at birth in Ghana: a barrier to safe motherhood. In: Economic and social research council. Centre for Population change working paper. 2012. Number 21.

Permissions

All chapters in this book were first published in P&C, by BioMed Central; hereby published with permission under the Creative Commons Attribution License or equivalent. Every chapter published in this book has been scrutinized by our experts. Their significance has been extensively debated. The topics covered herein carry significant findings which will fuel the growth of the discipline. They may even be implemented as practical applications or may be referred to as a beginning point for another development.

The contributors of this book come from diverse backgrounds, making this book a truly international effort. This book will bring forth new frontiers with its revolutionizing research information and detailed analysis of the nascent developments around the world.

We would like to thank all the contributing authors for lending their expertise to make the book truly unique. They have played a crucial role in the development of this book. Without their invaluable contributions this book wouldn't have been possible. They have made vital efforts to compile up to date information on the varied aspects of this subject to make this book a valuable addition to the collection of many professionals and students.

This book was conceptualized with the vision of imparting up-to-date information and advanced data in this field. To ensure the same, a matchless editorial board was set up. Every individual on the board went through rigorous rounds of assessment to prove their worth. After which they invested a large part of their time researching and compiling the most relevant data for our readers.

The editorial board has been involved in producing this book since its inception. They have spent rigorous hours researching and exploring the diverse topics which have resulted in the successful publishing of this book. They have passed on their knowledge of decades through this book. To expedite this challenging task, the publisher supported the team at every step. A small team of assistant editors was also appointed to further simplify the editing procedure and attain best results for the readers.

Apart from the editorial board, the designing team has also invested a significant amount of their time in understanding the subject and creating the most relevant covers. They scrutinized every image to scout for the most suitable representation of the subject and create an appropriate cover for the book.

The publishing team has been an ardent support to the editorial, designing and production team. Their endless efforts to recruit the best for this project, has resulted in the accomplishment of this book. They are a veteran in the field of academics and their pool of knowledge is as vast as their experience in printing. Their expertise and guidance has proved useful at every step. Their uncompromising quality standards have made this book an exceptional effort. Their encouragement from time to time has been an inspiration for everyone.

The publisher and the editorial board hope that this book will prove to be a valuable piece of knowledge for researchers, students, practitioners and scholars across the globe.

List of Contributors

Abel Mukengeshayi Ntambue and Françoise Kaj Malonga
Université de Lubumbashi: École de Santé Publique, Unité d'Epidémiologie et de Santé de la Mère, du Nouveau-né et de l'enfant, Lubumbashi, Democratic Republic of the Congo (DRC)

Michele Dramaix-Wilmet
Université Libre de Bruxelles: École de Santé Publique: Centre de recherche en Epidémiologie, Biostatistiques et recherche clinique, Brussels, Belgium

Roger Nlandu Ngatu
Graduate School of Health and Nursing Sciences & Disaster Nursing Global Leader doctoral program (DNGL), University of Kochi, Kochi, Japan

Philippe Donnen
Université Libre de Bruxelles: École de Santé Publique: Centre de recherche en Epidémiologie, Biostatistiques et recherche clinique, Brussels, Belgium
Université Libre de Bruxelles: École de Santé Publique: Centre de Recherche en Politiques et systèmes de santé-Santé internationale, Brussels, Belgium

Elizabeth Ekirapa-Kiracho and Suzanne N. Kiwanuka
Makerere University School of Public Health (MakSPH), Makerere University College of Health Sciences, Kampala, Uganda

Robert Wamala and Leonard K. Atuhaire
Department of Planning and Applied Statistics, Makerere University School of Statistics and Planning, Kampala, Uganda

Moses Tetui
Makerere University School of Public Health (MakSPH), Makerere University College of Health Sciences, Kampala, Uganda
Epidemiology and Global Health Unit, Department of Public Health and Clinical Medicine, Umeå University, Umeå, Sweden

Rornald Muhumuza Kananura
Makerere University School of Public Health (MakSPH), Makerere University College of Health Sciences, Kampala, Uganda
Department of Planning and Applied Statistics, Makerere University School of Statistics and Planning, Kampala, Uganda
Maternal and Newborn Centre of Excellence, Makerere University School of Public Health, Kampala, Uganda

Peter Waiswa
Makerere University School of Public Health (MakSPH), Makerere University College of Health Sciences, Kampala, Uganda
Global Health Division, Department of Public Health Sciences, Karolinska Institutet, Stockholm, Sweden
Maternal and Newborn Centre of Excellence, Makerere University School of Public Health, Kampala, Uganda

Lisa Howard-Grabman
Training Resources Group, Inc., 4301 Wilson Boulevard, Suite 400, Arlington, VA 22203, USA

Andrea Solnes Miltenburg
Institute of Health and Society, Department of Community Medicine and Global Health, Faculty of Medicine, University of Oslo, Blindern, 0316 Oslo, Norway

Cicely Marston
Faculty of Public Health and Policy, London School of Hygiene & Tropical Medicine, 15-17 Tavistock Place, London WC1H 9SH, UK

Anayda Portela
World Health Organization Department of Maternal, Newborn, Child and Adolescent Health, 20 Avenue Appia, 1211 Geneva, Switzerland

Tina Miller
Department of Social Sciences, Oxford Brookes University, Oxford OX3 0BP, UK

Helen Smith
Centre for Maternal and Newborn Health, Liverpool School of Tropical Medicine, L3 5QA, Liverpool, UK

Kazuyoshi Aoyama
Department of Anesthesia and Pain Medicine, The Hospital for Sick Children, University of Toronto, Toronto, Canada

Intensive Care Unit, Mount Sinai Hospital and University Health Network, University of Toronto, Toronto, Canada
Interdepartmental Division of Critical Care Medicine, University of Toronto, Toronto, Canada
Department of Anesthesiology and Pain Medicine, School of Medicine, Juntendo University, Tokyo, Japan
Institute of Health Policy, Management and Evaluation, University of Toronto, Toronto, Canada
555 University Ave, Room 2211, Toronto, ON M5G 1X8, Canada

Rohan D'Souza
Department of Obstetrics and Gynaecology, Division of Maternal-Fetal Medicine, Mount Sinai Hospital, University of Toronto, Toronto, Canada
Institute of Health Policy, Management and Evaluation, University of Toronto, Toronto, Canada

Eiichi Inada
Department of Anesthesiology and Pain Medicine, School of Medicine, Juntendo University, Tokyo, Japan

Stephen E. Lapinsky
Intensive Care Unit, Mount Sinai Hospital and University Health Network, University of Toronto, Toronto, Canada
Interdepartmental Division of Critical Care Medicine, University of Toronto, Toronto, Canada

Robert A. Fowler
Department of Critical Care Medicine, Sunnybrook Health Science Centre, University of Toronto, Toronto, Canada
Interdepartmental Division of Critical Care Medicine, University of Toronto, Toronto, Canada
Institute of Health Policy, Management and Evaluation, University of Toronto, Toronto, Canada

Godofreda V. Dalmacion
Department of Pharmacology and Toxicology, College of Medicine, University of the Philippines-Manila, Manila, Philippines
Department of Clinical Epidemiology, College of Medicine, University of the Philippines-Manila, Manila, Philippines
Institute of Clinical Epidemiology, National Institutes of Health, University of the Philippines-Manila, Manila, Philippines

Emmanuel S. Baja
Department of Clinical Epidemiology, College of Medicine, University of the Philippines-Manila, Manila, Philippines
Institute of Clinical Epidemiology, National Institutes of Health, University of the Philippines-Manila, Manila, Philippines

Lalaine Mae V. Cruz
Institute of Clinical Epidemiology, National Institutes of Health, University of the Philippines-Manila, Manila, Philippines

Ramon T. Reyles and Maricelle C. Chua
Department of Obstetrics and Gynecology, Makati Medical Center, Makati, Philippines

Antonia E. Habana
Department of Obstetrics and Gynecology, College of Medicine, University of the Philippines- Manila, Manila, Philippines

Analyn T. Ngo
Department of Obstetrics and Gynecology, Manila Doctors Hospital, Manila, Philippines

Milagros J. Tia-Jocson
Department of Obstetrics and Gynecology, College of Medicine, Manila Central University FDT Medical Foundation, Caloocan, Philippines

Chimezie Anyakora, Uchenna Ezedinachi, Adebola Adekoya and Jude Nwokike
Promoting the Quality of Medicines Program, USP, Rockville, MD, USA

Ibrahim Ali, Charles Nwachukwu, Victor Abiola and Yetunde Oni
National Agency for Food and Drug Administration and Control, Abuja, Nigeria

Charles Esimone
Faculty of Pharmacy, Nnamdi Azikiwe University, Awka, Nigeria

Nicola Vousden, Elodie Lawley, Hannah L. Nathan, Paul T. Seed, Lucy C. Chappell, Jane Sandall and Andrew H. Shennan
Department of Women and Children's Health, School of Life Course Sciences, Faculty of Life Sciences and Medicine, King's College London, London SE1 7EH, UK

Adrian Brown
Maternity Worldwide Community Base, 113 Queens Road, Brighton BN1 3XG, UK

Umesh Charantimath, Mrutyunjaya Bellad and Shivaprasad Goudar
Women's and Children's Health Research Unit, KLE Academy of Higher Education and Research Jawaharlal Nehru Medical College, Belgaum, Karnataka 590010, India

Tafadzwa Muchengwa
Morgenster Mission Hospital, Masvingo, Zimbabwe

Muchabayiwa Francis Gidiri
Department of Obstetrics and Gynaecology, College of Health Sciences, University of Zimbabwe, Harare, Zimbabwe

Fenling Fan, Yushun Zhang and Junbo Zhang
Department of Cardiovascular Medicine, the First Affiliated Hospital of Medical College, Xi'an Jiaotong University, Xi'an 710061, China

Yuliang Zou, Cai Liu, Jie Li, Meili Pei and Yu Jiang
Department of Gynaecology and Obstetrics, the First Affiliated Hospital of Medical College, Xi'an Jiaotong University, Xi'an 710061, China

Xiancang Ma
Department of Psychology and Psychiatry, the First Affiliated Hospital of Medical College, Xi'an Jiaotong University, Xi'an 710061, China

Anthony M. Dart
Department of Cardiovascular Medicine, The Alfred, Baker Heart and Diabetes Institute, Melbourne, Vic 3004, Australia

Sanni Yaya and Ghose Bishwajit
School of International Development and Global Studies, University of Ottawa, Ottawa, Canada

Olalekan A. Uthman
Warwick Centre for Applied Health Research and Delivery (WCAHRD), Division of Health Sciences, Warwick Medical School, University of Warwick, Coventry CV4 7AL, UK

Agbessi Amouzou
Bloomberg School of Public Health, Johns Hopkins University, Baltimore, MD, USA

Michael Ekholuenetale
Department of Epidemiology and Medical Statistics, Faculty of Public Health, College of Medicine, University of Ibadan, Ibadan, Nigeria

Katharine Bowker, Sophie Orton, Sue Cooper, Rachel Whitemore, Tim Coleman and Anne Dickinson
NIHR School for Primary Care Research and UK Centre for Tobacco and Alcohol Studies, Division of Primary Care, School of Medicine, University of Nottingham, Nottingham NG7 2RD, UK

Felix Naughton
School of Health Sciences, University of East Anglia, Edith Cavell Building, Norwich NR4 7TJ, UK

Sarah Lewis
Division of Epidemiology and Public Health and UK Centre for Tobacco and Alcohol Studies and, University of Nottingham, Clinical Sciences Building 2, Nottingham City Hospital, Hucknall Road, Nottingham NG5 1PB, UK

Linda Bauld and Lesley Sinclair
Institute for Social Marketing and UK Centre for Tobacco and Alcohol Studies, University of Stirling, Stirling FK9 4LA, UK

Michael Ussher
Institute for Social Marketing and UK Centre for Tobacco and Alcohol Studies, University of Stirling, Stirling FK9 4LA, UK
Population Health Research Institute, St George's, University of London, London SW17 0RE, UK

Gabriel Makuei, Mali Abdollahian and Kaye Marion
School of Science (Mathematical and Geospatial Sciences), College of Science, Engineering, and Health, RMIT University, Melbourne, VIC 3001, Australia

Zufan Abera Damtew and Chala Tesfaye Chekagn
Federal Ministry of Health of Ethiopia, Health Extension and Primary Health Service Directorate, Sudan Street, Addis Ababa, Ethiopia

Ali Mehryar Karim, Nebreed Fesseha Zemichael, Bantalem Yihun and Wuleta Betemariam
Last 10 Kilometers Project (L10K) 2020, JSI Research & Training Institute, Inc, Bole Sub-City, Kebele 03/05, Hs #, 2111 Addis Ababa, Ethiopia

Barbara A. Willey
Department of Infectious Disease Epidemiology, Faculty of Epidemiology and Population Health, London School of Hygiene and Tropical Medicine, Keppel Street, London WC1E 7HT, UK

Shankar Prinja, Aditi Gupta, Pankaj Bahuguna and Ruby Nimesh
School of Public Health, Post Graduate Institute of Medical Education and Research, Sector-12, Chandigarh 160012, India

Sofus Rabow
Department of Clinical Sciences Lund, Anaesthesiology and Intensive Care, Skåne University Hospital, Lund University, S-22185 Lund, Sweden
Department of Intensive and Perioperative Care, Skåne University Hospital, S-22185 Lund, Sweden

Ull Hjorth, Sofia Schönbeck and Per Olofsson
Department of Clinical Sciences Malmö, Obstetrics and Gynaecology, Skåne University Hospital, Lund University, Malmö, Sweden

Usman Gulumbe
Department of Mathematics and Statistics, Federal University, Birnin-Kebbi, Kebbi State, Nigeria

Olatunji Alabi and Olusola A. Omisakin
Department of Demography and Social Statistics, Federal University, Birnin-Kebi, Kebbi State, Nigeria

Semeeh Omoleke
Immunisation, Vaccines and Emergencies Unit, World Health Organisation, Abuja, Nigeria

Ingrid Hylander
Department of Neurobiology, Care Sciences and Society, Division of Family Medicine, Karolinska Institutet, Nobels allé 12, 141 83 Huddinge, Sweden

Ulrika Baker
Department of Public Health sciences, Global health - Health Systems and Policy Research, Widerströmska huset, Karolinska Institutet, Tomtebodavägen 18 A, 171 77 Stockholm, Sweden
Department of Neurobiology, Care Sciences and Society, Division of Family Medicine, Karolinska Institutet, Nobels allé 12, 141 83 Huddinge, Sweden

Farida Hassan and Fatuma Manzi
Ifakara Health Institute, Plot 463 Kiko Avenue, Mikocheni, Dar es Salaam, Tanzania

Claudia Hanson
Department of Public Health sciences, Global health - Health Systems and Policy Research, Widerströmska huset, Karolinska Institutet, Tomtebodavägen 18 A, 171 77 Stockholm, Sweden
Department for Disease Control, London School of Hygiene and Tropical Medicine (LSHTM), Keppel Street, London WC1E 7HT, UK

Tanya Marchant
Department for Disease Control, London School of Hygiene and Tropical Medicine (LSHTM), Keppel Street, London WC1E 7HT, UK

Stefan Swartling Peterson
Department of Public Health sciences, Global health - Health Systems and Policy Research, Widerströmska huset, Karolinska Institutet, Tomtebodavägen 18 A, 171 77 Stockholm, Sweden
International Maternal and Child Health, Uppsala University, Drottninggatan 4, 751 85 Uppsala, Sweden
Makerere School of Public Health, Kampala, Uganda

Pavel Dietz, Matteo C. Sattler, Wolfgang Ruf and Sylvia Titze
Department of Physical Activity and Public Health, Institute of Sports Science, University of Graz, Mozartgasse 14, Graz 8010, Austria

Estelle D. Watson
Centre for Exercise Science and Sports Medicine, School of Therapeutic Sciences, Faculty of Health Sciences, University of Witwatersrand, Private Bag 3, Johannesburg 2050, South Africa

Mireille van Poppel
Department of Physical Activity and Public Health, Institute of Sports Science, University of Graz, Mozartgasse 14, Graz 8010, Austria
Department of Public and Occupational Health, EMGO Institute for Health and Care Research, VU University Medical Centre, Van der Boechorststraat 7, Amsterdam 1081 BT, The Netherland

Sonja L. Myhre
Department of International Public Health, Norwegian Institute of Public Health, Nydalen N-0403, Oslo, Norway

Jane Kaye
Centre for Health, Law and Emerging Technologies, Nuffield Department of Population Health, University of Oxford, Rosemary Rue Building, Old Road Campus, Headington, Oxford OX3 7LF, UK

Lee A. Bygrave
Department of Private Law, Faculty of Law, University of Oslo, Postboks 6706St Olavs plass, 0130 Oslo, Norway

Margunn Aanestad
Department of Informatics, University of Oslo, Gaustadalléen 23 B, N-0373 Oslo, Norway

Buthaina Ghanem
Palestinian National Institute of Public Health, Qaddoura Street, Ministry of Health Building, 1st Floor, Ramallah, Palestine

Patricia Mechael
School of Advanced International Studies, Johns Hopkins University, 1717 Massachusetts Ave, NW, Washington, DC 20036, USA
HealthEnabled, Unit D11, Westlake Square, Westlake Drive, Westlake, Cape Town, South Africa7945

J. Frederik Frøen
Department of International Public Health, Norwegian Institute of Public Health, Nydalen N-0403, Oslo, Norway
Centre for Intervention Science in Maternal and Child Health, University of Bergen, Bergen, Norway

Jing Gu
School of Public Health, Sun Yat-sen University, No. 74 Zhongshan 2nd Road, Guangzhou 510080, People's Republic of China
Sun Yat-sen Global Health Institute, Sun Yat-sen University, No. 74 Zhongshan 2nd Road, Guangzhou 510080, People's Republic of China

Marisa Hofstee
Department of Global Health, University of Washington, 1510 N.E. San Juan Road, Seattle, WA 98195-7965, USA

Juan Nie
School of Public Health, Sun Yat-sen University, No. 74 Zhongshan 2nd Road, Guangzhou 510080, People's Republic of China
Sun Yat-sen Global Health Institute, Sun Yat-sen University, No. 74 Zhongshan 2nd Road, Guangzhou 510080, People's Republic of China
Department of Global Health, University of Washington, 1510 N.E. San Juan Road, Seattle, WA 98195-7965, USA
Health Alliance International, 1107 NE 45th Street, Suite 350, Seattle, WA 98105, USA

Jennifer Anna Unger
Department of Global Health, University of Washington, 1510 N.E. San Juan Road, Seattle, WA 98195-7965, USA
Department of Obstetrics & Gynecology, University of Washington, Harborview Medical Center, 325 Ninth Ave, Seattle, WA 98104, USA

Susan Thompson and Mary Anne Mercer
Department of Global Health, University of Washington, 1510 N.E. San Juan Road, Seattle, WA 98195-7965, USA
Health Alliance International, 1107 NE 45th Street, Suite 350, Seattle, WA 98105, USA

Henrietta Asante-Sarpong, Adobea Yaa Owusu and Ernest Appiah
Institute of Statistical Social and Economic Research, University of Ghana, Legon, Accra, Ghana

Sheela Saravanan
South Asia Institute, Im Neuenheimer Feld 330, 69120 Heidelberg, Germany

Mumuni Abu
Regional Institute for Population Studies, University of Ghana, Legon, Accra, Ghana

Index

N

O

P

Q

R

S

T

V

W

www.ingramcontent.com/pod-product-compliance
Lightning Source LLC
LaVergne TN
LVHW080911210926
848485LV00004B/631
* 9 7 8 1 6 3 9 2 7 1 5 5 9 *